PATHOLOGY
OF THE TESTIS
AND ITS ADNEXA

CONTEMPORARY ISSUES IN SURGICAL PATHOLOGY VOLUME 7

SERIES EDITOR
Lawrence M. Roth, M.D.

Professor of Pathology
Director, Division of Surgical Pathology
Indiana University School of Medicine
Indianapolis, Indiana

PATHOLOGY
OF THE TESTIS
AND ITS ADNEXA

Edited by

Aleksander Talerman, M.D., Ph.D., F.R.C.Path.

Professor of Pathology and Obstetrics and Gynecology
University of Chicago Pritzker School of Medicine
Chicago, Illinois

Lawrence M. Roth, M.D.

Professor of Pathology
Director, Division of Surgical Pathology
Indiana University School of Medicine
Indianapolis, Indiana

Churchill Livingstone
New York, Edinburgh, London, Melbourne 1986

Acquisitions editor: *Robert A. Hurley*
Copy editor: *Kamely Dahir*
Production designer: *Michiko Davis*
Production supervisor: *Sharon Tuder*
Compositor: *Kingsport Press*
Printer/Binder: *Halliday Lithograph*

Accurate indications, adverse reactions, and dosage
schedules for drugs are provided in this book, but
it is possible that they may change. The reader is
urged to review the package information data of the
manufacturers of the medications mentioned.

Distributed in the United Kingdom by Churchill Livingstone,
Robert Stevenson House, 1–3 Baxter's Place, Leith Walk,
Edinburgh EH1 3AF and by associated companies, branches
and representatives throughout the world.

First published 1986
Printed in U.S.A.

ISBN 0–443–08351–7

7 6 5 4 3 2 1

Library of Congress Cataloging in Publication Data
Main entry under title:

Pathology of the testis and its adnexa.

(Contemporary issues in surgical pathology; v. 7)
Includes bibliographies and index.
1. Testis—Cancer. 2. Testis—Diseases.
I. Talerman, Aleksander. II. Roth, Lawrence M.
III. Series. [DNLM: 1. Genital Diseases, Male—
pathology. 2. Testicular Neoplasms—pathology.
W1 C0769MS v. 7 / WJ 858 P2973]
RC280.T4P38 1986   616.99′463   85-24281
ISBN 0-443-08351-7

Manufactured in the United States of America

Dedicated to our wives
Margaretha and Ann-Katrin

Contributors

Ivan Damjanov, M.D.
Professor of Pathology, Hahnemann University School of Medicine, Philadelphia, Pennsylvania

John J. Gillespie, M.D.
Director of Surgical Pathology, Department of Laboratories, Edward W. Sparrow Hospital, Lansing, Michigan

Bernard Gondos, M.D.
Professor of Pathology, University of Connecticut Health Center School of Medicine, Farmington, Connecticut

F. Gonzalez-Crussi, M.D.
Professor of Pathology, Northwestern University Medical School; Division Head, of Anatomic Pathology, Children's Memorial Hospital, Chicago, Illinois

Nasser Javadpour, M.D.
Professor and Director of Urologic Oncology, University of Maryland School of Medicine, Baltimore, Maryland; Consultant to the National Naval Hospital, Bethesda, Maryland

R. Scott Klappenbach, M.D.
Assistant Professor of Pathology, Georgetown University School of Medicine, Washington, D.C.

Robert J. Kurman, M.D.
Associate Professor of Pathology and Obstetrics and Gynecology, Georgetown University School of Medicine, Washington, D.C.

W. Dwayne Lawrence, M.D.
Assistant Professor of Pathology, Wayne State University School of Medicine; Chief Anatomic Pathologist, Hutzel Hospital, Detroit, Michigan

Markku Miettinen, M.D.
Assistant Professor of Pathology, University of Helsinki, Finland

Maria Paoletti, M.D.
Resident, Department of Pathology, University of Chicago Pritzker School of Medicine, Chicago, Illinois

Lawrence M. Roth, M.D.
Professor of Pathology and Director, Division of Surgical Pathology, Indiana University School of Medicine, Indianapolis, Indiana

Robert E. Scully, M.D.
Professor of Pathology, Harvard Medical School; Pathologist, Massachusetts General Hospital, Boston, Massachusetts

Francis H. Straus II, M.D.
Professor of Pathology, University of Chicago Pritzker School of Medicine, Chicago, Illinois

Aleksander Talerman, M.D., Ph.D., F.R.C.Path.
Professor of Pathology and Obstetrics and Gynecology, University of Chicago Pritzker School of Medicine, Chicago, Illinois

Lyly Teppo, M.D.
Finnish Cancer Registry, Helsinki, Finland

Thomas M. Ulbright, M.D.
Associate Professor of Pathology, Indiana University School of Medicine, Indianapolis, Indiana

Ismo Virtanen, M.D.
Senior Research Fellow (MRS), Department of Pathology, University of Helsinki, Helsinki, Finland

Nicholas J. Vogelzang, M.D.
Assistant Professor of Medical Oncology, University of Chicago Pritzker School of Medicine, Chicago, Illinois

Robert H. Young, M.D., M.R.C.Path.
Assistant Professor of Pathology, Harvard Medical School; Assistant Pathologist, Massachusetts General Hospital, Boston, Massachusetts

Preface

In this volume we have endeavored to present an up-to-date review of the disease processes affecting the testis and its adnexa that are most commonly encountered by the pathologist, urologist, and medical oncologist. As testicular tumors and tumorlike conditions represent the most important aspect of testicular and paratesticular diseases encountered by this audience, and because of the remarkable progress in this field during the last decade, a considerable part of this volume is devoted to various aspects of testicular neoplasms.

Although we have attempted to present a complete review of the pathology of testicular and paratesticular neoplasms, we have tried to place emphasis on new developments in the field. In this regard, new or incompletely understood entities, recently developed diagnostic techniques, such as immunocytochemistry, analysis of intermediate filaments, measurement and application of tumor markers, and new trends in therapy are covered in depth. Tumorlike lesions and non-neoplastic diseases affecting the testis and its adnexa are also discussed in some detail.

It has been the intention of the editors to allow the contributors a free forum for their opinions. Thus the views of some contributors may differ from those expressed by others. As many aspects of this subject are still controversial, such differences are inevitable in a multiauthored book and provide a forum for discussion.

This volume is not intended to compete with standard textbooks on the subject. Instead we have attempted to discuss some aspects which perhaps have not received sufficient coverage elsewhere, and to emphasize the multidisciplinary approach to testicular disease which is so important at the present time. For these reasons this book may be of interest to investigators dealing with various aspects of the cancer problem in general, in addition to those concerned specifically with testicular neoplasms.

Although testicular disease is usually only encountered by the pathologist, urologist, and medical oncologist of large medical centers with a special interest and experience in this field, the great advances in treatment make it imperative to provide the exact diagnosis and to use the correct therapeutic approach when one encounters such patients. It is hoped that this volume will provide some guidance and help to achieve this goal as well as contribute in some measure toward a better understanding of testicular and paratesticular disease.

Finally we wish to thank all our colleagues for their excellent contributions. We also wish to thank Mrs. Cathy Regovic for her competent secretarial assistance, and Ms. Kim Loretucci and Ms. Kamely Dahir of Churchill Livingstone, our publishers, for their help and cooperation.

Aleksander Talerman
Chicago, Illinois

Lawrence M. Roth
Indianapolis, Indiana

Contents

PATHOLOGY
OF THE TESTIS
AND ITS ADNEXA

1

Epidemiology of Testicular Neoplasms

Lyly Teppo

Testicular tumors form an interesting group of malignant neoplasms with many exceptional and even unique epidemiologic features.[1] They occur mainly in young and middle-aged adults, and this suggests that their risk factors are different from those relevant to most other epithelial cancers. Moreover, it is believed that the origin of the great majority of testicular tumors is the germ cell. This may be of great importance because possible environmental risk factors in testicular cancer are liable to influence future generations.

The epidemiologic features of testicular cancer are outlined here. Special emphasis is placed upon germ cell tumors; other types of cancer will be mentioned only briefly.

INCIDENCE

There is substantial variation in the incidence of testicular cancer in different parts of the world. Table 1-1 lists the rates in selected countries.[2] High rates (4 to 6/100,000) are found in Denmark, Norway, and New Zealand, whereas Finland and some countries of eastern and southern Europe have low rates (1 to 2/100,000). Black populations in Africa seem to experience an extremely low risk of testicular cancer.[3] Similarly, the rate among blacks in the United States is much lower than that observed among whites.[4] Cancer of the testis is also rare in Asia.

Table 1-1. Age-Adjusted Incidence Rates ("World Standard Population") of Testis Cancer in Selected Countries and Areas in the mid 1970s

Country, Area	Incidence (/10⁵)
Denmark	6.7
New Zealand (non-Maori)	4.5
Norway	4.4
German Democratic Republic	4.0
United States, Bay Area (white)	4.0
Canada, Alberta	3.8
United States, Connecticut	3.6
United States, Los Angeles (white)	3.6
Canada, British Columbia	3.3
Sweden	3.0
United Kingdom, Birmingham	2.9
Israel (Jews)	1.9
Finland	1.7
Canada, Quebec	1.6
Colombia, Cali	1.5
Brazil, Sao Paolo	1.4
Hong Kong	1.4
United States, Bay Area (black)	1.4
China, Shanghai	0.9
India, Bombay	0.9
United States, Los Angeles (black)	0.9
Japan, Miyagi	0.8
Puerto Rico	0.8

1

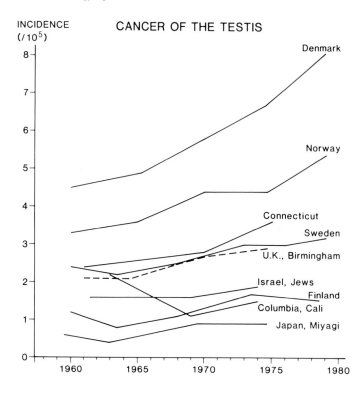

INCIDENCE ($/10^5$)

CANCER OF THE TESTIS

Denmark

Norway

Connecticut

Sweden

U.K., Birmingham

Israel, Jews

Finland

Columbia, Cali

Japan, Miyagi

1960   1965   1970   1975   1980

Fig. 1-1. Trends in the age-adjusted ("world standard population") incidence rate of testis cancer in selected countries. (Based on data in Waterhouse J, Muir C, Shanmugaratnam K, Powell J (eds): Cancer Incidence in Five Continents. Vol. IV. IARC Scientific Publications No. 42. International Agency for Research on Cancer, Lyon, 1982; Cancer Incidence in Denmark 1978, 1979 and 1980: Danish Cancer Registry, Copenhagen, 1983; Incidence of Cancer in Norway 1978, 1979, 1980, 1981. The Cancer Registry of Norway, Oslo, 1981, 1982, 1983; Cancer Incidence in Sweden 1976, 1977, 1978, 1979, 1980. National Board of Health and Welfare, The Cancer Registry, Stockholm, 1980, 1981, 1982, 1983.)

TRENDS

There has been a slight increase in the incidence of cancer of the testis in many areas (Fig. 1-1). The Danish Cancer Registry has reported a steady increase since the mid 1940s. The observed trends may be partly attributable to random variation of low rates or to more accurate reporting to cancer registries.

AGE DISTRIBUTION

The great majority of testicular cancers occur in young and middle-aged adults aged between 20 and 45 years of age. In addition, in many parts of the world there are peaks in young children (0 to 4 years) and in old age. This unique distribution reflects the variation in the incidence of different histologic types. Yolk sac tumors and mature teratomas occur in young children, while seminoma and

various other types of malignant germ cell tumors predominate in adults. In older persons, most of the tumors are lymphomas or sarcomas.

Figure 1-2 gives the age-specific incidence rates of testicular cancer in a high-risk, moderate-risk, and low-risk area (Denmark, Connecticut, and Finland, respectively).[2] The peak incidence in Denmark occurs 10 years later than that observed in Connecticut or Finland. In all these areas, prepubertal boys experience a very low risk of testicular cancer. It appears that the differences in the general risk are largely due to differences in the risks among young adults and middle-aged men. The variations in incidence among boys less than 5 years of age are not similar to those observed in adults. Similarly, the risks among elderly men show inconstant variation, which is at least partly due to differences in various cancer registries' coding of testicular lymphomas, namely, whether they are coded as testicular tumors or as malignant lymphomas.

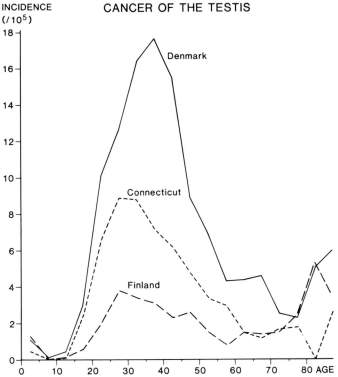

Fig. 1-2. Age-specific incidence rates of testis cancer in Denmark 1973 to 1976 (high-risk area), Connecticut 1973 to 1977 (moderate-risk area), and Finland 1971 to 1976 (low-risk area). (Based on data in Waterhouse J, Muir C, Shanmugaratnam K, Powell J (eds): Cancer Incidence in Five Continents, Vol. IV. IARC Scientific Publications No. 42. International Agency for Research on Cancer, Lyon, 1982.)

URBAN–RURAL DISTRIBUTION

In Finland, seminoma has a distinct urban preponderance (urban–rural ratio of the age-adjusted incidence rates is 1.5), whereas no difference between the urban and rural populations is found in the risk of other germ cell tumors (i.e., embryonal carcinoma, teratocarcinoma, choriocarcinoma and their different combinations, urban–rural ratio 1.1[5]). In this analysis the classification of the municipalities into "urban" and "rural" was based on the official definitions which do not always describe the municipalities' real character. A

more detailed picture of the situation was obtained in an analysis in which the 464 municipalities in Finland were divided into four or five categories according to the numerical value of different background variables describing the degree of urbanization and industrialization.[6] Within each of these groups the age-specific numbers of cases (and populations) of each municipality were added together, and age-adjusted incidence rates were calculated (Fig. 1-3). The increase in the total risk of testicular cancer coincided with an increasing percentage of the population living in urban-type centers and each inhabitant hav-

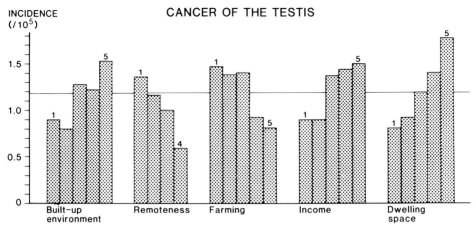

Fig. 1-3. Testicular cancer in Finland, 1955 to 1974: incidence rates (adjusted for age to the mean population of Finland) in classes of municipalities defined by the values of background variables referring to the degree of urbanization and standard of living. The horizontal line indicates the rate for the whole population. Definitions of the variables and their classes: Built-up environment; percentage of population living in urbanlike centers in 1970, 1, lowest, 5, highest; Remoteness; distance between the center of the municipality and the town center of the local economic area, 1, shortest, 4, longest; Farming; percentage of population in farming and forestry 1950, 1, lowest, 5, highest; Income; average monthly income per inhabitant in 1968, 1, lowest, 5, highest; Dwelling space; mean dwelling space per inhabitant in 1970, 1, lowest, 5, highest (Based on data in Teppo L, Pukkala E, Hakama M et al: Way of life and cancer incidence in Finland. A municipality-based ecological analysis. Scand J Soc Med Suppl 19:1, 1980.)

ing a higher mean income and larger dwelling space. A decrease in the total risk coincided with an increasing percentage of the population engaged in farming and forestry, and residing further from the center of the local economic area ("remoteness"). This shows that in the low risk area of Finland the association between the developed, urbanized environment and higher risk of testicular cancer is demonstrable even after an individual categorization of the living area. In Denmark both seminomatous and nonseminomatous tumors occur more frequently in persons living in towns.[7] No urban–rural difference in the risk of testicular cancer (all types) has been found in Norway.[2]

Talerman et al.[8] have reported an urban–rural ratio of 0.6 for seminoma and 0.5 for teratoma in the Netherlands, that is, a clear rural preponderance. A high risk of developing testicular cancer was also associated with

rural residence in the United States: the relative risk (rural vs. urban) was 2.3 for seminoma, 1.4 for other histologic types.[9] In England and Wales a slight rural preponderance has been found for seminoma (U–R ratio of the rates, 0.8), although no difference was recorded for nonseminomatous tumors.[10] In the area covered by the Birmingham Cancer Registry, the urban–rural ratio of the incidence rates of all testicular cancers taken together was 1.13 in 1964 to 1968, and 0.73 in 1969 to 1973. This change was due to a marked increase in the rural rate.

Consequently, no consistent risk pattern in urban–rural distribution is seen among the various types of testicular cancer. This can at least partly be attributable to differences in the character of the "urban" and "rural" environments between sparsely populated countries (such as Finland) and highly industrialized areas.

Table 1-2. Standardized Incidence Ratios (SIR) of Testis Cancer at Ages 35–69 Years in Finland in 1971–1975 in the Main Occupational Categories

Occupational Category	Observed	Expected	SIR
Technical, scientific, humanistic, and artistic	21	8.3	2.55[a]
Legal	2	0.2	10.98[b]
Teaching	7	1.9	3.66[c]
Technical	10	3.9	2.56[b]
Administration, managerial, and clerical	9	4.5	2.01
Administration	7	2.6	2.69[b]
Sales	5	4.1	1.21
Services	3	2.8	1.06
Transport, communication	7	8.0	0.88
Industry, manufacturing	18	28.4	0.63
Farming, forestry	11	18.3	0.60
Other or unspecified	10	9.6	1.04

From unpublished data of the Finnish Cancer Registry.
[a] $p < 0.001$
[b] $p < 0.05$
[c] $p < 0.01$

SOCIOECONOMIC STATUS, OCCUPATION, RELIGION

Several investigators have reported an association between the high risk of testicular cancer and high socioeconomic status, which is itself defined differently. Record linkage between the files of the Finnish Cancer Registry from 1971 to 1975 and the National Census records of Finland in 1970 revealed a clear association between social class defined by main occupational categories and the risk of testicular cancer (Table 1-2). A significantly elevated standardized incidence ratio (SIR) was found among "academic professions" and in those employed in administrative, managerial, and clerical work. On the other hand, low SIRs were encountered in persons working in manufacturing and in farming and forestry.

Davies[11] studied death rates specific to social groups in England and Wales and found high rates of testicular cancer among professionals and administrative and clerical workers. The differences between the social classes had already persisted for some 50 years. Ross et al.[12] in Los Angeles used census tract information in their analysis, and also showed that high risk was associated with high social class.

In the case–control analysis of Graham et al.,[9] based on testicular cancers reported to the New York State Tumor Registry, high risk was associated with professional occupations, rural residence, being native-born, having been married at some time, and being a Protestant. Each of these factors carried a higher risk, even when considered in the context of other traits. The risk was highest among those with several of the above-mentioned characteristics. The results were similar for both seminomas and nonseminomatous tumors. The authors concluded that part of the low rate of testicular cancer among the American black population may be attributable to difference in the socioeconomic status of whites and blacks.

Morrison[13] found a direct association between the level of education (duration of schooling) and risk of seminoma, but there was no such correlation with other tumor types, in his case–control study of men on active duty in the U.S. Army. Protestants ran a higher risk of seminoma than Catholics (risk ratio 1.5), whereas no difference was found between other histologic types (1.1). Those married at some time ran a relative risk of 1.5 for seminoma compared to those never married, while again no difference was found in the case of other types of testicular tumors.

According to Davies,[14] single men under 65 years of age in England and Wales had a higher death rate due to testicular cancer than married men, while among elderly men the reverse was true. An excess risk among single men was found also in the study of Ross et al.[12] in persons aged 25 to 55 years. Davies[14] has discussed in detail the possible reasons for the inconsistent findings regarding the association between marital status and the risk of testicular cancer. These reasons include, among others, difficulties related to use of mortality data, case-control design, and matching, particularly at younger ages. Her final conclusion is that single men run a higher risk, which is also easy to understand biologically: constitutional factors and testicular abnormalities (see below) are likely to lead to a higher than average rate of nonmarriage.

Mills et al.[15] found a sixfold increase in the risk of testicular cancer among farmers in Texas. This could not be confirmed by mortality data from England and Wales.[16] Neither was any difference in the risk of testicular cancer found between farmers and men with other occupations in Denmark.[17] There is no consistent pattern when studies on the association between occupational exposure and risk of testicular cancer are being evaluated.

Many studies have demonstrated risk differences according to religion. In general, Protestants experience a greater risk than Catholics.[13, 18, 19] This association may be at least partly attributable to differences in the socioeconomic conditions of Protestant and Catholic men.

PRENATAL AND CONSTITUTIONAL FACTORS

The occurrence of testicular cancer in children and young adults has stimulated studies on possible prenatal risk factors. Case–control studies in the United States[20, 21] have shown that hormone treatment of mothers during pregnancy increases the risk of testicular cancer in their offspring. The same is true of severe nausea, which is known to be associated with hyperestrogenism. Moreover, it has been claimed that administration of diethylstilbestrol during pregnancy has resulted in an increased risk of testicular cancer in the offspring,[22] but further careful case–control studies failed to confirm these findings.[23]

Cryptorchidism is a well-known risk factor in testicular cancer. In recent case–control studies the relative risk has varied between 3 and 10 times compared with normal subjects.[20-22, 24] Even a scrotal testis contralateral to an abdominal or inguinal testis carries an increased risk of cancer. Similarly, inguinal hernia has also been associated with an increased risk of testicular cancer.[22, 24]

Since we know that cryptorchidism and hernia have been induced in animal experiments by estrogen administration, hormonal medication and nausea of the mother and cryptorchidism of the offspring can be causally linked. It can be hypothesized that a major risk factor in testicular cancer is a relative excess of certain hormones (in particular estrogen) at the time of differentiation of the testes.[20]

Testicular dysgenesis and atrophy from different causes (e.g., mumps orchitis) have been associated with an increased risk of testicular cancer.[25, 26] The same is true of certain urogenital malformations.[27] It is interesting that some of these factors are related to estrogens. Similarly, severe acne at puberty, indicating enhanced secretion of androgens, has been considered to have a protective effect against testicular cancer.[21] In conclusion, a modified hormonal milieu affecting both the mother and her offspring appear to be important in the later development of testicular cancer.

HEREDITARY FACTORS

There are several reports on the occurrence of testicular cancer in twins and in both father and son.[7, 28-30] Frequently, the tumors have been histologically identical. These findings suggest that there may be some hereditary susceptibility to testicular cancer although the available data are insufficient to establish the real importance of heredity.

SUSPECTED RISK FACTORS

There are several suspected risk factors related to testicular cancer, mostly based on anecdotal, limited, or more or less nonconvincing clinical or other data. Tight trousers (jeans) and brief-type underwear[25] have been implicated as increasing the risk of testicular cancer. This hypothesis fits with the observed increase in the incidence among young men. Trauma has also been considered as a possible etiologic factor. The testis is, of course, easily affected by different types of trauma, and a testis with a tumor may be particularly vulnerable. The diagnosis of cancer could thus be enhanced by a trauma without any causal relationship. It is, however, interesting that in Denmark, where the incidence of testicular cancer is highest, people very frequently ride bicycles, which is likely to lead to occasional episodes of slight testicular trauma.

Maternal tuberculosis and epilepsy have been found to be risk factors in testicular cancer,[31] as is the use of LSD.[32] Finally, there has been speculation about the possible protective role of the sauna bath against testicular cancer. Some biological support exists for this hypothesis. High scrotal temperature is known to depress the activity of the spermatogenic epithelium, both in laboratory animals and in humans. This would explain the low incidence of testicular cancer in Finland, where it is customary to have a sauna bath once a week from early childhood to old age. There is, however, no direct evidence in favor of this hypothesis.

CONCLUDING REMARKS

The main characteristics of testicular cancer are the increase in its incidence in many areas, the rather wide geographical variation in its occurrence, and the specific age–incidence pattern, with a peak rate among young men. The etiology of testicular cancer is not well understood, but the hormonal milieu of the mother during pregnancy, and of the son during childhood and puberty, seem to be important. The risk of testicular cancer is associated with higher social class, and part of the increase in the incidence may be a reflection of the improvement in the standard of living. It is of interest that rural populations have higher rates in many places, although no consistent patterns have emerged.

Further studies on the epidemiology of testicular cancer should take into account the variation in histologic types.[33] Seminoma and nonseminomatous germ cell tumors are biologically different neoplasms. Their age–incidence patterns also refer to differences in the etiologic factors involved. The occurrence of these tumors in children and relatively young men is a challenge to epidemiologists and other cancer researchers, and should stimulate them to intensify their work in this field.

REFERENCES

1. Muir CS, Nectoux J: Epidemiology of cancer of the testis and penis. Nat Cancer Inst Monogr 53:157, 1979
2. Waterhouse J, Muir C, Shanmugaratnam K,

Powell J (eds): Cancer Incidence in Five Continents, Vol. IV. IARC Scientific Publications No. 42. International Agency for Research on Cancer, Lyon, 1982

3. Zimmerman RR, Kung'u A: Testicular neoplasms in Kenyan Africans. Cancer 41:2452, 1978

4. Berg JW, Godwin JD II, McKay FW, Percy CL: Testis cancer in Negroes. Lancet I:782, 1973

5. Teppo L: Histology of testicular cancer in Finland. p. 81. In Stalsberg H (ed): An International Survey of Distributions of Histologic Types of Tumours of the Testis and Ovary. UICC Technical Report Series, Vol. 75. International Union Against Cancer, Geneva, 1983

6. Teppo L, Pukkala E, Hakama M et al: Way of life and cancer incidence in Finland. A municipality-based ecological analysis. Scand J Soc Med, Suppl 19:1, 1980

7. Clemmesen J: Statistical studies in the aetiology of malignant neoplasms. III. Testis cancer. Basic tables, Denmark 1958–1962. Acta Pathol Microbiol Scand, Suppl 209, 15, 1969

8. Talerman A, Kaalen JGAH, Fokkens W: Rural preponderance of testicular neoplasms. Br J Cancer 29:176, 1974

9. Graham S, Gibson R, West D et al: Epidemiology of cancer of the testis in upstate New York. J Nat Cancer Inst 58:1255, 1977

10. Lipworth L, Dayan AD: Rural preponderance of seminoma of the testis. Cancer 23:1119, 1969

11. Davies JM: Testicular cancer in England and Wales: some epidemiological aspects. Lancet I:928, 1981

12. Ross RK, McCurtis JW, Henderson BE et al: al: Descriptive epidemiology of testicular and prostatic cancer in Los Angeles. Br J Cancer 39:284, 1979

13. Morrison AS: Some social and medical characteristics of army men with testicular cancer. Am J Epidemiol 104:511, 1976

14. Davies JM: Is testicular cancer incidence related to marital status? Int J Cancer 28:721, 1981

15. Mills PK, Newell GR, Johnson DE: Testicular cancer associated with employment in agriculture and oil and natural gas extraction. Lancet I:207, 1984

16. McDowall M, Balarajan R: Testicular cancer and employment in agriculture. Lancet I:510, 1984

17. Jensen OM, Olsen JH, Osterlind A: Testis cancer risk among farmers in Denmark. Lancet I:794, 1984

18. Grumet RF, MacMahon B: Trends in mortality from neoplasms of the testis. Cancer 11:790, 1958

19. Graham S, Gibson RW: Social epidemiology of cancer of the testis. Cancer 29:1242, 1972

20. Henderson BE, Benton B, Jing J et al: Risk factors for cancer of the testis in young men. Int J Cancer 23:598, 1979

21. Depue RH, Pike MC, Henderson BE: Estrogen exposure during gestation and risk of testicular cancer. J Nat Cancer Inst 71:1151, 1983

22. Schottenfeld D, Warshauer ME, Sherlock S, et al: The epidemiology of testicular cancer in young adults. Am J Epidemiol 112:232, 1980

23. Gill WB, Schumacher GFB, Bibbo M et al: Association of diethylstilbesterol exposure in utero with cryptorchidism, testicular hypoplasia and semen abnormalities. J Urol 122:36, 1979

24. Morrison AS: Cryptorchidism, hernia, and cancer of the testis. J Natl Cancer Inst 56:731, 1976

25. Lin RS, Kessler II: Epidemiologic findings in testicular cancer. Am J Epidemiol 110:357, 1979

26. Kaufman JJ, Bruce PT: Testicular atrophy following mumps. A cause of testis tumour? Br J Urol 35:67, 1963

27. Li FP, Fraumeni JR Jr: Testicular cancer in children: epidemiologic characteristics. J Natl Cancer Inst 48:1575, 1972

28. Simpson JL, Photopulos G: Hereditary aspects of ovarian and testicular neoplasia. Birth Defects Ser. 12:51, 1976

29. Wilbur HJ, Woodruff MW, Welch MS: Concomitant germ cell tumors in monozygotic twins. J Urol 121:538, 1979

30. Raghavan D, Jelihovsky T, Fox RM: Father–son testicular malignancy. Does genetic anticipation occur? Cancer 45:1005, 1980

31. Swerdlow AJ, Stiller CA, Kinnier Wilson LM: Prenatal factors in the aetiology of testicular cancer: an epidemiological study of childhood testicular cancer deaths in Great Britain, 1953–73. J Epidemiol Commun Health 36:96, 1982

32. Levick LJ, Levick SN: Testicular choriocarcinoma in LSD users. JAMA 217:475, 1971

33. Teppo L: Testicular cancer in Finland. Acta Pathol Microbiol Scand [A] Suppl 238:1, 1973

34. Cancer Incidence in Denmark 1978, 1979 and 1980. Danish Cancer Registry, Copenhagen, 1983

35. Incidence of Cancer in Norway 1978, 1979, 1980, 1981. The Cancer Registry of Norway, Oslo, 1981, 1982, 1983

36. Cancer Incidence in Sweden 1976, 1977, 1978, 1979, 1980. National Board of Health and Welfare, The Cancer Registry, Stockholm, 1980, 1981, 1982, 1983

2

Intratubular Germ Cell Neoplasia: Ultrastructure and Pathogenesis

Bernard Gondos

The significance of intratubular germ cell neoplasia, or carcinoma in situ of the testis, has only recently been recognized. Although the occurrence of intratubular proliferation of atypical germ cells in areas adjacent to invasive testicular tumors has been well known for many years, the existence of such a finding as a precursor to testicular cancer was first reported by Skakkebaek[1] in 1972. Similar observations of intratubular abnormalities in the absence of testicular enlargement were subsequently described by others.[2-6] The importance of the finding is indicated by the evidence of progression to typical malignant tumors, such as seminoma and embryonal carcinoma, in a significant number of cases.

The finding has generally been made in infertile men with testicular abnormalities of various types, including atrophy, cryptorchidism, and testicular feminization. The changes have also been identified in the contralateral testis of individuals with previously diagnosed testicular cancer.

The pathologic findings consist of germ cell abnormalities restricted to the seminiferous tubules. In the earliest stage, large atypical cells are seen at the periphery of the tubules. Later, the spermatogenic cells become completely replaced by the atypical cells which fill the seminiferous tubules. The atypical cells have large, round nuclei and prominent, often multiple, nucleoli closely resembling seminoma cells. They have ultrastructural characteristics of spermatogenic precursor cells and the malignant cells present in seminoma.[7, 8]

As in the latter, the DNA content of the nuclei demonstrates an aneuploid pattern.[9]

The lesion may progress to an invasive stage, with cells breaking through the tubular basement membrane into the surrounding interstitial tissue. The cells invade as small clusters or as single cells with the same cytologic features as the atypical intratubular cells. The early invasive lesions have been referred to as intratubular germ cell neoplasia with extratubular infiltration and microinvasive germ cell tumor.[10]

In spite of the increasing literature on the subject, there is still not wide recognition of the existence and clinical implications of intratubular neoplasia. Little is known regarding its pathogenesis. Some investigators, in fact, have been reluctant to accept this as a malignant condition rather than an atypical proliferative process.[11, 12] At a recent international symposium on testicular cancer, a committee of pathologists convened to discuss the classification and nomenclature of testicular tumors, with particular reference to intratubular germ cell neoplasia.[13] The consensus was that the intratubular abnormality is a preinvasive malignant condition. Descriptions of intratubular germ cell neoplasia subsequently have begun to appear in major pathology textbooks.[14, 15]

Previous reviews have focused on the histopathologic findings[13, 16] and clinical implications[17, 18] of intratubular neoplasia. This chapter summarizes these aspects with emphasis on the ultrastructure and pathogenesis of

11

Table 2-1. Characteristics of Developing Germ Cells in Human Testis

	Primitive Germ Cells	*Gonocytes*	*Prespermatogonia*	*Spermatogonia*
Period of development	Early fetal	Fetal	Late fetal/postnatal	Adult
Gonadal differentiation	Indifferent	Testis	Testis	Testis
Germ Cell differentiation	Prespermatogenesis	Prespermatogenesis	Prespermatogenesis	Spermatogenesis
Location	Indifferent gonad	Seminiferous cords, central	Seminiferous cords, peripheral	Seminiferous tubules, peripheral
Shape	Irregular ameboid	Spherical	Spherical	Spherical to ovoid[a]
Nucleus	Round to oval	Round	Round	Round to oval
Nucleolus	Central	Central	Central	Eccentric
Chromatin	Loose, evenly distributed	Loose, evenly distributed	Loose, evenly distributed	Dense, compact to coarse[b]
Glycogen	Abundant	Moderate	Minimal to absent	Minimal to absent
Intercellular bridges	Absent	Present	Present	Present
Cellular arrangement	Individual	Individual or pairs	Pairs or groups	Rows

[a] Type A spermatogonia flattened at base along basal lamina.
[b] Varies in type A and B spermatogonia.

the condition. Since studies thus far indicate that the pathogenesis of intratubular neoplasia relates directly to abnormalities in germ cell differentiation, an introductory section will include a review of current information on normal testicular germ cell differentiation.

GERM CELL DIFFERENTIATION

The principal features of developing germ cells in the human testis are summarized in Table 2-1. Primitive germ cells formed in the yolk sac endoderm migrate to the genital ridge at 4 to 5 weeks of gestation. These cells are characterized by large, round nuclei, prominent nucleoli and an irregular oval ameboid shape. The cytoplasm contains abundant glycogen and exhibits a positive response to alkaline phosphatase. The germ cells are individually arranged and are surrounded by somatic elements.

During the migratory phase, gonadal outgrowths from the genital ridges begin to project into the coelmic cavity. They are lined by a surface epithelial layer continuous with the mesothelial lining. By 6 weeks, a layer of connective tissue, the tunica albuginea, has formed in the male gonad, separating the epithelium and the underlying cellular aggregates. The latter consist of germ cells and Sertoli cells bounded by a basal lamina (Fig. 2-1). Within the developing seminiferous cords, the germ cells lose their ameboid appearance and become spherical. The glycogen content is decreased, and there is a general paucity of cytoplasmic organelles. The germ cells within the fetal testicular cords are referred to as gonocytes (Fig. 2-2).

Mitotic activity in the seminiferous cords involves both germ cells and Sertoli cells, maintaining a relatively equal number of the two cellular components in the fetal testis. During this time, there is no further differenti-

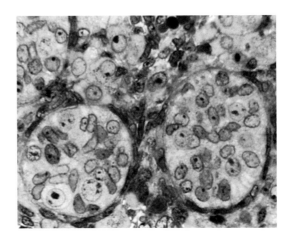

Fig. 2-1. Seminiferous cords, fetal testis, 12 weeks' gestation, including large round germ cells and elongated Sertoli cells. Toluidine blue, × 250.

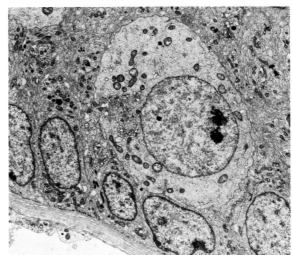

Fig. 2-2. Gonocyte and adjacent Sertoli cells, fetal seminiferous cord. Uranyl acetate and lead citrate, × 4,000.

ation of the testicular germ cells, which is in sharp contrast to the situation in the fetal ovary. Oogenesis begins late in the first trimester and continues throughout the remainder of gestation with oocytes progressing through the first meiotic prophase. Although relatively quiescent, the testicular germ cells do undergo certain changes. The gonocytes begin to move to the periphery where they become situated along the basal lamina (Fig. 2-3). The cells are now referred to as prespermatogonia because of their basal location, similar to that of spermatogonia. However, they lack certain morphologic features of spermatogonia, including cellular flattening along the basal la-

mina, marked chromatin condensation, and eccentric location of nucleoli.

Another noteworthy event associated with early germ cell differentiation is the formation of intercellular bridges between adjacent cells (Fig. 2-4). These broad cytoplasmic connections result from incomplete separation at the time of mitotic division. The phenomenon affects developing germ cells in both the ovary and testis and differs from other types of cell contacts in that open channels are maintained, allowing free exchange of organelles and other materials. Intercellular bridges of this type have been found only in germ cells and occur extensively in a wide variety of species.[19]

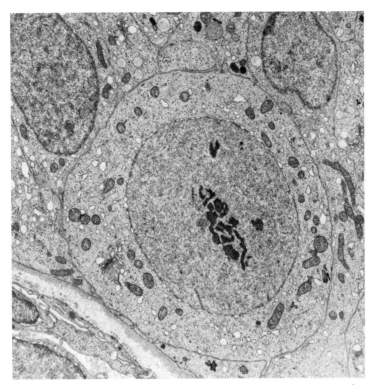

Fig. 2-3. Prespermatogonium adjacent to basal lamina. Note complex reticular nucleolus, evenly distributed chromatin, and scattered cytoplasmic organelles. Uranyl acetate and lead citrate, × 10,000.

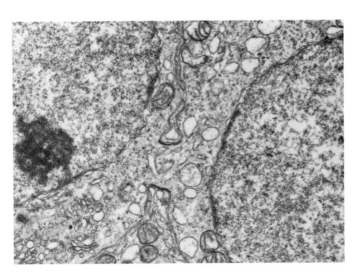

Fig. 2-4. Intercellular bridge connecting two spermatogonia. Open cytoplasmic channel allowing free exchange of organelles is evident. Uranyl acetate and lead citrate, × 14,000.

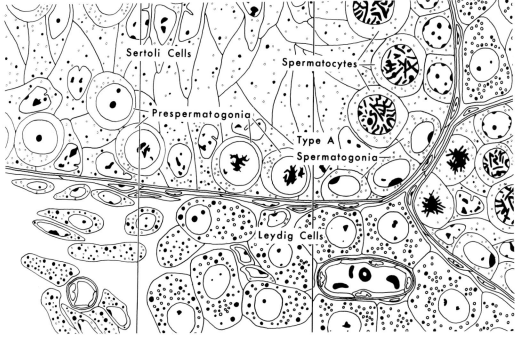

Fig. 2-5. Diagrammatic representation of stages of testicular development. Panel at left represents early postnatal testis, at center prepubertal testis, and at right initiation of spermatogenesis. (Gondos B: Testicular development. In Johnson AD, Gomes WR (eds): The Testis, Vol IV. Academic Press, New York, 1975.)

In the postnatal testis, mitotic activity in prespermatogonia is limited. Sertoli cells continue to divide actively, so that during childhood the relative proportion of germ cells decreases and there is an evident preponderance of Sertoli cells. The latter are primarily responsible for the progressive increase in diameter of the seminiferous cords. Germ cell number shows a steady but only slight increase. The typical appearance of the prepubertal testis is that of scattered single, paired, or small groups of germ cells lying along the basal lamina among the more numerous Sertoli cells.

Shortly before the onset of spermatogenesis, which generally occurs at 10 to 11 years of age, there is marked nucleolar enlargement in the prespermatogonia associated with increased RNA synthesis by the germ cells. Differentiation and proliferation of spermatogonia follow, indicating the initiation of spermatogenesis.

The process of spermatogenesis continues through adult life in a recurring, cyclic fashion. Spermatogonia constitute the pool of stem cells, a portion of which undergo differentiation as a new cycle begins, while the remainder represent the renewing stem cells for subsequent spermatogenic cycles. Differentiating spermatogonia proceed through a series of mitotic divisions associated with incomplete cytokinesis and, therefore, increasing numbers of persistent intercellular connections. The result is a syncytial pattern of organization which is reflected by the arrangement of spermatogonia in rows.

The next stage is that of spermatocyte formation in which the type of division shifts from mitosis to meiosis as the cells move away from the basal lamina. At this time, two other important events occur. First, the development of occlusive tight junctions between adjacent Sertoli cells results in the formation of a blood–testis barrier, dividing the tubules into a basal and adluminal compartment. Second, a central lumen begins to appear, indicating the transformation of seminiferous cords to tubules. Of the two meiotic divisions, the first, in which redistribution of genetic material occurs, is the longer. Cellular interconnection is maintained throughout the period of spermatocyte differentiation. Serial sections at the electron microscopic level have demonstrated that groups of as many as several hundred spermatocytes can be joined in this manner.[20]

During the spermatid stage, the final period of spermatogenesis, which is marked by maturation and elongation, acrosome formation occurs. As spermatogenesis is completed, individual spermatozoa are released into the tubular lumen and then transported to the excurrent ducts.

In considering this extensive process of cellular transformation, it is important to recognize that there is continuity from the primitive germ cells in the indifferent gonad to gonocytes and prespermatogonia in the prespermatogenic testis to spermatogonia involved in spermatogenesis (Fig. 2-5). The derivation of adult germ cells from gonocytes in the fetal testis is now well established, since there is no evidence of neoformation of germ cells at the time of spermatogenesis.[21] It is also significant that in contrast to the ovary, there is an arrest of differentiation and limited proliferation of germ cells in the developing testis. Only when spermatogenesis begins at the time of puberty do active mitotic division and progression through meiosis occur in the testis. This difference in timing may relate to the difference in age incidence of malignant germ cell tumors in the ovary and testis.[22]

TERMINOLOGY

The classification of testicular germ cell tumors is discussed in Chapter 3. The relationship of intratubular germ cell neoplasia to the invasive germ cell tumors is that of a precursor lesion. Those cases in which progression to

invasive tumors has occurred include seminomas, embryonal carcinomas, and teratomas. The general appearance of the intratubular lesions in these instances is similar, although distinctive patterns of differentiation can be identified. The designations intratubular seminoma and intratubular embryonal carcinoma have been used in such cases. The characteristic and most frequently observed lesion is classified nonspecifically as intratubular germ cell neoplasia.

The term carcinoma in situ of the testis is the designation initially proposed by Skakkebaek and colleagues.[1, 17] Based on priority and general usage, this would be the preferred terminology. However, existence of malignant potential in all cases has not been established. Furthermore, germ cells are not epithelial and, therefore, strictly speaking, carcinoma in situ is not an appropriate term. Nevertheless, it should be recognized that the histologic appearance and clinical implications are analogous to carcinoma in situ in other sites, and the appropriate connotation is clearly provided by this terminology.

According to the classification proposed by the Minneapolis study group, designation of intratubular germ cell neoplasia as a precursor of definite, but not necessarily uniform, malignant potential is recommended.[13, 14] The term intratubular germ cell neoplasia is noncommittal in regard to the type of tumor, which usually cannot be predicted at the intratubular stage. Subgroups of intratubular seminoma and intratubular embryonal carcinoma have been recognized. The most frequent form is intratubular germ cell neoplasia without further classification.

As additional information becomes available, the precise classification and nomenclature of this group of lesions will most likely need to undergo further revision.

CLINICAL FEATURES

Intratubular germ cell neoplasia occurring in the absence of a demonstrable testicular mass has been identified in testicular biopsy specimens from infertile men. The underlying conditions have included cryptorchidism,[2, 3, 18, 23, 24] severe oligospermia[1, 4, 7, 18, 25] and testicular feminization.[15, 26] It is difficult to know the precise incidence of intratubular neoplasia in these disorders since testicular biopsy is infrequently employed as a diagnostic method. Similarly, information on occurrence in an otherwise normal testis is not available. In studies involving large series of testicular biopsies in infertile men, intratubular germ cell neoplasia has been found in 0.5 to 1 percent of patients with severe oligospermia[4, 18] and in 2 to 8 percent of those with cryptorchidism.[24]

Detection generally occurs in young adults who are being evaluated for infertility. Five percent of patients who have previously undergone orchiectomy for testicular cancer have been found to have intratubular lesions in the remaining testis.[27] In individuals with both a unilateral testicular germ cell tumor and a history of maldescent, the risk for development of a lesion in the remaining testis may be as high[18] as 15 to 20 percent. Intratubular germ cell neoplasia has also, although infrequently, been diagnosed in children, including those with cryptorchidism[18, 23] and precocious puberty associated with unilateral Leydig cell proliferation.[28]

Experience with this lesion indicates that approximately half of the cases will progress to invasive carcinoma within 5 years if orchiectomy is not performed.[4, 17] Consequently, the precancerous potential is well established. For this reason, screening programs utilizing testicular biopsies for the detection of intratubular neoplasia in infertile men and those with previous tumors in the contralateral testis have been instituted in Denmark,[18] a country with a particularly high incidence of testicular cancer.

DIAGNOSIS

The diagnosis of intratubular neoplasia is made by testicular biopsy in patients at risk. This is contrary to the usual procedure in testicular neoplasms, for which biopsy is generally contraindicated. However, in this condition biopsy is the only available means of diagnosis.

Sampling represents a potential problem, which has been addressed by Skakkebaek et al.[29] By examining serial sections of entire testes in specimens containing intratubular germ cell neoplasia, they demonstrated that a 3-mm biopsy specimen has a high likelihood of detecting the abnormality if the volume of tubules involved is greater than 10 percent. Thus far, none of the individuals who had a negative biopsy on screening examination subsequently developed testicular neoplasia.

Use of serum markers, such as human chorionic gonadotropin (HCG) and alpha-fetoprotein (AFP), has not been of value in diagnosis.[30] This is reflected by corresponding negative results of immunohistochemical studies for these substances in most cases of intratubular neoplasia.[12, 31] The possibility that other tumor markers may be identified remains a subject for future investigation.

LIGHT MICROSCOPY

The histologic features of intratubular germ cell neoplasia have previously been reviewed in detail.[13, 16] In early stages, large atypical cells with prominent nuclei and abundant clear cytoplasm appear at the tubular periphery in sites where spermatogenesis may be present. Characteristically, there is extensive replacement of the normal tubular components by accumulations of large atypical cells (Fig. 2-6). At higher magnifications, enlarged, often multiple, irregular nucleoli are seen (Fig. 2-7). Mitotic figures, including abnormal forms, are commonly present.

Immunohistochemical studies and other special staining techniques have indicated the presence of both alkaline phosphatase[32] and ferritin[12, 33] in the cytoplasm of the neoplastic cells. The former is a typical germ cell marker, and both have been found in seminomas and other germ cell tumors.[34, 35] Generally, as

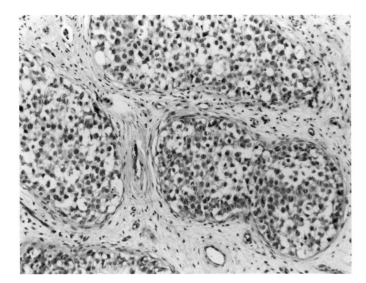

Fig. 2-6. Light micrograph of intratubular germ cell neoplasia shows replacement of spermatogenic elements by large atypical cells. H & E. × 150.

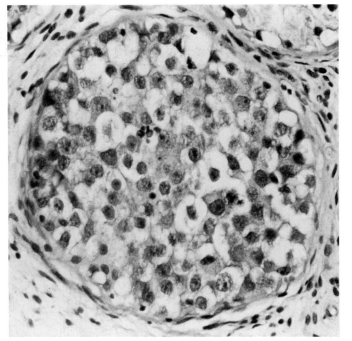

Fig. 2-7. Higher magnification demonstrates large nuclei and prominent nucleoli. Extratubular infiltration is not seen. H & E. × 500.

noted above, neither HCG nor AFP is present in intratubular neoplasia,[12, 31] although occasional staining with HCG has been reported.[36] The presence of glycogen in the cytoplasm of the abnormal cells is noteworthy in that this finding is characteristic of early stages of germ cell differentiation.

ELECTRON MICROSCOPY

Ultrastructural studies of intratubular neoplasia have indicated a close resemblance of the tumor cells to germ cells in the fetal and postnatal testis.[7, 8, 12, 37-39] The electron microscopic features are characteristic of pres-

Table 2-2. Comparison of Ultrastructural Features in Normal and Neoplastic Germ Cells

	Prespermatogenic Germ Cells	*Intratubular Germ Cell Neoplasia*	*Seminoma/ Dysgerminoma*
Nucleus	Large, round	Large, round	Large, round
Nucleolus	Large, irregular, occasionally multiple	Large, irregular, occasionally multiple	Large, irregular, occasionally multiple
Chromatin	Loose, diffuse	Loose, diffuse	Loose, diffuse
Mitochondria	Round, eccentric cristae	Round, eccentric cristae	Round, eccentric cristae
Glycogen	Depends on stage	May be abundant	Usually present
Nuage material	Present	Present	Present
Dense-core vesicles	Present	Present	Present
Intercellular bridges	Present	Absent	Absent

permatogenic cells, including gonocytes and prespermatogonia (Table 2-2).

Nuclei of the neoplastic cells are symmetrical with evenly distributed chromatin (Fig. 2-8). The pattern is diffusely granular without evidence of peripheral margination. Nucleoli demonstrate an elaborate reticular pattern, most prominent in cells with multiple nucleoli (Fig. 2-9). The nucleoli are usually centrally located, resembling the appearance in prespermatogonia. Occasional cells with single eccentric nucleoli characteristic of type A spermatogonia have also been observed. Chromatin and nucleolar patterns found in type B spermatogonia have not been described nor have synaptinemal complexes or other evidence of spermatocyte differentiation. Thus, the nuclear characteristics are predominantly those of prespermatogenic germ cells.

Cytoplasmic features are variable, including abundant glycogen in some cells and a general paucity of organelles in others. Aggregates of

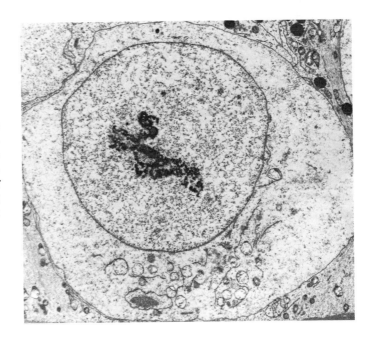

Fig. 2-8. Electron micrograph of intratubular germ cell neoplasia demonstrates elaborate reticular nucleolus, loose chromatin pattern, and paucity of cytoplasmic organelles. Uranyl acetate and lead citrate, × 5,100.

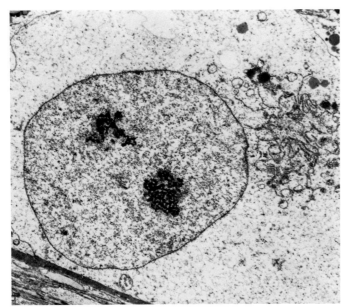

Fig. 2-9. Ultrastructural findings in intratubular neoplasia include multiple nucleoli and polarization of cytoplasmic organelles. Uranyl acetate and lead citrate, × 3,200.

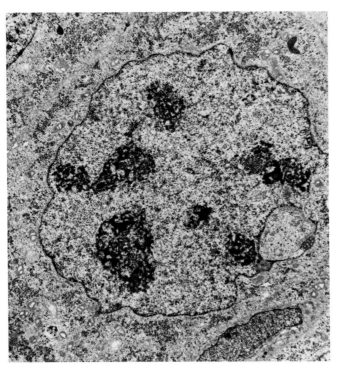

Fig. 2-10. Extensive nucleolar proliferation and diffuse accumulation of glycogen are evident. Uranyl acetate and lead citrate, × 14,000.

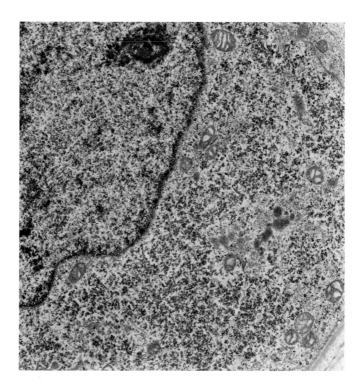

Fig. 2-11. Abnormal germ cell at tubular periphery with dense aggregates of glycogen, scattered mitochondria, and group of dense-core vesicles. Uranyl acetate and lead citrate, × 17,000.

glycogen granules may be particularly abundant, filling much of the cytoplasm (Fig. 2-10). This finding is reminiscent of the appearance of primitive germ cells. Many other cells have a loose cytoplasmic content with only scattered mitochondria, strands of endoplasmic reticulum, and occasional smooth vesicles. Regional clustering of organelles characteristic of later stages of prespermatogenic germ cell differentiation is frequently seen. Dense-core vesicles and annulate lamellae, ultrastructural features associated with germ cells, have also been noted (Fig. 2-11). The appearance of mitochondria provides further evidence of germ cell origin, particularly the eccentric location of cristae and the presence of intermitochondrial granular material. Similar granular material, referred to as nuage, is often found elsewhere in the cytoplasm of the tumor cells. This material is considered a morphologic marker of germ cells since it is characteristically found in differentiating germ cells in a wide variety of animal species.[40]

Cell membranes are generally smooth and regular. Occasional microvillus-like projections can be seen around intercellular spaces. Where adjacent tumor cells are closely apposed, recognizable intercellular junctions are not evident except for scattered loose attachment plaques (Fig. 2-12). No desmoplastic attachments have been observed between neoplastic cells and remaining Sertoli cells. Intercellular bridges of the type connecting normal developing germ cells have not been identified. Because this is such a characteristic feature of prespermatogenic germ cells, we have made a particularly careful search for bridges but have been unable to find any intercellular connections. This appears to be the only significant ultrastructural difference between the neoplastic cells and normal prespermatogenic germ cells.

PATHOGENESIS

Ultrastructural analysis indicates a close resemblance of the neoplastic cells within the tubules to germ cells at early stages of differen-

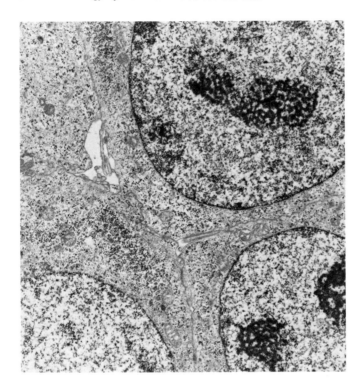

Fig. 2-12. Group of cells characteristic of intratubular germ cell neoplasia. Note close approximation of adjacent cell membranes. Uranyl acetate and lead citrate, × 14,000.

tiation. Most of the cells have electron microscopic features characteristic of prespermatogenic germ cells. Comparison with developing germ cells in the human testis[41-43] and other mammalian species[44] reveals a fundamental similarity of the abnormal intratubular cells to gonocytes and prespermatogonia found in the fetal and prepubertal testis.

Thus, origin of the lesions from germ cells at an early stage of differentiation is likely. The neoplastic cells have larger nuclei and somewhat greater nucleolar complexity than normal developing germ cells but are otherwise comparable in general contour, nuclear structure, and cytoplasmic organization. The fact that occasional cells resembling type A spermatogonia may also be present suggests that some degree of maturation can take place, but it is limited since cells with features of type B spermatogonia are not seen.

A particular point of interest is the lack of intercellular bridges between adjacent tumor cells. Germ cell interconnections are normally present in large numbers in the developing and adult testis.[19, 45] Although the original descriptions of such bridges were in groups of spermatocytes and spermatids,[46, 47] subsequent studies have demonstrated their presence at spermatogonial and prespermatogonial stages of differentiation.[48, 49] Thus, their absence in intratubular neoplasia represents a significant departure from the usual appearance of developing germ cells.

A similar situation exists in invasive testicular germ cell tumors. Ultrastructural studies of these tumors have demonstrated resemblance of the neoplastic cells to germ cells at early stages of differentiation, but intercellular bridges have not been described.[37, 50-55] The only exception is the spermatocytic seminoma in which characteristic intercellular bridges have been observed.[56] The neoplastic cells in these tumors have ultrastructural features of spermatocytes rather than prespermatogenic cells, suggesting that spermatocytic seminomas have a different pathogenesis from other germ cell tumors.[57] In an extensive ultrastructural analysis of typical seminomas,[53] it

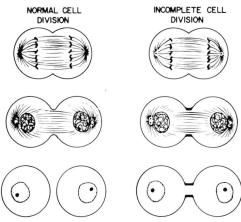

NORMAL CELL DIVISION

INCOMPLETE CELL DIVISION

Fig. 2-13. Comparison of normal mitotic division and incomplete division leading to intercellular bridge formation. (Gondos B, Zamboni L: Ovarian development: the functional importance of germ cell interconnections. Fertil Steril 20:176, 1969.)

was noted that intercellular bridges were absent in all of the tumors. Bridges identified in adjacent uninvolved tubules were much wider than usual and abnormally formed. These findings suggest a possible association of defective intercellular bridge formation and germ cell neoplasia.

In this regard, it is of interest to review the formation and function of germ cell interconnections in the normal developing testis.[19, 45] The intercellular bridges between adjacent germ cells originate from incomplete mitotic division resulting from failure of daughter cells to separate at telophase (Fig. 2-13). The shape and location of the bridges as well as the inclusion within them of microtubules consistent with residual spindle fibers indicate that they represent residual midbodies that persist after the completion of the cell division.

The pattern of incomplete cytokinesis begins during the phase of active mitotic proliferation of gonial cells. Primitive germ cells undergoing mitosis during their migration to the genital ridges are evidently able to complete cytokinesis in the usual manner since intercellular bridges are not present at this stage. Bridges appear in the fetal testis shortly after formation of the seminiferous cords. In the human testis, germ cell interconnections are seen as early as the 3rd month of gestation.[41]

During development, the arrangement and number of intercellular bridges undergo changes related to the pattern of germ cell division. Because there is limited mitotic activity in the fetal and prepubertal testis, pairs and small groups of cells connected by bridges remain. With the onset of spermatogenesis, mitotic activity is greatly increased, and there is a corresponding increase in the number of bridges. It appears that once the pattern of incomplete cytokinesis is initiated, all subsequent divisions result in a similar persistence of cellular connection (Fig. 2-14). This produces an ever-enlarging syncytium, with the interconnected cells differentiating as a unit.

The most likely and widely supported function of intercellular bridges is the coordination and synchronization of germ cell differentiation.[19, 45, 49, 58] It has been consistently observed that cells joined by intercellular bridges are at the same stage of development and have identical ultrastructural features.[19, 47] Studies of spermatogenic development utilizing serial sections have revealed that hundreds of cells may be linked together, all at the same stage of differentiation.[59] Since the open cytoplasmic connections allow free intercellular communication, the extensive pattern of interconnection is responsible for establishing a common cytoplasmic milieu for large numbers of cells.

It has also been suggested that intercellular bridges may function in restricting the number of germ cell divisions.[19, 60] There is normally a fixed number of mitotic divisions before meiosis begins. How the number of divisions is regulated is unknown. One possibility is that once a maximal number of interconnections has formed, no further mitosis can occur and the cells proceed into meiosis. If this is so, then failure of intercellular bridge formation might lead to continued, uncontrolled mitotic division or neoplasia.

Support for this hypothesis comes from both clinical and experimental observations.

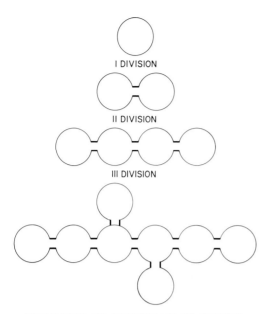

FORMATION OF INTERCELLULAR BRIDGES

Fig. 2-14. Diagram illustrating pattern of repeated incomplete mitotic division resulting in increasing cellular interconnection. (Gondos B: Germ cell relationships in the developing rabbit ovary. In Butt WR, Crooke AC, Ryle M (eds): Gonadotrophins and Ovarian Development. E & S Livingstone, Edinburgh, 1970.)

The consistent absence of intercellular bridges in a variety of germ cell tumors examined by electron microscopy is particularly noteworthy. Tumors derived directly from germ cells, including testicular seminomas, ovarian dysgerminomas, and extragonadal germinomas otherwise share ultrastructural features with developing germ cells, but lack bridges. The same findings pertain to intratubular testicular neoplasia. Since the latter represents a precursor to the commonly seen testicular germ cell tumors, the implication is that lack of intercellular bridges may be associated with early stages of germ cell neoplasia.

It is interesting that bridges were described in a report of a mixed germ cell sex cord stromal tumor occurring in an otherwise normal adult man.[61] The precise nature and histogenesis of such tumors is unclear, but they have all showed a benign clinical course without

the emergence of a corresponding malignant form. If this proves to be the case in other similar tumors, the presence of intercellular bridges may be an indicator of benign behavior. Conversely, absence of bridges may provide a clue to malignant potential.

Further evidence bearing on the role of intercellular bridges in germ cell neoplasia is provided by studies on a mutant species of *Drosophila* in which absence of germ cell connections is associated with spontaneous germ cell tumors.[62] The mutations can be readily produced, and there is a consistent occurrence of neoplasms when the bridges are not formed. Investigators working in this area have proposed that a class of genes exists which regulates the incomplete cytokinesis associated with normal germ cell development.[63] These genes would only be activated in germ cells and would function to arrest the advance of the cleavage furrow and stabilize the cellular bridges. Mutations in these genes could lead to a high incidence of complete cytokinesis, resulting in excessive mitotic division and germ cell tumors.

This intriguing hypothesis would substantiate the proposed function of intercellular bridges in limiting mitosis and thereby preventing unrestricted germ cell proliferation. The natural consequence of unlimited proliferation would be neoplasia. Whether lack of intercellular bridge formation leads to tumor development is a question that needs to be resolved. Investigators considering the role of intercellular communication in carcinogenesis have suggested that a genetic correlation exists between coupling and tumorigenicity, and that the loss or interruption of communication could be a key event in some forms of cancer.[64, 65] These comments derive from work done principally on epithelial tumors but may apply with equal relevance to germ cell neoplasms.

While the precise pathogenesis of intratubular germ cell neoplasia remains to be clarified, electron microscopic studies have clearly demonstrated its origin from germ cells at early stages of differentiation. The findings suggest that excessive, uncontrolled proliferation of spermatogenic precursors related to interruption of cellular communication may be responsible for the abnormality. Further work in this area is needed.

SUMMARY

The existence of intratubular germ cell neoplasia as a precursor to invasive germ cell tumors is now well established. The high association of untreated lesions with subsequent evidence of invasion indicates the malignant potential of the intratubular process. Whether all germ cell tumors go through an intratubular phase remains to be determined, but the frequent finding of abnormal germ cells in tubules adjacent to invasive lesions suggests that this is likely.

Ultrastructural studies support this view. There is a close similarity in the cytologic features of intratubular lesions and their invasive counterparts. This is evident on examination by light microscopy, but is particularly well demonstrated by electron microscopy. Furthermore, the resemblance of the neoplastic cells to developing germ cells implies that the process originates from spermatogenic precursors within the tubules. The initial growth phase presumably occurs within tubules, followed by an early or microinvasive stage and, finally, diffuse infiltration of the testicular parenchyma.

This indicates that the intratubular lesion is extremely important, both from a clinical and basic science point of view. Clinically, the implication is that detection of the most common forms of testicular cancer can be accomplished at a preinvasive stage and, therefore, prior to the opportunity for metastasis. The extent to which this information can be utilized to diagnose early stages of disease and reduce the need for aggressive therapy remains to be established.

From the point of view of basic science, it would follow that much is to be learned about the pathogenesis of invasive germ cell tumors from studies on intratubular neoplasia. Such investigations might include, in addition to the electron microscopic studies described here, histochemical, immunologic, chromosomal, cell kinetic, and culture studies. In addition, it is possible that insights can be gained into other pathologic processes affecting germ cells such as developmental abnormalities and effects of exogenous physical and chemical factors. The lesion of intratubular neoplasia, therefore, represents a useful model for studying abnormalities in germ cell growth and differentiation.

As recognition of the practical and theoretical importance of intratubular neoplasia becomes more widespread, additional information should become available. Reevaluation and refinement of concepts regarding the pathogenesis of germ cell cancers should follow. The existence of an intratubular neoplastic lesion with ultrastructural features of developing germ cells confirms earlier experimental observations on the origin of germ cell neoplasms. The opportunity for further studies on the precursor intratubular lesion and its relationship to invasive testicular tumors offers special challenges to the pathologist, clinician, and developmental biologist alike.

ACKNOWLEDGMENTS

Appreciation is expressed to Drs. Niels E. Skakkebaek and Jørgen C. Berthelsen for providing specimens utilized in this study. Dr. Robert E. Scully kindly provided prepublication material. Research performed in the author's laboratory was supported by grants from the National Institutes of Health (HD-12918) and Connecticut Research Foundation.

REFERENCES

1. Skakkebaek NE: Possible carcinoma-in-situ of the testis. Lancet 2:516, 1972
2. Waxman M: Malignant germ cell tumor in situ

in a cryptorchid testis. Cancer 38:1452, 1976

3. Williams TR, Brendler H: Carcinoma in situ of the ectopic testis. J Urol 117:610, 1977

4. Nüesch-Baumann IH, Hedinger C: Atypische Spermatogonien als Präkanzerose. Schweiz Med Wochenschr 107:795, 1977

5. Andres TL, Trainer TD, Leadbetter GW: Atypical germ cells preceding metachronous bilateral testicular tumors. Urology 15:307, 1980

6. Ishida H, Isurugi K, Niijima T et al: Carcinoma in situ of germ cells and subsequent development of an invasive seminoma in a hyperprolactinaemic man. Int J Androl 6:229, 1983

7. Nielsen H, Nielsen M, Skakkebaek NE: The fine structure of a possible carcinoma-in-situ in the seminiferous tubules in the testis of four infertile men. Acta Path Microbiol Scand [A] 82:235, 1974

8. Gondos B, Berthelsen JG, Skakkebaek NE: Intratubular germ cell neoplasia (carcinoma in situ): a preinvasive lesion of the testis. Ann Clin Lab Sci 13:185, 1983

9. Müller J, Skakkebaek NE: Microspectrophotometric DNA measurements of carcinoma-in-situ germ cells in the testis. Int J Androl [suppl] 4:211, 1981

10. von Eyben FE, Mikulowski P, Busch C: Micro-invasive germ cell tumors of the testis. J Urol 126:842, 1981

11. Sigg C, Hedinger C: Atypical germ cells in testicular biopsy in male sterility. Int J Androl [suppl] 4:163, 1981

12. Sigg C, Hedinger C: Atypical germ cells of the testis: Comparative ultrastructural and histochemical investigations. Virchows Arch Pathol [A] 402:439, 1984

13. Scully RE: Intratubular germ cell neoplasia (carcinoma in situ): What it is and what should be done about it. World Urol Update Ser 1:17, 1982

14. Rosai J: Ackerman's Surgical Pathology, 6th Ed, Vol I. CV Mosby, St. Louis, 1981

15. Scully RE: The testis. In Albores-Saavedra J, Henson D (eds): Incipient Neoplasia. WB Saunders, Philadelphia, in press

16. Skakkebaek NE: Carcinoma-in-situ of the testis: frequency and relationship to invasive germ cell tumours in infertile men. Histopathology 2:157, 1978

17. Skakkebaek NE, Berthelsen JG, Visfeldt J: Clinical aspects of testicular carcinoma-in-situ. Int J Androl, [suppl] 4:153, 1981

18. Skakkebaek NE, Berthelsen JG, Müller J: Carcinoma-in-situ of the undescended testis. Urol Clin North Am 9:377, 1982

19. Gondos B: Intercellular bridges and mammalian germ cell differentiation. Differentiation 1:177, 1973

20. Moens PB, Hugenholtz AD: The arrangement of germ cells in the rat seminiferous tubule: an electron-microscope study. J Cell Sci 19:487, 1975

21. Courot M, Hochereau-de Reviers MT, Ortavant R: Spermatogenesis. In Johnson AD, Gomes WR, Vandemark NL (eds): The Testis, Vol I. Academic Press, New York, 1970

22. Erickson RP, Gondos B: Alternative explanations of the differing behaviour of ovarian and testicular teratomas. Lancet 1:407, 1976

23. Dorman S, Trainer TD, Lefke D, Leadbetter G: Incipient germ cell tumor in a cryptorchid testis. Cancer 44:1357, 1979

24. Krabbe S, Skakkebaek NE, Berthelsen JG et al: High incidence of undetected neoplasia in maldescended testis. Lancet 1:999, 1979

25. Skakkebaek NE: Abnormal morphology of germ cells in two infertile men. Acta Path Microbiol Scand [A] 80:374, 1972

26. Skakkebaek NE: Carcinoma-in-situ of testis in testicular feminization. Acta Path Microbiol Scand [A] 87:87, 1979

27. Berthelsen JG, Skakkebaek NE, von der Maase H, Sorensen BL: Screening for carcinoma in situ of the contralateral testis in patients with germinal testicular cancer. Br Med J 285:1683, 1982

28. Wurzel R, Gondos B, Ratzan SK, Walzak MP: Intratubular germ cell neoplasia associated with precocious puberty. J Androl 5:28P, 1984

29. Berthelsen JG, Skakkebaek NE: Value of testicular biopsy in diagnosing carcinoma in situ testis. Scand J Urol Nephrol 15:165, 1981

30. von Eyben F, Krabbe S, Skakkebaek NE: Alpha-fetoprotein and human chorionic gonadotropin in men with maldescended testis. Br J Cancer 42:156, 1980

31. Jacobsen GK, Jacobsen M, Clausen PP, Pedersen NS: Immunohistochemical demonstration of tumor associated antigens in carcinoma-in-situ of the testis. Int J Androl [suppl] 4:203–210, 1981

32. Beckstead JH: Alkaline phosphatase histochemistry in human germ cell neoplasms. Am J Surg Pathol 7:341, 1983

33. Jacobsen GK, Jacobsen M, Clausen PP: Ferritin as a possible marker protein of carcinoma-in-situ of the testis. Lancet 2:533, 1980

34. Uchida T, Shimoda T, Miyata H et al: Immunoperoxidase study of alkaline phosphatase in testicular tumor. Cancer 48:1455, 1981

35. Jacobsen GK, Jacobsen M: Ferritin (FER) in testicular germ cell tumours. Acta Path Microbiol Scand [A] 91:177, 1983

36. Jacobsen GK, Jacobsen M: Alpha-fetoprotein (AFP) and human chorionic gonadotropin (HCG) in testicular germ cell tumours. Acta Pathol Microbiol Scand [A] 91:165, 1983

37. Schulze C, Holstein AF: On the histology of human seminoma: development of the solid tumor from intratubular seminoma cells. Cancer 39:1090, 1977

38. Akhtar M, Sidiki Y: Undifferentiated intratubular germ cell tumor of the testis: light and electron microscopic study of a unique case. Cancer 42:2332, 1979

39. Albrechtsen R, Nielsen MH, Skakkebaek NE, Wewer U: Carcinoma in situ of the testis: some ultrastructural characteristics of germ cells. Acta Path Microbiol Scand [A] 90:301, 1982

40. Eddy EM: Germ plasm and the differentiation of the germ cell line. Int Rev Cytol 43:229, 1975

41. Gondos B, Hobel CJ: Ultrastructure of germ cell development in the human fetal testis. Z Zellforsch 119:1, 1971

42. Wartenberg H, Holstein AF, Vossmeyer J: Zur Cytologie der pränatalen Gonadenentwicklung beim Menschen. II. Elektronenmikroskopische Untersuchungen über die Cytogenese von Gonocyten und fetalen Spermatogonien im Hoden. Z Anat Entwickl 134:165, 1971

43. Fukuda T, Hedinger C, Groscurth P: Ultrastructure of developing germ cells in the fetal human testis. Cell Tissue Res 161:55, 1975

44. Gondos B: Testicular development. In Johnson AD, Gomes WR (eds): The Testis, Vol IV. Academic Press, New York, 1975

45. Fawcett DW: Intercellular bridges. Exp Cell Res (suppl) 8:174, 1961

46. Burgos MH, Fawcett DW: Studies on the fine structure of the mammalian testis. I. Differentiation of the spermatids in the cat (*Felis domestica*). J Biophys Biochem Cytol 1:287, 1955

47. Fawcett DW, Ito S, Slautterback D: The occurrence of intercellular bridges in groups of cells exhibiting synchronous differentiation. J Biophys Biochem Cytol 5:453, 1959

48. Gondos B, Zemjanis R: Fine structure of spermatogonia and intercellular bridges in *Macaca nemestrina*. J Morphol 131:431, 1970

49. Gondos B: Differentiation and growth of cells in the gonads. In Goldspink G (ed): Differentiation and Growth of Cells in Vertebrate Tissues. Chapman and Hall, London, 1974

50. Pierce GB, Beals TF: The ultrastructure of primordial germinal cells of the fetal testes and of embryonal carcinoma cells of mice. Cancer Res 24:1553, 1964

51. Pierce GB: Ultrastructure of human testicular tumors. Cancer 19:1963, 1966

52. Pierce GB. Stevens LC, Nakane PK: Ultrastructural analysis of the early development of teratocarcinomas. J Natl Cancer Inst 39:755, 1967

53. Holstein AF, Körner F: Light and electron microscopical analysis of cell types in human seminoma. Virchows Arch Pathol [A] 363:97, 1974

54. Bjersing L, Cajander S: Ultrastructure of gonadoblastoma and disgerminoma (seminoma) in a patient with XY gonadal dysgenesis. Cancer 40:1127, 1977

55. Janssen M, Johnston WH: Anaplastic seminoma of the testis: ultrastructural analysis of three cases. Cancer 41:538, 1978

56. Rosai J, Khodadoust K, Silber I: Spermatocytic seminoma. II. Ultrastructural study. Cancer 24:103, 1969

57. Skakkebaek NE, Berthelsen JG: Carcinoma in situ of the testis and invasive growth of different types of germ cell tumours: a revised germ cell theory. Int J Androl, suppl 4:26–34, 1981

58. Togawa Y: Occurrence and structure of intercellular bridges between the human spermatogonia. Arch Histol Jpn 33:301, 1971

59. Dym M, Fawcett DW: Further observations on the numbers of spermatogonia, spermatocytes, and spermatids connected by intercellular bridges in the mammalian testis. Biol Reprod 4:195, 1971

60. King RC, Akai H: Spermatogenesis in *Bombyx mori*. I. The canal system joining sister spermatocytes. J Morphol 134:47, 1971

61. Bolen JW: Mixed germ cell-sex cord stromal tumor: a gonadal tumor distinct from gonado-blastoma. Am J Clin Pathol 75:565, 1981

62. Gollin SM, King RC: Studies of fs(1)1621, a mutation producing ovarian tumors in *Drosophila melanogaster.* Dev Genet 2:203, 1981

63. King RC: Ovarian Development in *Drosophila melanogaster.* Academic Press, New York, 1970

64. Loewenstein WR: Communication through cell junctions. Implications in growth control and differentiation. Dev Biol 19 (suppl) 2:151–183, 1968

65. Azarnia R, Larsen WJ: Intercellular communication and cancer. In DeMello WC (ed): Intercellular Communication. Plenum, New York, 1977

3

Germ Cell Tumors

Aleksander Talerman

Germ cell tumors form by far the largest group of testicular neoplasms. They make up from 86.6[1] to 93 percent[2] of all testicular neoplasms and therefore hold the most important place in testicular tumor pathology.

Testicular germ cell tumors show a remarkable homology with ovarian and extragonadal germ cell neoplasms and, with the exception of spermatocytic seminoma, all the histologic types of germ cell tumors occurring in the testis are found in the ovary and in extragonadal sites, although the incidence of the various histologic types shows considerable differences.

In the testis, germ cell tumors form approximately 90 percent of all testicular neoplasms[1, 2] while only 20 percent of ovarian neoplasms are of germ cell origin.[3]

Another major difference between testicular and ovarian germ cell tumors is the fact that benign tumors are very rare in the testis and occur almost exclusively during infancy and early childhood,[4] while the great majority of ovarian germ cell tumors (92 percent) are mature cystic teratomas, which are benign.[3]

Testicular germ cell tumors are encountered from infancy to old age, but the majority occur in persons between the ages of 15 and 50 years.[1, 2, 4] Because of this specific age incidence, these tumors are considered among the more common malignant neoplasms in the postpubertal and young adult male.

HISTOGENESIS

Although the germ cell origin of seminoma has been accepted for a very long time, the origin of other histologic types of tumors forming this group of neoplasms has been a matter of dispute and controversy. While some investigators[5-8] considered that all these tumors were of germ cell origin, others considered that they originated from blastomeres displaced during embryonal development,[9] or were of indeterminate or uncertain origin.[10]

Over the last two decades the germ cell theory of origin has received strong support from the experimental studies of Stevens[11] and of Pierce and his collaborators,[12, 13] as well as from studies emphasizing both the homology and frequent admixture of the various neoplastic germ cell elements present in germ cell neoplasms, occurring in both gonadal and extragonadal sites.[14] As a result of these studies, the germ cell origin of the whole group of these neoplasms has become generally accepted. The histogenesis and interrelationship of germ cell neoplasms are represented in Figure 3-1. According to this concept,[15] seminoma is a very primitive germ cell neoplasm which has not acquired the potential for further differentiation, while embryonal carcinoma is a germ cell tumor composed of primitive multipotential cells capable of further differentiation. The embryonal carcinoma

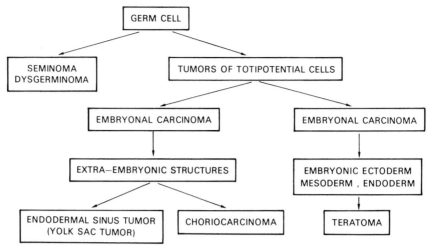

Fig. 3-1. Histogenesis and interrelationship of germ cell neoplasms. (Modified from Teilum G: Classification of endodermal sinus tumor (mesoblastoma vitellinum) and so-called embryonal carcinoma of the ovary. Acta Pathol Microbiol Scand 64:407, 1965.)

cells are capable of differentiating in the embryonal or somatic direction, forming teratomatous neoplasms with varying degrees of maturity from very immature to fully mature. All these neoplasms are composed of tissues originating from the three primitive germ layers: ectoderm, mesoderm, and endoderm. The embryonal carcinoma cells are also capable of differentiating in the extraembryonal direction along two separate pathways, either the vitelline forming endodermal sinus (yolk sac) tumor, or the trophoblastic pathway differentiating into a choriocarcinoma. The process of differentiation of the embryonal carcinoma cells is dynamic and this helps to explain why the resulting neoplasms may contain various germ cell elements at different stages of differentiation. According to this concept endodermal sinus tumor (EST) or yolk sac tumor (YST) and choriocarcinoma are well-differentiated neoplasms like the mature teratoma, but differ from the latter by being highly malignant.[15] However, there is now evidence that occasionally seminoma cells are also capable of further differentiation either into embryonal carcinoma, or possibly even further into EST (YST), choriocarcinoma, or tera-

toma. The presence of tumors exhibiting very intimate admixture of seminoma and EST (YST), or embryonal carcinoma or various teratomatous structures, as well as seminoma containing syncytiotrophoblastic giant cells, lends strong supportive evidence to these views. Additional evidence has been recently provided by the presence of occasional cytokeratin reactive cells in 40 percent of classic seminomas studied, thus indicating the presence of occasional more differentiated cells (see Chapter 9).

CLASSIFICATION

Although different types of testicular neoplasms have been recognized for many years, the first successful attempt at classifying them was made in 1946, when Friedman and Moore proposed a new classification based on studies performed on nearly 1,000 testicular tumors collected from United States military personnel during the Second World War.[7] The material on which this classification was based was larger by far than any of this type examined previously. Friedman and Moore[7] considered that the majority of testicular tumors were derived from germ cells, and they classified testicular germ cell tumors into five types:

1. Seminoma
2. Teratoma
3. Embryonal carcinoma
4. Choriocarcinoma
5. Teratocarcinoma

Friedman and Moore[7] were aware of the fact that many testicular germ cell neoplasms were combined or mixed and were composed of a number of these tumor types in various combinations resulting in tumors exhibiting many different histologic patterns. One such combination represented by embryonal carcinoma and teratoma was particularly common and was included in the classification as a specific entity under the term of teratocarcinoma.

Some years later the classification of Friedman and Moore[7] was modified by Dixon and Moore[8] whose studies were based on the same material and the same histologic criteria, but included follow-up data and thus provided not only histologic but also prognostic information. This classification[8] was as follows:

1. Seminoma (pure)
2. Embryonal carcinoma pure or with seminoma
3. Teratoma pure or with seminoma
4. Teratoma with either embryonal carcinoma or choriocarcinoma or both with or without seminoma
5. Choriocarcinoma pure or with either seminoma or embryonal carcinoma or both

The most favorable prognosis was observed in the pure seminoma (group 1). This was followed by group 3 (teratoma pure or with seminoma). The worst prognosis was seen in group 5 followed by group 2. Dixon and Moore[8] noted that if embryonal carcinoma or choriocarcinoma was associated with teratoma (group 4) the prognosis was more favorable than when there were no teratomatous elements present. Over the years this classification[8] has become very well established, especially in the United States, and is still being used today. One of the drawbacks of these two classifications[7, 8] was that they were based on material obtained from service personnel and therefore testicular neoplasms occurring in infants and children as well as those observed in the elderly were not represented. This deficiency was rectified in the classification proposed by Mostofi and Price,[2] which was a modification of the classifications of Friedman and Moore[7] and Dixon and Moore[8] and was intended to embrace all the histologic types of testicular tumors.

Some years earlier, in 1964, another classification of testicular tumors was proposed by the British Testicular Tumor Panel.[10] This panel[10] did not accept the concept of embryonal carcinoma and classified testicular germ cell tumors into seminoma and teratoma. The seminoma group was classified into classic and spermatocytic types and the teratoma group was subclassified as follows:

1. Teratoma differentiated (TD)
2. Malignant teratoma intermediate
   (a) with organoid differentiation (MTI_A)
   (b) without organoid differentiation (MTI_B)
3. Malignant teratoma anaplastic (MTA)
4. Malignant teratoma trophoblastic (MTT)

This classification,[10] like the classification of Dixon and Moore,[8] was based both on the histologic nature of the tumor and on prognostic considerations. The prognosis in the teratoma group was progressively worse from group 1 to group 4.

As a result of further studies related to prognosis, the British Testicular Tumor Panel in 1976[1] modified its original classification of the teratoma group into the following:

1. Teratoma differentiated (TD)
2. Malignant teratoma intermediate (MTI) (previously MTI_A)

Table 3-1. Comparison of British and American Classifications of Testicular Tumors

Modified British Testicular Tumor Panel Classification[1] (1976)	American Classifications Friedman and Moore[7] (1946) Mostofi and Price[2] (1973)
Seminoma	Seminoma
Teratoma differentiated (TD)	Teratoma mature
Malignant teratoma intermediate (MTI)	Teratoma immature
Malignant teratoma undifferentiated (MTU)	Embryonal carcinoma
Malignant teratoma trophoblastic (MTT)	Choriocarcinoma

3. Malignant teratoma undifferentiated (MTU) (previously MTI_B and MTA)

4. Malignant teratoma trophoblastic (MTT)

Apart from being based on a larger number of cases and better prognostic information, this classification was also an attempt to produce a degree of uniformity with the classifications of Friedman and Moore[7] and Mostofi and Price[2] as shown in Table 3-1.

The classifications evolved by the British Testicular Tumor Panel[1, 10] have made considerable impact and have become accepted in Great Britain and in parts of Europe, but have received little recognition in the United States.

A further attempt at formulating an acceptable, all-embracing, and simple classification of testicular neoplasms was made by the World Health Organization in 1978. This classification,[16] which was based solely on histologic findings, was intended to include all the different histologic tumor types known to occur in the testis, including newly established entities such as the EST (YST), which were not included in the previous classifications.

The World Health Organization (WHO) classification[16] divides testicular germ cell tumors as follows:

1. Tumors of one histologic type
   (a) Seminoma
   (b) Spermatocytic seminoma
   (c) Embryonal carcinoma
   (d) Yolk sac tumor (embryonal carcinoma infantile type, endodermal sinus tumor)
   (e) Polyembryoma
   (f) Choriocarcinoma
   (g) Teratomas
       (i) Mature
       (ii) Immature
       (iii) With malignant transformation
2. Tumors of more than one histologic type
   (a) Embryonal carcinoma and teratoma (teratocarcinoma)
   (b) Choriocarcinoma and any other type (specify type)
   (c) Other combinations (specify)

This classification[16] classifies seminoma into two types, the well-recognized classic type and the more recently established spermatocytic type. It recognizes the existence in the testis of EST, although the synonym of embryonal carcinoma infantile type is considered to be confusing because tumors of this histologic type are not infrequent components of combined testicular germ cell tumors occurring in adults.[17, 18] The WHO classification[16] also recognizes other less common histologic types, and emphasizes that testicular germ cell tumors are frequently composed of more than one histologic type. Recent studies have shown that some components, such as EST and choriocarcinoma, are detected more frequently within testicular tumors when the tumor is carefully sampled, and that testicular germ cell tumors are more frequently mixed or combined than has been noted previously.[4, 17, 18] This could also be partly due to a changing incidence of testicular neoplasms.[19]

Apart from spermatocytic seminoma, which only occurs in pure form, all the other histologic types of germ cell tumors are frequently mixed or combined.[4]

The WHO classification[16] classifies teratoma into mature and immature types, and includes a third category: the mature teratoma with malignant transformation. The distinction between the first two types is fully justifiable and is important from the prognostic point of view since the presence of mature elements implies that the tumor is benign, while the presence of immature elements indicates that the tumor is malignant or at least potentially malignant. Mature testicular teratomas occur almost exclusively during infancy or early childhood and immature teratomas or combined mature and immature teratomas are seen in young adults.[4] However, tumors showing features similar to mature teratomas with malignant transformation observed in the ovaries of postmenopausal women[3] have not been documented in the testis. Therefore the inclusion of this subgroup in the classification of teratoma is not considered justifiable.

EXAMINATION OF THE SPECIMEN

It has been mentioned above that recent studies based on more careful and extensive sampling indicate that testicular germ cell tumors are more frequently mixed or combined than has been hitherto believed.[17-19] It is therefore considered that every tumor should be carefully examined and judiciously sampled to facilitate the examination of numerous sections. This enables the examiner to provide not only the exact histologic diagnosis, but also an approximate quantification of the different components present within the tumor. The whole tumor should be sectioned and that at least one whole cross section of the tumor over its central area should be taken for histologic examination. In addition to this, sections

should be taken from every part of the tumor showing different macroscopic appearances from those seen in the central parts of the tumor, including hemorrhagic areas. Parts of the tumor showing obvious necrosis however should be avoided. Therefore, many more sections should be taken from tumors showing varied macroscopic appearances than from those showing a uniform pattern.

Sections should also be taken from unaffected testicular tissue both adjoining the tumor and located more distantly, as well as from the epididymis, spermatic cord (proximal, middle, and the highest point at the resection margin), and from parts of the tumor adjoining the tunica albuginea and the rete testis. The presence of tumor deposits within lymphatic and blood vessels should be mentioned in the report, but only if accurate assessment of this feature could be made. If lymph node dissection is also performed, the specimen must be very carefully sampled to determine the presence, extent, and type of metastases.

SPECIFIC FINDINGS

CLASSIC SEMINOMA

The term seminoma was first introduced in 1906 by Chevassu,[20] who provided the first detailed description of this neoplasm. Chevassu[20] considered that seminoma originated from the seminiferous epithelium and thus from the germ cell component of the seminiferous tubule. Although this view met with some opposition at the time, the concept that this neoplasm originates from germ cells had achieved universal acceptance long ago. The term classic seminoma came into use more recently when spermatocytic seminoma became established as a specific histopathologic entity.

Classic seminoma is the most common testicular neoplasm.[1, 2] In its pure form it accounts for approximately 40 percent of all testicular neoplasms.[1] It also forms a major component of mixed or combined testicular germ cell tumors and in these cases it may be admixed with any other neoplastic germ cell element.[1, 2, 4, 10] While the classic seminoma present in these tumors may be observed macroscopically and quantitatively forms a major or a considerable part of the tumor, based on their behavior and recommended therapy, these tumors have to be included with the nonseminomatous testicular germ cell neoplasms. Tumors of this type account for approximately 15 percent of testicular germ cell neoplasms.[1] In addition, small foci of seminoma may be observed microscopically in all types of testicular germ cell tumors. They are usually found at the periphery of the tumor.[1, 10]

Pure classic seminoma occurs most frequently in patients between the ages of 25 and 55 years.[1] It is very rare before puberty, but is not uncommon after the age of 55 years, although its incidence shows a marked decline with age.[1] Pure classic seminoma shows a slight predilection for the right testis, and is bilateral in 2 percent of cases.[1] Bilaterality is usually asynchronous. In 8.5 percent of cases, classic seminoma occurs in undescended testes.[1] By far the most frequent clinical presenting symptom is testicular enlargement; this has been noted in more than 70 percent of cases.[1] In 4 percent of cases there were no symptoms.[1]

Macroscopically, pure classic seminoma forms a solid, firm, round, or oval tumor, which usually produces symmetrical enlargement of the affected testis. On sectioning, the tumor presents a uniform white to pink, sometimes coarsely lobulated surface, due to the presence of fibrous bands. Although the tumor is not encapsulated it appears to be sharply demarcated from the surrounding testicular tissue. It varies in consistency from soft to firm and the firmness is associated with an increased amount of fibrous tissue. In large tumors, necrosis and hemorrhage may alter the appearance of the tumor. The size of the tumor varies from a small nodule, measuring a few centimeters, to large masses replacing

the whole testis. Most seminomas lead to considerable enlargement of the testis.[1, 2]

Microscopically, classic seminoma exhibits very distinctive appearances. It is composed of aggregates, islands, cords, or strands of large uniform cells, surrounded by varying amounts of connective tissue stroma, which invariably contains lymphocytes (Fig. 3-2), and usually contains plasma cells, histiocytes, and eosinophils. A granulomatous reaction, manifesting itself as collections of histiocytes surrounded by lymphocytes, plasma cells, and occasional giant cells, both of the Langhans' and foreign body type, is also seen in a considerable number of tumors (Fig. 3-3). The extent of lymphocytic infiltration varies from tumor to tumor as well as within different parts of the same tumor. The tumor cells are large, oval or rounded, and measure from 15 to 25 μm. The cellular boundaries are usually visible. The cytoplasm is pale, slightly granular, eosinophilic, or clear. The nucleus, which is centrally located, is large and occupies nearly half of the cell. It is oval or round and has a sharp nuclear membrane and a considerable amount of somewhat unevenly distributed finely granular chromatin. It contains usually one, but sometimes two, prominent nucleoli. Although the cells are generally very uniform, there is some variation in the cell and nuclear size, as well as in the amount of nuclear chromatin (Fig. 3-4). Occasional larger but otherwise typical seminoma cells may be seen. Mitotic activity is almost always present and varies from slight to brisk. The variation in mitotic activity is seen not only in different tumors but also in different parts of the same tumor.

The cytoplasm of the tumor cells contains an ample amount of glycogen, demonstrable by the periodic acid–Schiff (PAS) reaction, although the glycogen is less evident after long fixation, especially in formalin. Seminoma cells also contain lipid, which can be demonstrated in frozen tissue by lipid stains. Alkaline phosphatase is found within seminoma cells, and is present beneath the cytoplasmic rim. All these substances are also found in primi-

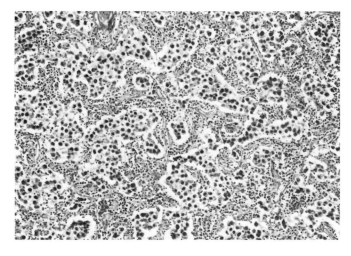

Fig. 3-2. Typical appearances of classic seminoma. The tumor is composed of nests or aggregates of uniform tumor cells surrounded by connective tissue septa containing lymphocytes. H & E. × 150.

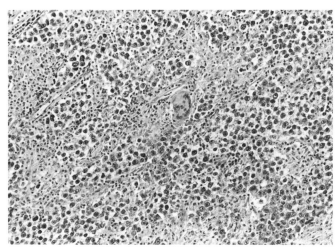

Fig. 3-3. Classic seminoma exhibiting granulomatous reaction. Histiocytes and chronic inflammatory cells surround nests of tumor cells. A Langhans giant cell is seen in the center. H & E. × 150.

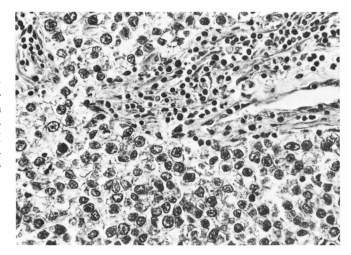

Fig. 3-4. Classic seminoma. Cellular and nuclear appearances. H & E. × 460. (Talerman A: Germ cell tumors of the testis. In Fenoglio CM, Wolff M (eds): Progress in Surgical Pathology, Vol. 1, Masson, New York, 1980.)

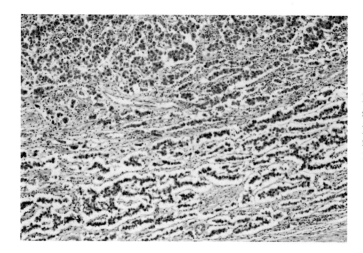

Fig. 3-5. Classic seminoma showing different patterns depending on the amount of connective tissue present. H & E. × 90.

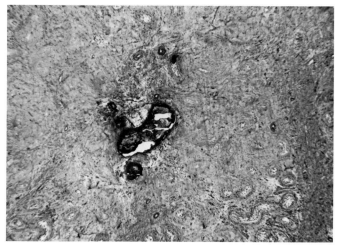

Fig. 3-6. Classic seminoma affected by hyalinization and containing a calcified nodule ("calcified scar"). H & E. × 60.

tive germ cells and are observed in the same locations within the cytoplasm. These findings further support the germ cell origin of seminoma cells. The amount of connective tissue stroma present within the tumor is variable and tends to determine the histologic appearances of the tumor. The connective tissue varies in amount from scanty to abundant and in appearance from a fine fibrovascular network to large fibrous bands or septa, which are often hyalinized. Thus a tumor may be composed of small nests, islands, cords, or strands of tumor cells widely separated by broad fibrous bands, or it may be very cellular containing only an imperceptible amount of fine fibrovascular connective tissue (Fig. 3-5).

In some tumors the amount of connective tissue is so abundant that the tumor cells are difficult to discern, or the whole tumor may be affected by fibrosis and hyalinization, with the only sign of the previous existence of a seminoma being a fibrous, sometimes calcified, scar (Fig. 3-6). Foci of necrosis and hemorrhage are sometimes found, especially in large tumors where they may be abundant. The extent of lymphocytic infiltration and granulomatous reaction also varies and differs from tumor to tumor as well as within the same tumor. Some parts of a tumor may be very cellular, exhibit cellular and nuclear pleomorphism, brisk mitotic activity, an imperceptible amount of connective tissue, and only slight

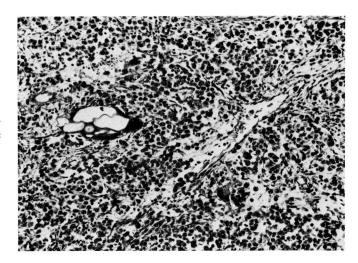

Fig. 3-7. Classic seminoma containing syncytiotrophoblastic giant cells. H & E. × 90.

lymphocytic infiltration. This pattern may be present in conjunction with less cellular areas, or it may be predominant. The term "anaplastic seminoma" has been applied to tumors of the latter type,[21-23] but in view of the fact that this pattern is frequently seen in conjunction with other patterns observed in classic seminoma, and since there is no good evidence that patients with tumors showing this histologic pattern tend to have a worse prognosis, it is considered that the use of the term "anaplastic seminoma" is confusing and not justifiable. It is also important to note that tumors of this type are not infrequently confused with embryonal carcinoma showing a solid pattern, and because of the important therapeutic and prognostic implications these tumors must be differentiated from each other. Detailed histologic examination of the tumor cells and their patterns would lead the observer to the correct diagnosis (see section on embryonal carcinoma for differential diagnosis). It should be noted in this context that embryonal carcinoma may occasionally exhibit lymphocytic infiltration and that the presence of this feature is not diagnostic of seminoma.

In 6 to 8 percent of classic seminomas multinucleated giant cells are present,[4] varying in appearance from a mass of cytoplasm containing a few small nuclei to large irregular, frequently vacuolated, cytoplasmic masses containing numerous nuclei, or collections of dense chromatin (Fig. 3-7). These giant cells have been shown to represent syncytiotrophoblastic cells which are capable of producing human chorionic gonadotropin (HCG) and its beta subunit (β-HCG) in the same way as syncytiotrophoblastic cells of choriocarcinoma.[24] Although originally it was suggested that patients with seminomas containing these cells may have a worse prognosis, there is no evidence that this is the case.[25, 26] It is important to distinguish these giant cells from foreign body and Langhans' giant cells (Fig. 3-3), which are associated with a granulomatous reaction. The presence of syncytiotrophoblastic giant cells explains why some pure seminomas are associated with elevated levels of serum HCG and β-HCG.

In a number of classic seminomas, at the edge of the tumor are seminiferous tubules containing numerous seminoma cells which may completely fill the lumen of the tubule, while showing no evidence of involvement of the interstitium. This has been described as intratubular seminoma or seminoma in situ. Sometimes slight focal invasion of the interstitial tissue may be observed as the presence of isolated seminoma cells in the interstitium. In addition, seminiferous tubules unaffected by the tumor may contain at least occasional highly atypical germ cells showing features

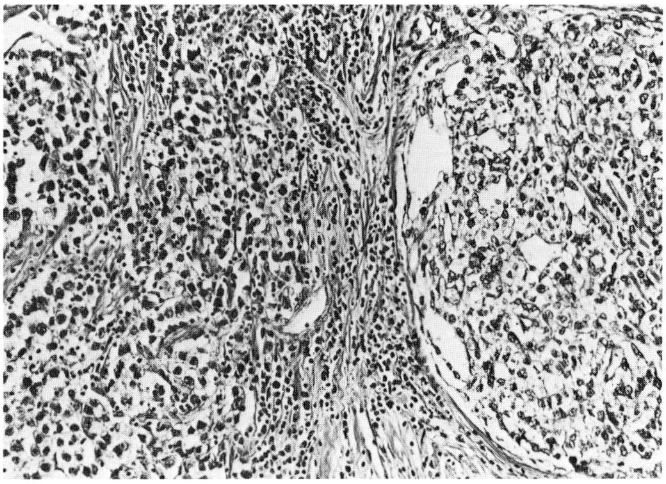

Fig. 3-8. Classic seminoma (left) associated with endodermal sinus (yolk sac) tumor (EST) (right). H & E. × 90.

of malignancy and usually resembling cells of classic seminoma. This has been observed in every case in a personal series of 186 classic seminomas and also in a series of 148 nonseminomatous or combined germ cell tumors. The subject of intratubular malignant germ cells is discussed in detail in Chapter 2.

Classic seminoma is not infrequently associated with other neoplastic germ cell elements (Fig. 3-8), and it may be associated with any one specific histologic type or with the whole spectrum of germ cell neoplasia. In view of this, each tumor must be carefully examined. A pure classic seminoma, which is the most radiosensitive tumor known, must be differentiated from one containing other neoplastic germ cell elements that are not radiosensitive, to facilitate prescription of the appropriate mode of therapy.

Classic seminoma metastasizes first via the lymphatics to the paraaortic and parailiac lymph nodes. From these locations further spread takes place to the mediastinal and supraclavicular lymph nodes. Hematogenous spread occurs much later and affects the lungs, liver, bones, and other organs.[27, 28] Because of the lymphatic spread of the tumor, lymphangiography is of considerable value as a diagnostic procedure for detection of metastases in patients with seminoma. Although in most cases of pure seminoma the metastases

are composed of classic seminoma, in 20 to 25 percent of cases the metastases do not reflect the appearance of the primary tumor and contain other neoplastic germ cell elements.[2, 27] Since the prognosis of patients with pure seminoma is very good, due to the remarkable radiosensitivity of the tumor, the presence of other neoplastic germ cell elements in the metastases has very important prognostic implications, requires a different mode of therapy, and is associated with a poorer prognosis.

SPERMATOCYTIC SEMINOMA

Spermatocytic seminoma was first described as a specific histopathologic entity by Masson[29] in 1946. He considered this tumor to be derived from spermatogonia and to represent a better-differentiated type of seminoma than the very much more common classic type. In spite of Masson's masterly description, spermatocytic seminoma did not become recognized as a specific histopathologic entity until two decades later when a number of investigators[30-35] reported additional cases and attested to the distinctive nature of this neoplasm.

One of the most important features differentiating spermatocytic seminoma from classic seminoma, as well as from any other germ cell neoplasm, and thus further supporting the view that it is a specific histopathologic entity and a unique germ cell neoplasm, is that spermatocytic seminoma is the only testicular germ cell neoplasm that does not have a homologous counterpart in the ovary, or in other locations where germ cell tumors are commonly found: the mediastinum, and the parapineal, sacrococcygeal, and retroperitoneal regions. Another important feature differentiating spermatocytic seminoma from the classic variety is that the former tumor is always seen in its pure form and is not admixed with any other neoplastic germ cell elements. Spermatocytic seminoma does not exhibit transitions to the classic type.

Spermatocytic seminoma is an uncommon tumor but more than 100 cases have been reported,[36, 37] accounting for 3.5 to 7.4 percent of all seminomas.[36] It shows a slight predilection for the right testis. In 10 percent of cases the tumor is bilateral, and is therefore more frequently bilateral than classic seminoma (1 to 2 percent). Although bilateral tumors are occasionally seen at the same time, bilaterality is usually asynchronous.[36] The tumor has only been reported to occur in normally descended testes.[36] Clinically, the main difference between spermatocytic and classic seminoma is the age incidence. Although the reported age of patients with spermatocytic seminoma ranges from 30 to 87 years, patients with spermatocytic seminoma are older than those with classic seminoma, and the great majority are older than 40 years.[36] In a personal series of 23 cases, 20 patients were older than 40 years; this was also seen in 80 percent of cases from the literature.[36] All patients with spermatocytic seminoma seen personally since 1980 (14 cases) were older than 40 years. In contrast the majority of patients with classic seminoma are aged 25 to 50 years.[1] Although classic seminoma is seen in patients older than 60 years, in a considerable proportion of elderly patients with seminoma, the tumor is of the spermatocytic type.

The macroscopic appearances of spermatocytic seminoma are very characteristic and differ from those of classic seminoma and other testicular tumors. The size of the tumor varies from a small round or oval nodule a few centimeters across to a large mass measuring 15 cm in the greatest diameter, weighing more than 500 g, and completely replacing the whole testis.[36] Some tumors may be lobulated and nodular. On cross section, the tumors are homogenous, solid, pale gray, soft, friable, and edematous. The edema may be very marked, and some tumors may be described as gelatinous or mucoid and may contain small cysts with clear fluid in the center (Fig. 3-9). Occasional small foci of necrosis may be seen in larger tumors, but necrosis is not a common feature. Hemorrhagic areas are infrequent and are only seen in large tumors. The tumors are usually well-circumscribed, and some may appear to be encapsulated (Fig. 3-9), although this is only apparent. In some cases the tumors appear to consist of a number of coalescing nodules. Occasionally a small tumor nodule may be present some distance from the main tumor mass.[1, 36] The tumor is usually confined to the testis, but when it is very large there may be penetration of the tunica and replacement of the epididymis.

Microscopically, spermatocytic seminoma also shows very distinctive and characteristic appearances. It is composed of solid sheets of tumor cells with little or no intervening stroma (Fig. 3-10). The cytoplasm of the tumor cells contains little or no glycogen. The connective tissue strands are fine and surround collections of tumor cells, forming lobules that vary in size (Figs. 3-10 and 3-11). The tumor cells may be widely dispersed in the edematous stroma, or form pseudoalveolar or pseudoglandular pattern. (Fig. 3-11). The edema fluid forms small cystic spaces or larger pools (Fig. 3-11). At the periphery of the tumor, spermatocytic seminoma shows two different patterns of infiltration.

The predominant pattern is intratubular, consisting of seminiferous tubules distended with either individual or small collections of tumor cells (Fig. 3-12), including giant cells,

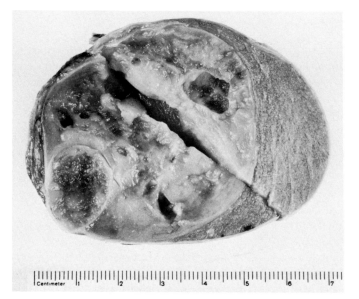

Fig. 3-9. Testis containing spermatocytic seminoma. The tumor is solid and well-demarcated from surrounding testicular tissue. It shows slight lobulation and contains a few small cysts. It presents a glistening mucoid or gelatinous surface.

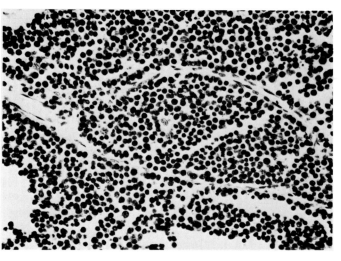

Fig. 3-10. Typical appearances of spermatocytic seminoma. The tumor is composed of solid aggregates of tumor cells, which in places form lobules (center) with little intervening stroma. H & E. × 150.

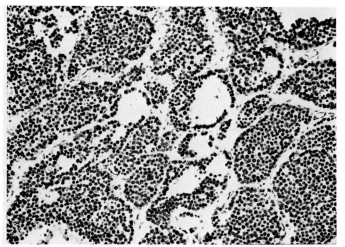

Fig. 3-11. Spermatocytic seminoma forming a lobular pattern. Note also a pseudoglandular pattern produced due to accumulation of edema fluid. H & E. × 75.

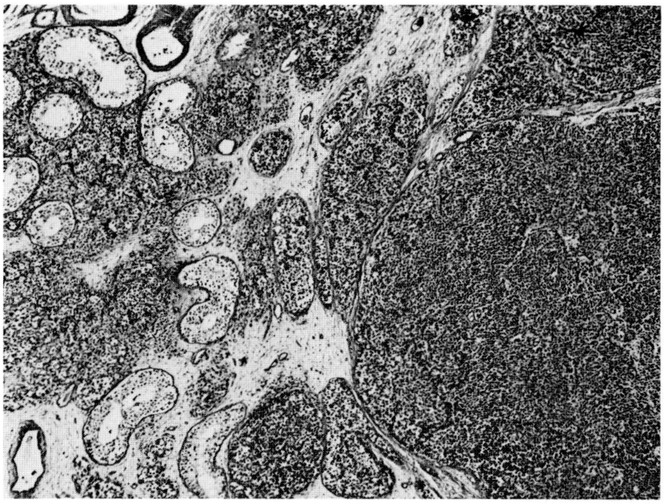

Fig. 3-12. Spermatocytic seminoma showing intralobular and interstitial patterns of growth. H & E. × 60.

Fig. 3-13. Spermatocytic seminoma. Note the involvement of seminiferous tubules at some distance from the main tumor mass. H & E. × 60.

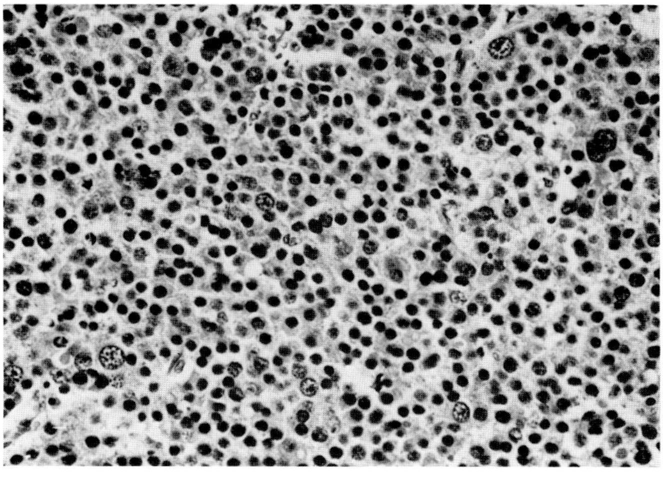

Fig. 3-14. Spermatocytic seminoma. Note the uniform shape of the cells and nuclei and their marked variation in size. H & E. × 230.

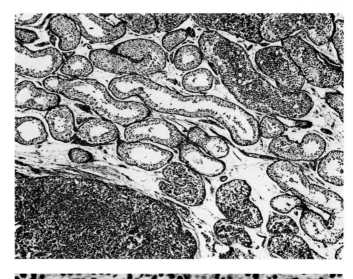

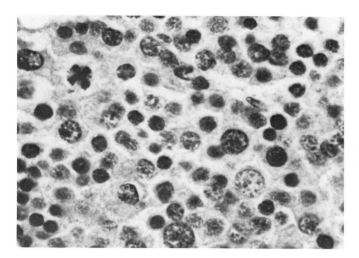

Fig. 3-15. Spermatocytic seminoma. Note the cellular and nuclear appearances. A large quadripolar mitosis is seen (top left). H & E. × 600.

and the involvement may persist for a considerable distance from the main tumor mass (Fig. 3-13). Interstitial infiltration, although sometimes less obvious, is also present in most tumors (Fig. 3-12). The cells of spermatocytic seminoma vary little in shape, being either round or oval, and contain perfectly round or slightly oval nuclei (Figs. 3-10 and 3-14). They can basically be classified into three main cell types according to their size.

The most common type consists of medium-sized cells measuring 15 to 20 μm. These cells contain a perfectly round nucleus with finely granular chromatin pattern, which is surrounded by a rim of dense eosinophilic or amphophilic cytoplasm.

A small cell type consists of cells measuring 6 to 8 μm, with a narrow rim of eosinophilic cytoplasm and a small, round, very dark hyperchromatic nucleus with an evenly spread chromatin pattern resembling lymphocytes.

A giant cell type consists of large uninucleated or multinucleated round, oval, or polygonal cells measuring 50 to 100 μm with abundant cytoplasm which varies from pale to deeply eosinophilic. Many of these cells are uninucleated, but multinucleated cells containing two or more nuclei are not infrequently found. The nuclei are usually round, but some are oval and show three characteristic chromatin patterns (Figs. 3-8 and 3-10):

1. Granular, forming small, regular clumps
2. Spireme, forming long filaments
3. Even, with very dark evenly spread chromatin

Nucleoli are prominent in some nuclei, showing the granular pattern, but are not observed in the nuclei exhibiting the spireme and even patterns.

Mitotic activity is evident in all tumors, although less marked in edematous areas, and abnormal forms are not infrequently found (Fig. 3-15). The number of mitotic figures varies not only from tumor to tumor but also within an individual tumor, and may be large.

Spermatocytic seminoma shows biologically less malignant behavior than classic seminoma, and although the tumor may become very large there is, to date, no well-documented case of spermatocytic seminoma associated with metastatic disease.[36] Although it has been suggested that spermatocytic seminoma is a tumor of spermatogonia or spermatocytes,[38] a recent study based on microspectrophotometric analysis and ultrastructural observations revealed that although spermatocytic seminoma is a better differentiated tumor than the classic type, it has not yet reached spermatocytic differentiation.[39] The differences between spermatocytic and classic seminoma are summarized in Table 3-2.

Table 3-2. Differential Features of Spermatocytic and Classic Seminoma

	Spermatocytic Seminoma	*Classic Seminoma*
Incidence (%)	3.5–7.5	92.5–96.5
Usual age on presentation (years)	Over 40	25–50
Site	Testis only	Testis, ovary, mediastinum, retroperitoneum, and pineal region
Bilaterality (%)	10	2
Occurrence in undescended testis (%)	No documented case	8.5
Associated tumor elements	None	Other neoplastic germ cell elements present in 25% of cases
Gross appearance	Solid, gray-yellow, soft gelatinous, mucoid	Solid, pink-yellow, firm, trabeculated
Histologic features		
Cell nuclei	Perfectly round and dark, marked variation in size, variable chromatin pattern	Ovoid, vesicular, little variation in size and chromatin pattern
Cytoplasm	Dense, scanty, acidophilic, glycogen scanty or absent	Clear or slightly granular, abundant, rich in glycogen
Edema	Present, often marked, may cause pseudoglandular or microcystic pattern	Absent
Stroma	Scanty and fine	More prominent often abundant, and dense
Lymphocytes	Absent	Present, may be abundant
Granulomas	Absent	Present, may be abundant
Type of growth	Intratubular more common, interstitial less common	Interstitial more common, intratubular less common
Metastases	No documented case	Metastases common
Radiosensitivity	Very sensitive	Very sensitive
Prognosis	Excellent; better than classic seminoma	Very good with adequate treatment

EMBRYONAL CARCINOMA

In this section embryonal carcinoma is described mainly as a morphologic entity, but it is also considered as a conceptual entity according to the descriptions and definitions of Teilum,[5, 6] Friedman and Moore,[7] and Dixon and Moore.[8] Thus from the conceptual point of view embryonal carcinoma is considered to be the least-differentiated germ cell neoplasm definitively capable of further differentiation. It may differentiate in the direction of somatic structures (teratomatous tumors in various stages of maturation) or toward extraembryonal structures along the vitelline path-way forming EST (YST), or along the trophoblastic pathway forming choriocarcinoma.[15]

Morphologically, embryonal carcinoma is a common testicular germ cell neoplasm. It does occur in pure form, but is frequently admixed with other neoplastic germ cell elements. It may be combined with teratoma, EST (YST), classic seminoma, or choriocarcinoma, either singly or in combination. Embryonal carcinoma and teratoma are frequently encountered in testicular germ cell tumors and this combined tumor has been designated as teratocarcinoma.[7] Embryonal carcinoma is common and is observed in up to 40 percent

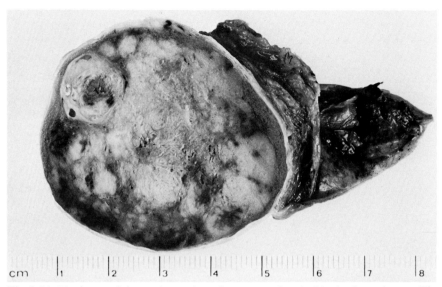

Fig. 3-16. Testis containing embryonal carcinoma associated with choriocarcinoma. The tumor is solid and produces relatively slight enlargement. There is distortion of testicular contour. The hemorrhagic areas (bottom) contain choriocarcinoma. Necrosis and hemorrhage are also seen (center and right).

of testicular germ cell neoplasms either in pure form or in combination. It occurs most frequently between the ages of 15 and 35 years, and its peak incidence is a decade earlier than that of classic seminoma.[1, 2, 10] It is uncommon above the age of 50 years and is rare in children before puberty.

Macroscopically pure embryonal carcinoma presents usually as a small tumor, replacing parts of, or the whole, testis without producing pronounced enlargement, but frequently distorting the testicular contour (Fig. 3-16). On cross section it is solid, gray-white, variegated, soft, and does not appear to be encapsulated. It is frequently associated with hemorrhage and necrosis (Fig. 3-16). When embryonal carcinoma is associated with teratoma or classic seminoma, the tumor may be larger, and in the case of teratoma may be partly cystic. Invasion of the tunica albuginea, epididymis, and spermatic cord is not infrequent.

Microscopically, embryonal carcinoma is composed of aggregates of epithelial-like medium to large polygonal or ovoid cells containing an ample amount of pale, eosinophilic, granular cytoplasm with poorly discernible cytoplasmic borders (Fig. 3-17). The nuclei are large, prominent, irregular, and somewhat vesicular, with a fine nuclear membrane, or they may be hyperchromatic. They frequently contain more than one nucleolus. Mitotic activity is brisk, and abnormal mitotic figures are frequently present. The tumor cells usually exhibit marked cellular and nuclear pleomorphism (Fig. 3-17).

The cells may form a solid or syncytial pattern (Fig. 3-17), or, in slightly better differentiated tumors, tend to line clefts and spaces and form papillae (Fig. 3-18). The papillary pattern may be very pronounced in some cases. When the tumor is better-differentiated, the cells appear to be even more epithelial and there is a suggestion of glandular formation (Fig. 3-18), but true glandular differentiation is absent. The papillae are composed of solid collections of cells surrounding a small cystic space or a small vessel. Very primitive mesenchymal tissue may be present in conjunction with the epithelial component. Iso-

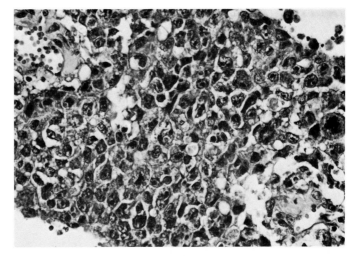

Fig. 3-17. Embryonal carcinoma showing solid and syncytial patterns. H & E. × 460.

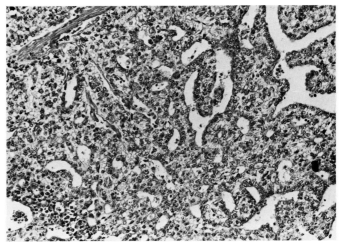

Fig. 3-18. Embryonal carcinoma showing solid, papillary and pseudoglandular, or pseudoalveolar patterns. H & E. × 230.

lated syncytiotrophoblastic giant cells may be present, and are by no means uncommon. Necrosis and hemorrhage are frequent findings. The amount of connective tissue stroma is usually small. Occasionally the stroma may contain lymphocytes, and the tumor may be confused with classic seminoma, which is composed of smaller, much more uniform cells with more easily discernible cellular boundaries, vesicular nuclei, more prominent and sharply defined nuclear membranes, usually a single nucleolus, and less brisk mitotic activity.

When embryonal carcinoma is combined with other neoplastic germ cell elements, their presence should be noted and, if possible, quantitated. Embryonal carcinoma is a highly malignant neoplasm. It is frequently associated with metastases on presentation, and the prognosis in these cases is worse.

Embryonal carcinoma metastasizes first to the paraaortic and parailiac lymph nodes. Sometimes enlargement of supraclavicular lymph nodes may be the initial presenting sign. Later metastases appear in the lungs, liver, bones, and gastrointestinal tract.[27] The metastases frequently reflect the appearances of the primary tumor, but other elements, such as endodermal sinus tumor, teratoma, or choriocarcinoma, may also be present in the metastases. It has been recognized for some time that when embryonal carcinoma is combined with teratoma, the prognosis is better than when the tumor is in pure form or combined with other neoplastic germ cell elements.[1, 8, 10]

Embryonal carcinoma is not radiosensitive and metastasizing embryonal carcinoma is treated with combination chemotherapy, which has become more effective in recent years and has considerably improved prognosis.

ENDODERMAL SINUS (YOLK SAC) TUMOR

The terminology and histogenesis of EST (YST) have been the subject of much debate. This tumor has been recognized for some time as a specific clinicopathologic entity occurring in the testes of infants and young children and is now considered the most common malignant neoplasm occurring in this age group.[1, 40-43] In older patients, this tumor was previously diagnosed as embryonal carcinoma, but in the last 10 years it has finally become fully recognized and accepted as a specific type of testicular neoplasm in adults.[1, 2, 7, 8, 10, 16-18]

Teilum described EST as a specific type of germ cell neoplasm occurring in the ovary, testis, and extragonadal locations.[5, 6, 14, 15, 41, 44] It is frequently admixed with other neoplastic germ cell elements forming a mixed or combined germ cell tumor.[14, 17, 18, 41] Teilum[5, 6, 14, 15, 41, 44] considered EST an extraembryonal derivative of embryonal carcinoma, which differentiates in the vitelline or yolk sac direction. This interpretation has received further support from recent studies linking the production of alpha-fetoprotein (AFP) with the presence of EST elements within a testicular tumor, and the demonstration that AFP is a very useful tumor marker for the presence of EST.[41, 45-50]

In infants and young children, EST nearly always occurs in pure form, and is only occasionally combined with other neoplastic germ cell elements.[1, 2, 14, 40, 43, 51] It occurs from birth to the age of 5 years.[1, 2, 10, 14, 40-43, 51, 52] In adults EST is invariably combined with other neoplastic germ cell elements and is usually found between the ages of 17 and 40 years,[17, 18, 51] but may sometimes occur in older men and has been described in an 85-year old man.[53]

Although the presence of EST elements has been considered to be very rare in testicular tumors in adults,[14, 53] recent studies indicate that EST elements are present in a considerable number of such tumors, pure seminomas being excluded.[17, 18, 51, 54] EST elements were noted in 44.4 percent of tumors in a prospective study, when the tumor was extensively sampled and numerous sections were examined.[18] An incidence of 38 percent was observed in combined prospective and retrospective studies[17, 55] and an incidence of 28.7 percent was noted when a retrospective study was undertaken[18] (Fig. 3-19). This indicates that EST elements are present relatively frequently in testicular germ cell tumors in adults and helps to explain why serum AFP levels are frequently elevated in patients with such tumors.

Macroscopically, a tumor occurring in an infant may be either firm or soft with cystic areas. The tumor tends to replace most of the testis and may invade the epididymis. It is not encapsulated, white–yellow, and measures 2 to 6 cm. In adults the tumor is solid, usually soft and somewhat mucoid, or slimy (Fig. 3-20). It is gray–white and frequently contains hemorrhagic and necrotic areas (Fig. 3-20). It shows considerable variation in size and its appearance may vary due to the presence of other neoplastic germ cell elements.

The histologic appearances of EST have been described in detail by Teilum.[5, 6, 14, 15, 41, 44] The tumors occurring in adults and children show similar histologic patterns although some patterns may be observed more frequently in one group than in the other.[4]

The Incidence of E.S.T. (Y.S.T.) elements in testicular germ cell tumours in adults (pure seminoma excluded).

Retrospective study

21 of 73 cases.   1950 – 1968   –   28.7%

Retrospective and

Prospective study

26 of 68 cases.   1969 – 1974   –   38%

Prospective study

27 of 61 cases.   1974 – 1979   –   44.4%

Fig. 3-19. Incidence of endodermal sinus (yolk sac) tumor elements in testicular germ cell tumors in adults. Comparison of retrospective and prospective studies. (Modified from Talerman A: Endodermal sinus (yolk sac) tumor elements in testicular germ cell tumors in adults. Comparison of prospective and retrospective studies. Cancer 46:1213, 1980.)

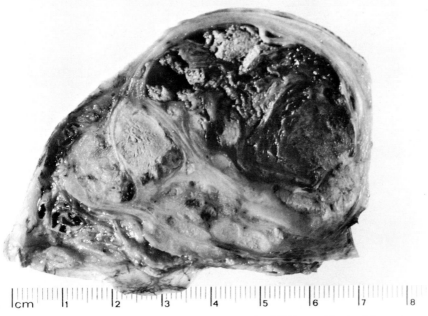

Fig. 3-20. Testis nearly completely replaced by EST (YST) combined with seminoma and embryonal carcinoma. Note the enlargement of the testis, necrosis and hemorrhage.

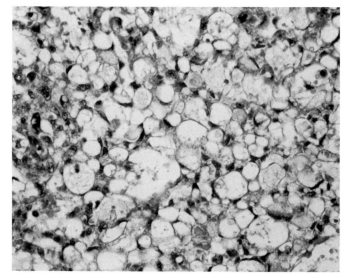

Fig. 3-21. EST (YST) showing microcystic pattern. H & E. × 230.

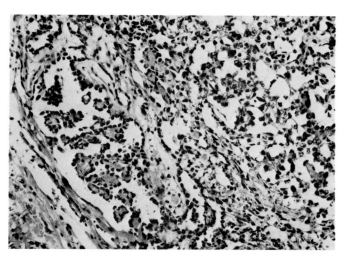

Fig. 3-22. EST (YST) showing papillary pattern. Note hyalinization in some of the papillary cores. H & E. × 150.

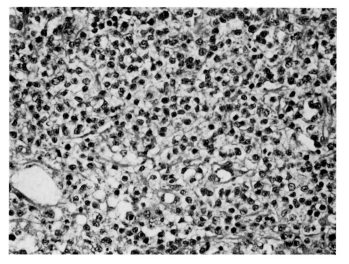

Fig. 3-23. EST (YST) showing solid pattern; note that a considerable number of microcysts is also present. H & E. × 230.

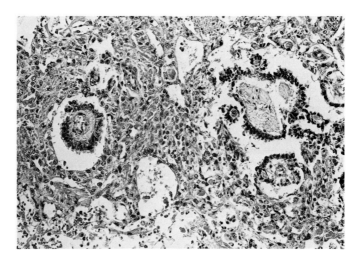

Fig. 3-24. EST (YST) showing solid pattern associated with endodermal sinus pattern containing numerous perivascular formations (Schiller-Duval bodies). H & E. × 185.

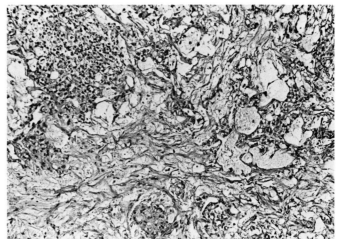

Fig. 3-25. EST (YST) Showing myxomatous and macrocystic patterns. Solid pattern is also seen (top left). H & E. × 75.

EST exhibits the following histologic patterns:

1. Endodermal sinus
2. Microcystic
3. Papillary
4. Solid
5. Glandular–alveolar
6. Myxomatous
7. Macrocystic
8. Polyvesicular vitelline
9. Hepatoid

These patterns are usually seen in combination and although one or two patterns may predominate, it is unusual for a tumor to exhibit a single histologic pattern. The microcystic (Fig. 3-21), papillary (Fig. 3-22), and solid (Fig. 3-23) patterns, the latter often admixed with endodermal sinus pattern composed of numerous perivascular formations (Schiller-Duval bodies) (Fig. 3-24), as well as macrocystic and myxomatous patterns (Fig. 3-25), are frequently observed in testicular tumors.[4] The solid pattern with the presence of perivascular formations (Fig. 3-24), or in combination with the microcystic pattern (Figs. 3-23 and 3-26), is frequently observed in testicular tumors of adults,[4, 17, 18] while the papillary, microcystic, macrocystic, and glandular–alveolar patterns

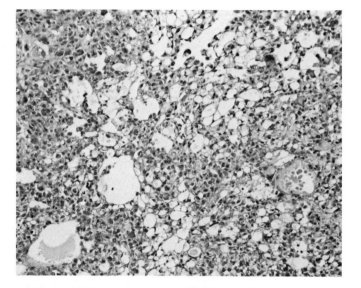

Fig. 3-26. EST (YST) showing solid and microcystic patterns. H & E. × 150.

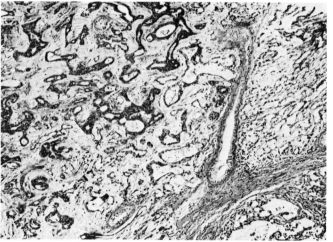

Fig. 3-27. EST (YST) showing glandular–alveolar pattern and composed of primitive endodermal glands and alveolar spaces. Note distorted and atrophic seminiferous tubule (right of center). H & E. × 60.

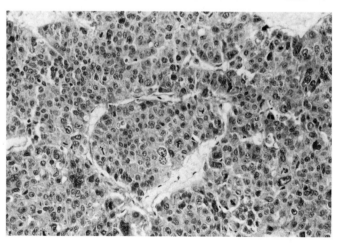

Fig. 3-28. EST (YST) showing hepatoid pattern, which may be considered as a variant of the solid pattern. H & E. × 185.

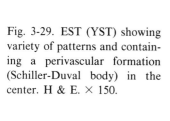

Fig. 3-29. EST (YST) showing variety of patterns and containing a perivascular formation (Schiller-Duval body) in the center. H & E. × 150.

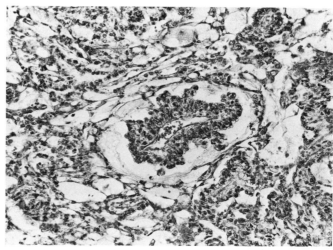

Fig. 3-30. EST (YST) showing a perivascular formation (Schiller-Duval body) and intra- and extracellular hyaline bodies. H & E. × 600.

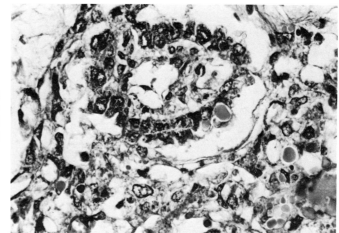

(Fig. 3-27) are seen somewhat more frequently in infantile EST.[4] The solid pattern associated with occasional microcysts (Figs. 3-23 and 3-26) may be confused with classic seminoma, as the tumor cells more closely resemble seminoma cells than embryonal carcinoma cells. The microcysts, which are not observed in classic seminoma differentiate between the two entities. The polyvesicular vitelline pattern[15] is only occasionally seen in testicular tumors, and the newly described hepatoid pattern,[56] which may be considered as a variant of the solid pattern (Fig. 3-28), is also observed infrequently. On the whole, EST exhibits an admixture of the above described patterns in various combinations. Perivascular formations (Schiller–Duval bodies) (Figs. 3-29 and 3-30), which are considered a hallmark of EST, are often present and may be abundant, but in a considerablenumber of tumors they may be very scanty or absent. Their absence does not preclude the diagnosis.

Endodermal sinus tumor usually contains small, round, PAS-positive, diastase-resistant hyaline globules which may be numerous (Fig. 3-30). These globules have been demonstrated to contain AFP. Although the presence of these globules was formerly considered to be diagnostic of EST, this is not the case, since similar hyaline globules are found in many other malignant, often poorly differentiated, neoplasms.[57]

Endodermal sinus tumor metastasizes via the lymphatics; the paraaortic and parailiac lymph nodes are affected first. From there the tumor spreads to the mediastinal and supraclavicular lymph nodes. Hematogenous spread, most frequently to the lungs and liver, is common. Metastases are frequently observed at the initial presentation.

A marked difference between the behavior of the tumors in infants and children under the age of 2 years and those occurring in older children has been noted for a long time. The former tend to have a much better prognosis and survival than the latter. However, this situation has been altered since the introduction of effective combination chemotherapy and there has been marked improvement in prognosis in the older children.[51] The duration of symptoms prior to diagnosis also bears a relationship to survival.[51, 52] The stage of the disease is even more important in this respect and patients with more extensive involvement have a worse prognosis.[58]

In adults, EST is invariably admixed with other neoplastic germ cell elements[17, 18, 55] (Fig. 3-8). The amount of EST within a tumor may vary from a few small microscopic foci to tumors composed nearly entirely of EST.[17, 18, 55] It may be admixed with classic seminoma (Fig. 3-8), embryonal carcinoma, teratoma, and choriocarcinoma. The presence of EST within a tumor is considered to be a poor prognostic feature[17, 18] because EST is a highly malignant neoplastic germ cell element. This is a radioresistant neoplasm,[14] which, until recently, showed little response to chemotherapy. During the last decade very much better therapeutic results have been obtained using cis-diaminoplatinum, vinblastine, and bleomycin combination chemotherapy, as well as other newer chemotherapeutic regimens (see Chapter 11).

CHORIOCARCINOMA

Choriocarcinoma, which is histologically indistinguishable from gestational choriocarcinoma occurring in the uterus and from nongestational choriocarcinoma of germ cell origin found in the ovary, also occurs in the testis. The diagnosis of choriocarcinoma can only be made if the tumor contains syncytiotrophoblast combined with cytotrophoblast. The presence of a villuslike arrangement is a further supporting feature, but since choriocarcinoma is frequently affected by hemorrhage and necrosis, this arrangement is not necessary for diagnosis. The presence of syncytiotrophoblastic giant cells, which may be encountered in any testicular germ cell tumor, except for spermatocytic seminoma and pure mature teratoma, is not regarded as choriocarcinoma.

Pure choriocarcinoma of the testis is very rare. Not a single example was encountered in the series of 2,739 testicular tumors reviewed by the British Testicular Tumor Panel.[1] The Armed Forces Institute of Pathology listed 18 pure choriocarcinomas among 6,000 testicular tumors registered there.[2] Since their series consists mainly of referred material, it is not unlikely that this figure is too high.

Although pure choriocarcinoma affecting the testis is extremely rare, it is present as a component in mixed or combined testicular tumors more frequently than had been previously believed. It is usually observed in testicular tumors in young adults, but may occasionally be seen in older men.

Macroscopically, tumors containing choriocarcinoma are usually hemorrhagic (Fig. 3-31) and the appearance of the tumor is dependent upon the presence of other neoplastic germ cell elements with which it is combined. The tumors vary in size, but when choriocarcinoma predominates, the tumors are usually small.

Histologically, choriocarcinoma is composed of two components, the first being a centrally located cytotrophoblast composed of medium-sized, polygonal, round, or oval cells with clear cytoplasm, sharp cellular borders, and centrally located small, round, hyperchromatic, or larger vesicular, nuclei containing nucleoli and exhibiting mitotic brisk activity.

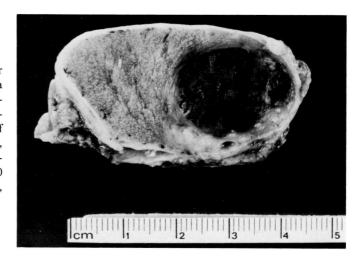

Fig. 3-31. Testicular tumor composed of choriocarcinoma admixed with teratoma. The tumor is very hemorrhagic. (Talerman A: germ cell tumors of the testis. In Fenoglio CM, Wolff M (eds): Progress in Surgical Pathology, vol. 1. 1980 Masson Publishing USA, Inc., New York.)

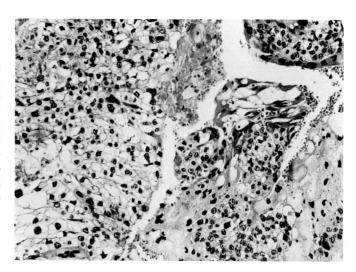

Fig. 3-32. Choriocarcinoma composed of centrally located epithelial-like cytotrophoblastic component and peripherally located syncytiotrophoblast with large vacuolated multinucleated cells. (Talerman A: germ cell tumors of the testis. In Fenoglio CM, Wolff M (eds): Progress in Surgical Pathology, vol 1. Masson, New York, 1980.) H & E. × 150.

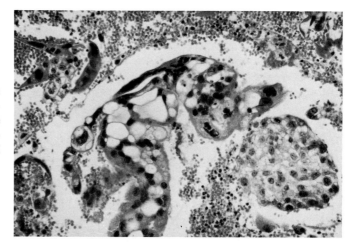

Fig. 3-33. Higher magnification of choriocarcinoma demonstrating the two components, the vesicular arrangement, and association with hemorrhage. H & E. × 380.

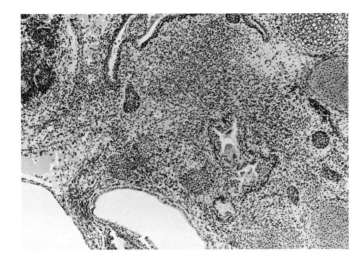

Fig. 3-34. Immature teratoma composed of various tissues in a haphazard arrangement. H & E. × 75.

The cytotrophoblastic cells are surrounded by the second component: syncytiotrophoblastic cells, which have irregular outlines, are large, basophilic, show vacuolation, and may contain many hyperchromatic nuclei varying in shape and size, or irregular masses of chromatin (Figs. 3-32 and 3-33). There may be a considerable variation in the amounts of the two components. Vesicular arrangement (Fig. 3-33) may or may not be present. These features together with hemorrhage and necrosis lead to marked variation in the appearance of the tumor. Hemorrhage is an invariable finding and it is always important to examine carefully the hemorrhagic areas for viable trophoblastic tissue. The latter is not infrequently completely destroyed or ablated by the hemorrhage. The presence of occasional atypical cells within the hemorrhagic areas may provide an explanation for elevated levels of serum HCG and β-HCG seen in some patients with testicular tumors without demonstrable choriocarcinoma, and for the presence of choriocarcinoma in metastatic deposits. It has been shown that the syncytiotrophoblast is the differentiated component of the tumor and originates from the cytotrophoblast.[13] Only the syncytiotrophoblast is capable of synthesizing HCG.[13, 50] Synthesis of HCG and its β-subunit by the tumor provides a very good and specific tumor marker for this neoplasm.

Choriocarcinoma is a highly malignant neoplasm, which metastasizes early through the lymphatic and hematogenous routes.[27] The prognosis of patients with choriocarcinoma depends on the amount of choriocarcinoma within the tumor and the presence or absence of metastases at the time of diagnosis. In recent years the prognosis, which was usually very poor, has improved due to the availability of more effective combination chemotherapy.

TERATOMA

Teratomas are germ cell neoplasms differentiating along the somatic pathway (Fig. 3-1) and composed of derivatives of the three primitive germ layers: endoderm, ectoderm, and mesoderm. They exhibit varying degrees of maturity and may be composed of fully mature tissues or may exhibit only slight somatic differentiation. Between these two extremes many intermediate types are seen, and they represent the majority of testicular teratomas. The maturity of the tumor may vary from area to area and the tumor is frequently composed of both immature and mature tissues. Teratomatous elements of different degrees of maturity may be closely admixed with each other, usually without any organoid arrangement (Fig. 3-34), although this may be observed in parts of the tumor. Testicular teratoma is frequently combined with other neoplastic germ cell elements, and its combination with embryonal carcinoma is particularly frequent, such tumors having been designated as teratocarcinoma.[7] It is now generally accepted that fully mature teratomas are associated with benign behavior, while the presence of immature tissue implies malignant potential.

The terms "mature" and "immature" teratoma are preferable to the terms "malignant" and "benign" teratoma because they are much more precise and describe the histologic appearances of the tumor. Testicular teratomas are usually partly solid and partly cystic, and either of these components may predominate. They show considerable variation in size from small to large. They are usually well-demarcated from the surrounding testicular tissue, and are not encapsulated. On sectioning, depending on their composition, they may be soft containing cysts filled with sebaceous or mucinous material, or very hard due to the presence of spicules of bone or fragments of ossifying cartilage.

Testicular teratomas occur in infancy and early childhood, and then become very rare until after puberty. Postpubertal testicular teratoma has a similar age incidence to other nonseminomatous germ cell neoplasms, which have their peak incidence one decade earlier than classic seminoma.

There is a considerable difference between the histologic appearances and the behavior of teratomas occurring in infants and children and those encountered in adults. While testicular tumors composed entirely of mature tissues are exceedingly rare in adults, nearly all teratomas occurring in infants and young children are composed entirely of mature tissues.[1] It should be added that a few cases have been encountered in which teratomatous tumors in infants and children contained some immature elements.[1] The number of such cases is very small, and none of them has been associated with metastases.[1] The immature elements observed in these cases were mostly neural,[1] although in two personal cases of infants aged 4½ and 9 months, respectively, immature mesenchymal and epithelial elements were

also encountered. Both patients are well and disease-free more than 5 years after diagnosis. On the other hand, in the author's experience of a number of teratomas occurring in adults in whom the primary tumor was diagnosed as a mature teratoma, metastases were already present and were composed of embryonal carcinoma, EST, or immature teratoma. Careful review of the original material revealed the presence of immature tissues. Similar findings were encountered in cases in which metastases were absent or occurred later. It is therefore considered that in a testicular tumor occurring in an adult, the diagnosis of mature teratoma must be based on the examination of the entire tumor and the well-documented absence of any immature elements. The diagnosis of mature teratoma carries with it a very good prognosis, and does not require further treatment beyond orchiectomy, while the presence of immature elements not only alters the diagnosis but also necessitates a different therapeutic approach. In view of this, every diagnosis of mature testicular teratoma in an adult should be viewed with a considerable degree of caution, and the presence of immature elements must be very carefully excluded.[4, 54]

Mature cystic teratoma with malignant transformation is a well-recognized entity in the ovary.[3, 59] In common with the WHO classification of ovarian neoplasms,[60] this entity has been included in the WHO classification of testicular neoplasms.[16] Due to the paucity of mature teratomas in adult men, tumors of this type are not observed in the testis. Therefore there seems to be no justification for the inclusion of this histologic type as a specific entity in the classification of testicular teratomas.

POLYEMBRYOMA

Polyembryoma is defined as a germ cell neoplasm composed entirely of embryoid bodies, resembling morphologically normal presomite embryos, which never reach beyond the 18-day stage. Such tumors in pure form have not been encountered to date, but polyembryoma may be observed as a component of mixed

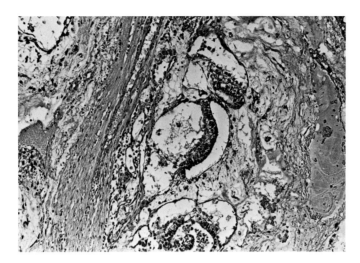

Fig. 3-35. Polyembryoma composed of embryoid bodies surrounded by loose myxomatous connective tissue. Teratomatous structures and embryonal carcinoma were present elsewhere. H & E. × 150.

or combined germ cell tumors. Tumors containing embryoid bodies are seen more frequently in the testis than in the ovary.

The histogenesis of polyembryoma is still a matter of dispute. Some investigators consider that it arises by parthenogenetic development from primitive germ cells present within a germ cell tumor.[61-63] Others consider that embryoid bodies develop by bizarre differentiation as a result of local release of organizers and persist only transiently.[9] Another view, based on experimental evidence in strain 129 mice, is that embryoid bodies originate from multipotential malignant embryonal cells present within the tumor, and not directly from germ cells.[11, 12, 64] This view supports the concept that embryoid bodies persist only transiently within the tumor, and while some are being formed others undergo further differentiation. This latter view appears to be the most favored at the present time.

Microscopically, polyembryoma is composed of numerous embryoid bodies which, when well-formed, are composed of an embryonic disk, which lies in the center separating the amniotic cavity from the yolk sac (Fig. 3-35). The embryoid body is surrounded by primitive extraembryonic mesenchyme and loose myxomatous tissue (Fig. 3-35). Less well formed embryoid bodies are composed of medullary plate and amnion associated with blastocystic space or extraembryonic mesenchyme. These atypical embryoid bodies may

contain two or more amniotic cavities and share a single yolk sac, or vice versa. The two cavities may vary in size and may be distorted. The embryoid bodies themselves may vary in size and show bizarre appearances. The embryonic disk is lined on one side by cuboidal epithelial cells resembling endoderm and on the other by tall columnar cells resembling ectoderm, which merge with low cuboidal epithelium lining the amniotic cavity. Teratomatous structures in various stages of differentiation are frequently seen in the vicinity of some of the embryoid bodies. Isolated syncytiotrophoblastic giant cells are also frequently found in the vicinity of the embryoid bodies, but there is no cytotrophoblast unless the tumor is combined with choriocarcinoma.

Tumors containing polyembryoma are considered to be highly malignant, are frequently associated with metastases and have a poor prognosis, although this outlook has been radically altered by more effective combination chemotherapy.

MONODERMAL OR SPECIALIZED TERATOMAS

Epidermoid Cyst

Epidermoid cyst is an uncommon testicular tumor. It consists of a cyst lined by keratinizing stratified squamous epithelium. The cystic space contains keratin and necrotic debris. Cutaneous adnexal structures are absent, and there are no other neoplastic germ cell elements present. The lesion is benign and is considered a one-sided development of a teratoma. The lesion is soft and well-demarcated from the surrounding testicular tissue. It is considered to be present since infancy, to develop before puberty, and to cease growing after reaching maturity.[65-67] None of the 70 cases observed by Price and Mostofi,[66] including 4 cases in children, contained immature elements or were associated with metastases, which confirmed that the lesion is benign.[66, 67]

Carcinoid

Carcinoid tumors occur in the testis either in pure form or combined with other elements present within a teratoma. Only 30 cases have been reported in the literature.[68, 69] In the majority of these cases the tumor was present in pure form, and only in five cases did the carcinoid originate in a teratoma. Eight cases of carcinoid tumors metastatic to the testis have been recorded.[68]

The histogenesis of the carcinoid tumors present within a teratoma is readily apparent, but the origin of pure primary testicular carcinoid tumors is uncertain. Two possible modes of origin have been suggested:

1. One-sided development of a teratoma
2. Origin from argentaffin or enterochromaffin cells which may be present in the testis, although such cells have never been detected in this location.

The ages of patients with primary testicular carcinoid ranged from 26 to 71 years, but the majority were between 40 and 60 years.[69] Therefore the patients were older than the majority of patients with testicular germ cell tumors. In all the reported cases the tumor was unilateral.[68, 69] Symptoms of the carcinoid syndrome were noted only in a single case, and even in this case which was the largest testicular carcinoid tumor recorded they were

minimal.[70] The direct relationship between the size of the tumor and the presence of the carcinoid syndrome has been noted in patients with primary carcinoid tumors of the ovary, which are associated with definite evidence of the syndrome in one-third of the cases.[71]

All primary carcinoid tumors observed in the testis showed the insular pattern typical of carcinoid tumors of midgut derivation.[71] They were composed of islands, nests, or aggregates of cells separated by fine or sometimes wider fibrous strands (Fig. 3-36). The cells forming the islands or nests exhibited a solid pattern, but small acini were also present (Fig. 3-36). Many of the cells at the periphery of the islands or nests, as well as some cells within the islands, contained orange–red granules when stained with hematoxylin and eosin. These granules stained black with the Masson-Fontana method and orange with the diazo method, indicating that they were argentaffin. Argyrophil granules demonstrable by the Grimelius stain were even more numerous (Fig. 3-37). Formalin-fixed, paraffin-processed tissue sections subjected to ultraviolet light using Enerback's method[72] exhibited marked yellow fluorescence, which is considered to be specific for serotonin and can be further confirmed by immunoperoxidase stains. Ultrastructural studies have revealed the presence of membrane-bound dense pleomorphic granules, which were similar to the granules found in cells of carcinoid tumors of midgut derivation.[69, 71]

Carcinoid tumor of the testis is rarely associated with metastatic disease. Metastases have been observed in only three cases.[68, 73] Two of these patients died of disseminated metastatic disease.[68, 73] All other patients, except for two patients who died of intercurrent disease, were well and disease-free for periods of 4 months to 28 years.[68, 69]

The treatment of choice is inguinal orchiectomy. Careful follow-up examination is advisable. Serial determinations of urinary 5-hydroxy-indoleacetic acid (5-HIAA) or of serum serotonin are of value in the follow-up of patients and further therapy can be withheld unless levels of these substances are elevated.

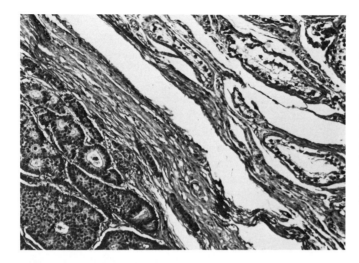

Fig. 3-36. Insular carcinoid tumor of the testis. Note the solid nests and small acini. Unaffected testicular tissue is seen on the right. H & E. × 185. (Talerman A: Germ cell tumors of the testis. In Fenoglio CM, Wolff M (eds): Progress in Surgical Pathology. Vol. 1. 1980 Masson Publishing USA, Inc., New York.)

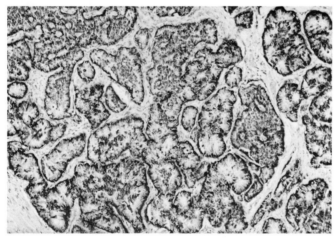

Fig. 3-37. Insular carcinoid tumor of the testis showing the argyrophil reaction. Grimelius stain × 90.

When the carcinoid tumor forms a part of a teratoma, the treatment and the prognosis will depend on the type of teratomatous elements present, as well as on the stage of the disease.

Retinal Anlage Tumor or Melanotic Hamartoma

Retinal anlage tumor is a rare, pigmented lesion, which may be a component of a teratoma or present in pure form, and it very rarely occurs in the testis. It is composed of nests of epithelial-like cells, some of which are small and dark-staining, with vesicular nuclei, while others are larger have eosino-philic cytoplasm, larger nuclei, and contain melanin pigment. The cells are surrounded by dense and hyalinized connective tissue stroma. The tumors are usually small, and are similar to those observed in the ovary. In the testis they have not been associated with metastases.[2]

MIXED OR COMBINED GERM CELL TUMORS

Due to more extensive and better sampling, the incidence of mixed or combined malignant germ cell tumors of the testis has been found to be higher than was previously believed. In fact, tumors composed of various combinations of these elements, including all but spermatocytic seminoma, make up approximately 50 percent of all testicular germ cell neoplasms. It is now evident that the poor prognosis of some patients with classic seminoma was due to the fact that other neoplastic germ cell elements were also contained within the primary tumor. If thorough sectioning and sampling is undertaken, however, detection of all elements present within a tumor is possible and can be of benefit in both correlating the findings with the presence of tumor markers in the serum and instituting the most appropriate therapy. Provision of appropriate therapy has become even more important with the discovery of more effective combination chemotherapy against specific, highly malignant neoplastic germ cell elements such as EST, choriocarcinoma, and embryonal carcinoma.

TUMORS COMPOSED OF GERM CELLS AND SEX CORD STROMA DERIVATIVES

Tumors composed of germ cells intimately admixed with sex cord stroma derivatives are uncommon. They can be classified into two types: gonadoblastoma and mixed germ cell sex cord stroma tumor.

Gonadoblastoma

Although 80 percent of gonadoblastomas occur in phenotypic females, the remaining 20 percent occur in phenotypic males who most frequently show pseudohermaphroditism and, less commonly, mixed gonadal dysgenesis.[74] These patients almost always have cryptorchidism, hypospadias, and internal female secondary sex organs.[74] In the majority of these patients gonadoblastoma is found in an inguinal location, or intraabdominally, usually at the site of the normal ovary.[74] Gonadoblastoma has been described in true hermaphrodites[75, 76] and in two patients with

normally descended scrotal testes,[77, 78] one of whom has subsequently fathered a child.[77] All the phenotypic males with gonadoblastoma were chromatin negative, and while two patients had 45X/46XY mosaicism,[74] the great majority had 46XY karyotype. Some patients exhibited gynecomastia.[74] The gonad of origin was in all cases a testis, and the contralateral gonad was a testis, or a streak, or was of indeterminate nature.[74] In at least one-third of the cases gonadoblastoma was bilateral and in 60 percent it was associated with malignant neoplastic germ cell elements, mostly seminoma, but sometimes with embryonal carcinoma or endodermal sinus tumor.[74, 78]

Gonadoblastomas occurring in phenotypic males are very small, unless they are overgrown by other neoplastic germ cell elements.

Microscopically, gonadoblastoma presents a very characteristic appearance and is composed of collections of cellular nests surrounded by connective tissue stroma (Figs. 3-38 and 3-39). The nests are composed of germ cells and sex cord derivatives resembling immature Sertoli and granulosa cells. The latter are arranged within the cell nests in three typical patterns (Fig. 3-39):

1. They line the periphery of the nests in a coronal pattern
2. They surround individual or collections of germ cells
3. They surround small spaces containing amorphous, hyaline, eosinophilic, PAS-positive material resembling Call-Exner bodies.

The germ cells exhibit mitotic activity, but mitoses are not observed in the immature sex cord derivatives. The surrounding connective tissue, which is usually dense, frequently contains collections of cells indistinguishable from Leydig cells, or luteinized cells of ovarian stromal origin. The number of these cells is variable. Reinke crystalloids have never been demonstrated in these cells.

The basic pattern of gonadoblastoma is frequently altered by hyalinization, calcification (Fig. 3-38), and overgrowth by other neoplas-

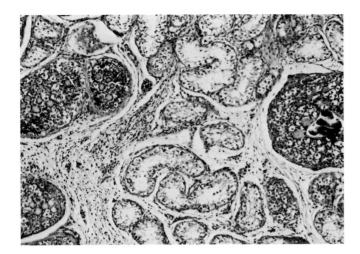

Fig. 3-38. Testis containing gonadoblastoma nests surrounded by seminiferous tubules. Note the hyaline bodies and calcification within one of the nests (right). H & E. × 60.

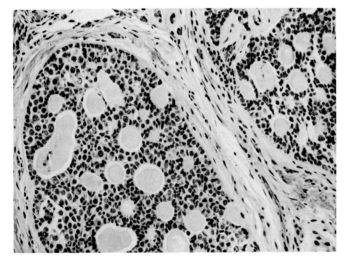

Fig. 3-39. Gonadoblastoma nests composed of larger round germ cells closely admixed with smaller sex cord derivatives. There are numerous Call-Exner-like hyaline bodies present within the nests. Occasional somewhat distorted Leydig-like cells are seen in surrounding connective tissue. H & E. × 150.

tic germ cell elements, usually seminoma. All these processes may be present at the same time and may lead to distortion and obliteration of the gonadoblastoma nests. The result may be round, smooth, calcified concretions, or foci of hyalinization with calcific concretions surrounded by seminoma. The histologic picture of gonadoblastoma has never been observed outside the gonads. The prognosis of patients with pure gonadoblastoma is excellent, and that of gonadoblastoma associated with seminoma is favorable; in the latter case metastases are infrequent.[74] On the other hand, when gonadoblastoma is overgrown by other malignant neoplastic germ cell elements, the prognosis is poor,[78] although it has im-

proved with the availability of more efficacious combination chemotherapy.

Since gonadoblastoma is frequently bilateral, careful investigation of the patient and excision of the contralateral gonad is mandatory because it may harbor a minute gonadoblastoma, which may become the source of a malignant germ cell tumor.

Mixed Germ Cell Sex Cord Stroma Tumor

Mixed germ cell sex cord stroma tumor is a recently established entity. Like gonadoblastoma, it is composed of germ cells intimately admixed with sex cord derivatives, however

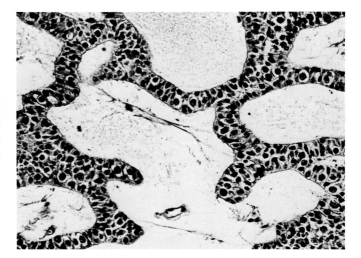

Fig. 3-40. Mixed germ cell/sex cord stroma tumor showing the cordlike pattern. Note the larger pale round germ cells and the smaller sex cord elements which surround them. H & E. × 320.

it differs from gonadoblastoma histologically, clinically, genetically, and endocrinologically.[79-81]

Mixed germ cell sex cord stroma tumor is most frequently seen in the normal ovaries of phenotypically and genetically normal female infants and children, but it also occurs in normally descended testes of phenotypically, anatomically, and genetically normal adult men, who are often elderly.[81, 82] No evidence of endocrine abnormalities has been encountered in male patients with this tumor.[81, 82]

Macroscopically, the testicular tumors are often large, especially when compared with gonadoblastomas, measuring up to 12 cm in maximum diameter. They are solid, firm, gray–white, and form a circumscribed nodule or mass within the testis. Large tumors may replace the whole testis and invade the epididymis.

Microscopically, the mixed germ cell sex cord stroma tumor is composed of germ cells intimately admixed with sex cord derivatives which show a greater resemblance to Sertoli cells than to granulosa cells. The tumor may exhibit three different histologic patterns and is composed of:

1. Long narrow ramifying cords or trabeculae (Fig. 3-40), which in places expand, form-

ing large, round, or oval cellular aggregates, or wide columns, which are surrounded by connective tissue stroma varying from loose and edematous to dense and hyalinized

2. Solid, tubules devoid of a lumen and surrounded by fine connective tissue septa (Fig. 3-41)

3. Large aggregates of germ cells and sex cord derivatives devoid of any specific arrangement (Fig. 3-42)

All these patterns may be observed in the same tumor and may intermingle with each other. The two components, the germ cells and the sex cord derivatives, are intimately admixed with each other. Although in some areas the sex cord derivatives may predominate, in others there is a preponderance of the germ cells. The tumor shows active proliferation, and mitotic activity is seen not only in the germ cells but also in the sex cord derivatives. There are no regressive changes such as hyalinization and calcification, and Call-Exner-like hyaline bodies are seen only occasionally. Cystic spaces lined by flattened epithelium, or by sex cord elements, and containing pale eosinophilic secretion, have been seen in some ovarian tumors, but were not observed in testicular tumors.

To date, there has been no association or

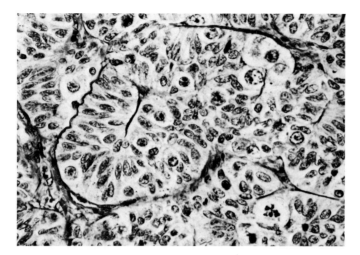

Fig. 3-41. Mixed germ cell/sex cord stroma tumor showing the tubular pattern and composed of solid tubules. Note the large germ cells and smaller sex cord derivatives. An abnormal mitosis is seen (bottom right). H & E. × 600.

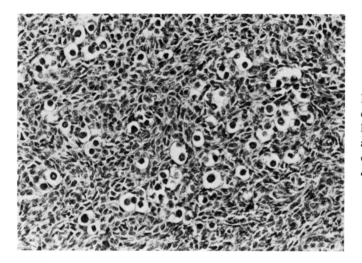

Fig. 3-42. Mixed germ cell/sex cord stroma tumor showing large aggregates of germ cells and sex cord derivatives devoid of any specific arrangement. H & E. × 380.

overgrowth by seminoma, or any other neoplastic germ cell elements in testicular tumors of this type.[81, 82] Metastases have not been encountered, although this has been observed in occasional ovarian tumors of this type.[3, 81] Mixed germ cell sex cord stroma tumor has never been observed in extragonadal locations.[3, 81]

The treatment of choice is inguinal orchiectomy. All the patients with mixed germ cell sex cord stroma tumor of the testis are well and disease-free for up to 15 years following orchiectomy.[80-82] The contralateral gonad in every case was a normal testis.

REFERENCES

1. Pugh RCB (ed): Pathology of the Testis. Blackwell Scientific Publications, Oxford, 1976
2. Mostofi FK, Price EB Jr: Tumors of the male genital system. Atlas of Tumor Pathology, 2nd series, Fasc. 8. Armed Forces Institute of Pathology, Washington, D.C., 1973
3. Talerman A: Germ cell tumors of the ovary. In Blaustein A (ed): The Pathology of the Female Genital Tract, 2nd Ed. Springer Verlag, New York, 1982
4. Talerman A: Germ cell tumors of the testis. In Fenoglio CM, Wolff M (eds): Progress in

Surgical Pathology, vol. 1. Masson, New York, 1980

5. Teilum G: Homologous tumours in ovary and testis: contribution to classification of gonadal tumours. Acta Obstet Gynecol Scand 24:480, 1944

6. Teilum G: Gonocytoma; homologous ovarian and testicular tumours; 1; with discussion of "Mesonephroma ovarii" (Schiller: Am J Cancer, 1939). Acta Pathol Microbiol Scand 23:242, 1946

7. Friedman NB, Moore RA: Tumors of the testis. A report of 922 cases. Milit Surg 99:573, 1946

8. Dixon FJ, Moore RA: Tumors of the Male Sex Organs. Atlas of Tumor Pathology, Sec. VIII, Fasc 31b and 32. Armed Forces Institute of Pathology, Washington, D.C., 1953

9. Willis RA: Pathology of Tumours, 4th Ed. Butterworths, London, 1967

10. Collins DH, Pugh RCB: Pathology of testicular tumours. Br J Urol 36:Suppl 1964

11. Stevens LC: Embryonic potency of embryoid bodies derived from transplantable testicular teratoma of the mouse. Dev Biol 2:285, 1960

12. Pierce BG, Dixon FJ: Testicular teratomas 1. Demonstration of teratogenesis by metamorphosis of multipotential cells. Cancer 12:573, 1959

13. Pierce GB, Midgley AR Jr: The origin and function of human syncytiotrophoblastic giant cells. Am J Pathol 43:153, 1963

14. Teilum G: Special Tumors of Ovary and Testis. Comparative Pathology and Histological Identification. Munksgaard, Copenhagen, 1971

15. Teilum G: Classification of endodermal sinus tumor (mesoblastoma vitellinum) and so-called "embryonal carcinoma" of the ovary. Acta Pathol Microbiol Scand 64:407, 1965

16. Mostofi FK, Sobin LH: Histological Typing of Testis Tumours, International Histological Classification of Tumours No. 16. World Health Organization, Geneva, 1977

17. Talerman A: The incidence of yolk sac tumor (endodermal sinus tumor) elements in germ cell tumors of the testis in adults. Cancer 36:211, 1975

18. Talerman A: Endodermal sinus (yolk sac) tumor elements in testicular germ cell tumors in adults. Comparison of prospective and retrospective studies. Cancer 46:1213, 1980

19. Oliver RTD, Hope-Stone HF, Blandy JP. Justification of the use of surveillance in the management of Stage 1 germ cell tumours of the testis. Br J Urol 55:760, 1983

20. Chevassu M: Tumeurs du Testicule. G Steinhall, Paris, 1906

21. Johnson DE, Gomez JJ, Ayala AG: Anaplastic seminoma. J Urol 114:80, 1975

22. Kademian M, Bosch A, Caldwell WL: Anaplastic seminoma. Cancer 40:3082, 1977

23. Percarpio B, Clements JC, McLeod DG et al: Anaplastic seminoma. An analysis of 77 patients. Cancer 43:2510, 1979

24. Kurman RJ, Scardino PT, McIntire KR et al: Cellular localization of alpha-fetoprotein and human chorionic gonadotropin in germ cell tumors of the testis by indirect immunoperoxidase technique. A new approach to classification utilizing tumor markers. Cancer 40:2136, 1977

25. Kuber W, Kratzik C, Schwartz HP et al: Experience with beta-HCG positive seminoma. Br J Urol 55:555, 1983

26. Bartsch G, Scheiber K, Mikuz G et al: HCG-positive seminoma: is this special type of seminoma with poor prognosis? (Abstr 480). J Urol 131:223A, 1984

27. Bredael JJ, Vugrin D, Whitmore WF Jr: Autopsy findings in 154 patients with germ cell tumors of the testis. Cancer 50:548, 1982

28. Huben RP, Williams PD, Pontes JE et al: Seminoma at Roswell Park 1970 to 1979. An analysis of treatment failures. Cancer 53:1451, 1984

29. Masson P: Etude sur le séminome. Rev Can Biol 5:361, 1946

30. Scully RE: Spermatocytic seminoma of the testis. A report of 3 cases and review of the literature. Cancer 14:788, 1961

31. Thackray AC: Seminoma. p. 12. In Collins DH, Pugh RCB (eds): Pathology of testicular tumours. Br J Urol Suppl 36, 1964

32. Jackson JR and Magner D: Spermatocytic seminoma. A variant of seminoma with specific microscopical and clinical characteristics. Cancer 18:751, 1965

33. Fox JE, Abell MR: Spermatocytic seminoma. J Urol 100:757, 1968

34. Rosai J, Silber I, Khodadoust K: Spermatocytic seminoma. Clinicopathologic study of six cases and review of the literature. Cancer 24:92, 1969

35. Talerman A: Spermatocytic seminoma. J Urol 112:212, 1974

36. Talerman A: Spermatocytic seminoma. Clinicopathological study of 22 cases. Cancer 45:2169, 1980

37. Farivari A, Mostofi FK: Spermatocytic seminoma (Abstr 491). J Urol 131:226A, 1984

38. Rosai J, Khodadoust J, Silber I: Spermatocytic seminoma II. Ultrastructural study. Cancer 24:103, 1969

39. Talerman A, Fu YS, Okagaki T: Spermatocytic seminoma. Ultrastructural and microspectrophotometric observations. Lab Invest 51:343, 1984.

40. Brown NJ: Yolk sac tumor (orchioblastoma) and other testicular tumours of childhood. p. 356. In Pugh RCB (ed): Pathology of the Testis. Blackwell Scientific Publications, Oxford, 1976

41. Teilum G: Special Tumors of Ovary and Testis. Comparative Pathology and Histological Identification, 2nd Ed. Munksgaard, Copenhagen, 1976

42. Gonzalez-Crussi F: The human yolk sac and yolk sac (endodermal sinus) tumor. A review. Perspect Pediatr Pathol 5:179, 1979

43. Wold LE, Kramer SA, Farrow GM: Testicular yolk sac and embryonal carcinomas in pediatric patients: comparative immunohistochemical and clinicopathologic study. Am J Clin Pathol 81:427, 1984

44. Teilum G: Endodermal sinus tumours of the ovary and testis. Comparative morphogenesis of the so-called mesonephroma ovarii (Schiller) and extraembryonic (yolk-sac allantoic) structures of the rat's placenta. Cancer 12:1092, 1959

45. Talerman A, Haije WG: Alpha fetoprotein and germ cell tumors: a possible role of yolk sac tumor in production of alpha fetoprotein. Cancer 34:1722, 1974

46. Talerman A, Haije WG, Baggerman L: Alpha-l-antitrypsin (AAT) and alpha-foetoprotein (AFP) in sera of patients with germ cell neoplasms. Value as tumour markers in patients with endodermal sinus tumour (yolk sac tumour). Int J Cancer 19:741, 1977

47. Teilum G, Albrechtsen R, Norgaard-Pedersen B: Immunofluorescent localization of alpha-fetoprotein synthesis in endodermal sinus tumor (yolk sac tumor). Acta Pathol Microbiol Scand [A] 82:586, 1974

48. Talerman A, Haije WG, Baggerman L: Serum alphafetoprotein (AFP) in patients with germ cell tumors of the gonads and extragonadal sites. Correlation between endodermal sinus (yolk sac) tumor and raised serum AFP. Cancer 46:380, 1980

49. Talerman A, Haije WG, Baggerman L: Serum alpha-fetoprotein (AFP) in diagnosis and management of endodermal sinus (yolk sac) tumor and mixed germ cell tumor of the ovary. Cancer 41:272, 1978

50. Fowler JE, Sesterhenn I, Stutzman RE et al: Localization of alpha-fetoprotein and human chorionic gonadotropin to specific histologic types of nonseminomatous testicular cancer. Urology 22:649, 1983

51. Woodtli W, Hedinger C: Endodermal sinus tumor or Orchioblastoma in children and adults. Virchows Arch [Pathol Anat] 364:93, 1974

52. Young PG, Mount BM, Foote FW Jr et al: Embryonal adenocarcinoma in the prepubertal testis. A clinicopathologic study of 18 cases. Cancer 26:1065, 1970

53. Pierce GB, Bullock WK, Huntington RW: Yolk sac tumors of the testis. Cancer 25:644, 1970

54. Von Hochstetter AR, Hedinger CE: The differential diagnosis of testicular germ cell tumors in theory and practice. A critical analysis of two major systems of classification and review of 389 cases. Virchows Arch [Pathol Anat] A 396:247, 1982

55. Wurster K, Hedinger C, Meienberg O: Orchioblastomatous foci in testicular teratoma in adults. Virchows Arch [Pathol Anat] 357:231, 1972

56. Jacobsen GK, Jacobsen M: Possible liver cell differentiation in testicular germ cell tumours. Histopathology 7:537, 1983

57. Talerman A: Hyaline globules in ovarian mixed mesodermal (mullerian) tumors. Hum Pathol 14:562, 1983

58. Kaplan GW, Cromie WJ, Kelalis PP et al: Preliminary report of the Prepubertal Testicular Registry (Abstr 369). J Urol 131:196A, 1984

59. Scully RE: Tumors of the Ovary and Maldeveloped Gonads. Atlas of Tumor Pathology, 2nd Series Fasc 16. Armed Forces Institute of Pathology, Washington, D.C. 1979

60. Serov SF, Scully RE, Sobin LH: Histological Typing of Ovarian Tumours. International His-

tological Classification of Tumours, No 9. World Health Organization, Geneva, 1973

61. Peyron A: Faits nouveaux relatifs à l'origine et à l'histogenèse des embryomes. Bull Assoc Fr Cancer 28:658, 1939

62. Simard LC: Polyembryonic embryoma of the ovary of parthenogenetic origin. Cancer 10:215, 1957

63. Marin-Padilla M: Origin, nature and significance of the "embryoids" of human teratomas. Virchows Arch [Pathol Anat] 340:105, 1965

64. Evans RW: Histological Appearances of Tumours, 2nd Ed. Livingstone Ltd., Edinburgh and London, 1967

65. Abell MR and Holtz F: Testicular tumors in adolescents. Cancer 17:881, 1964

66. Price EB Jr., Mostofi FK: Epidermoid cysts of the testis in children: a report of four cases. J Pediatr 77:676, 1970

67. Shah KH, Maxted WC, Chun B: Epidermoid cysts of the testis. A report of three cases and an analysis of 141 cases from world literature. Cancer 47:577, 1981

68. Berdjis CC, Mostofi FK: Carcinoid tumors of the testis. J Urol 118:777, 1977

69. Talerman A, Gratama S, Miranda S et al: Primary carcinoid tumor of the testis. Case report, ultrastructure and review of the literature. Cancer 42:2696, 1978

70. Wurster K, Brodner O, Rossner JA et al: A carcinoid occurring in the testis. Virchows Arch [Pathol Anat] 370:185, 1976

71. Talerman A: Carcinoid tumors of the ovary. J Cancer Res Clin Oncol 107:125, 1984

72. Enerback L: Specific methods for detection of 5-Hydroxytryptamine in carcinoid tumors. Virchows Arch [Pathol Anat] 358:35, 1973

73. Hosking DH, Bowman DM, McMorris SL et al: Primary carcinoid tumor of the testis with metastases. J Urol 125:255, 1981

74. Scully RE: Gonadoblastoma. A review of 74 cases. Cancer 25:1340, 1970

75. Park IJ, Pyeatte JC, Jones HW et al: Gonadoblastoma in a true hermaphrodite with 46 XY Karyotype. Obstet Gynecol 40:466, 1972

76. Talerman A, Jarabak J, Amarose AP: Gonadoblastoma and dysgerminoma in a true hermaphrodite with a 46,XX Karyotype. Am J Obstet Gynecol 140:475, 1981

77. Hughesdon PE, Kumarasamy T: Mixed germ cell tumours (gonadoblastomas) in normal and dysgenetic gonads. Virchows Arch [Pathol Anat] 349:258, 1970

78. Talerman A, Delemarre JFM: Gonadoblastoma associated with embryonal carcinoma in an anatomically normal male. J Urol 113:355, 1975

79. Talerman A: A mixed germ cell sex cord stroma tumor in a normal female infant. Obstet Gynecol 40:473, 1972

80. Talerman A: A distinctive gonadal neoplasm related to gonadoblastoma. Cancer 30:1219, 1972

81. Talerman A: The pathology of gonadal neoplasms composed of germ cells and sex cord stroma derivatives. Pathol Res Pract 170:24, 1980

82. Bolen JW: Mixed germ cell-sex cord stroma tumor: a gonadal tumor distinct from gonadoblastoma. Am J Clin Pathol 75:565, 1981

4

Sex Cord-Stromal Tumors

W. Dwayne Lawrence, Robert H. Young, and Robert E. Scully

In 1977 the World Health Organization[1] (WHO) adopted a classification of sex cord-stromal tumors of the testis (Table 4-1), which will be followed in this chapter; however, categories B and C, which are often difficult to differentiate and hard to separate when evaluating cases in the literature, will be considered as a group. Additionally, several specific entities recognized since adoption of the WHO classification will be discussed separately.

The term "sex cord-stromal tumors," which had been chosen previously by the WHO to describe homologous ovarian tumors,[2] refers to neoplasms containing cells that resemble Sertoli cells, Leydig cells, granulosa cells, and theca cells, as well as fibroblasts, in varying combinations and varying degrees of differentiation. The terminology used to describe these tumors has been controversial for more than 25 years. In 1944, Teilum[3] was the first investigator to focus attention on them, pointing out their resemblance to ovarian tumors composed of similar cell types. He designated tumors containing Sertoli cells and Leydig cells as "androblastomas," to emphasize their apparent recapitulation of testicular development. Although this term gained widespread acceptance, its unintentional connotation of androgen production is misleading. In 1952, Laskowski[4] reported an estrogenic granulosa cell tumor of the testis, the existence of which Teilum accepted and explained on the basis of the common origin of Sertoli and granulosa cells.[5] In 1959, Mostofi and his co-workers[6] introduced the term "tumors of specialized gonadal stroma," subsequently abbreviated to "gonadal stromal tumors," to include both androblastomas and granulosa cell tumors of the testis; these authors emphasized the frequent admixture of Sertoli cells, granulosa cells, Leydig cells, and theca cells within individual specimens. Their designation implies origin of all tumors in this category from a specific cell within the primitive gonadal "stroma." Although the term "gonadal stromal tumor" is still widely used, its identification of "stroma" as the source of granulosa and Sertoli cells as well as theca and Leydig cells is controversial and unacceptable according to modern teaching in embryology. In 1976 Symington and Cameron[7] designated neoplasms of obvious Sertoli cell nature as Sertoli cell tumors, but preferred the term "Sertoli cell mesenchyme tumors" for the larger and more heterogeneous group of neoplasms that contain both Sertoli cell and stromal elements.

Sex cord-stromal tumors account for approximately 4 percent of testicular neoplasms. Most of the reported cases have been Leydig cell tumors; smaller numbers of Sertoli cell tumors and rare granulosa cell tumors have also been described in the literature. The remaining neoplasms in this category contain cells of both male and female types or cells that cannot be specifically identified as male or female. Each of these four groups of tumor will be discussed separately.

LEYDIG CELL TUMORS

Leydig cell tumors account for 1 to 3 percent of all testicular neoplasms; approximately

Table 4-1. WHO Histologic Classification of Testicular Sex Cord-Stromal Tumors

Well-differentiated forms
Leydig cell tumor
Sertoli cell tumor
Granulosa cell tumor
Mixed forms
Incompletely differentiated forms

250 cases have been reported.[8-18] These tumors may be diagnosed at any age, but are most common in persons between 20 and 50 years. Adult patients usually complain of testicular swelling, but gynecomastia is the presenting symptom in about 15 percent of the cases; occasional patients complain of both testicular swelling and gynecomastia.[14] The gynecomastia is synchronously bilateral in about 90 percent of the cases, and is of more than 1 year's duration in approximately half of them. In 3 percent of the reported cases, an operation for gynecomastia had been performed before the testicular tumor was detected.[14] About one-quarter of the patients with gynecomastia also have a decrease in libido, potency, or both. In one case a Leydig cell tumor presented as a metastatic mass in a cervical lymph node.[19] About 10 percent of the patients have had no symptoms, and their tumors were discovered incidentally on physical examination or at autopsy.

With one possible exception,[20] all 50 children with a Leydig cell tumor whose cases have been reported in the literature have presented with isosexual pseudoprecocity.[21-26] In addition, two adults had a history of precocity.[14, 27] The precocious development typically appears between the ages of 5 and 9 years. Ten percent of the patients with sexual precocity also had gynecomastia.[14] The duration of the sexual precocity has varied greatly; in 70 percent of the cases it had been present for more than 1 year and in 15 percent for more than 5 years before the discovery of the tumor. In 5–10 percent of the cases the tumor has arisen in an undescended testis or one that had been previously cryptorchid. Leydig cell tumors occur almost always in genotypically normal males, but in three cases have developed in patients with Klinefelter's syndrome.[18, 28, 29]

Testosterone is the major androgen produced by Leydig cell tumors, but secretion of androstenedione and dehydroepiandrosterone has also been recorded.[30-32] Urinary 17-ketosteroid levels may be normal or high. Elevated estrogen levels have been documented in patients with gynecomastia and also in patients without it, and estradiol has been recovered in high concentration from the spermatic vein blood in several cases.[33] Testosterone levels have been reported to be low or normal in patients with gynecomastia and high estradiol levels[34]; in a few patients with gynecomastia, plasma progesterone or urinary pregnanediol levels have been elevated.[35]

Approximately 3 percent of Leydig cell tumors are bilateral. The tumor has extended beyond the testis at the time of presentation in 10 to 15 percent of the cases.[14] Pathologic examination reveals a mass that usually ranges between 3 and 5 cm in diameter. Sectioning typically reveals sharp circumscription and lobulation of the tumor by fibrous septa (Fig. 4-1). The neoplastic tissue is uniformly solid and usually yellow or yellow-tan, but occasionally it is gray, grayish white, brown, or greenish brown (Fig. 4-2). Foci of hemorrhage, necrosis, or both are present in 25 percent of the cases (Fig. 4-3).

The most common microscopic pattern is diffuse, but insular, trabecular, solid–tubular, and ribbonlike arrangements of the tumor cells are also encountered. The neoplastic cells are most often large and polygonal with abundant eosinophilic, slightly granular cytoplasm (Fig. 4-4); occasionally the cytoplasm is extensively vacuolated or foamy as a result of lipid accumulation (Fig. 4-5). Rarely the cells are spindle-shaped or are small with scanty cytoplasm and nuclei containing grooves (Fig. 4-6). Crystalloids of Reinke (Fig. 4-7) have been identified in 25 to 40 percent of the cases, and lipochrome pigment[14] in 10 to 15 percent. Nuclear atypicality is usually absent or of mi-

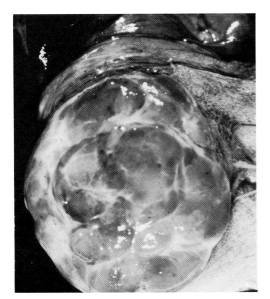

Fig. 4-1. Leydig cell tumor. The tumor is lobulated and was yellow in the fresh state. (Kim I, Young RH, Scully RE: Leydig cell tumor of the testis. A clinicopathological analysis of 40 cases and review of the literature. Am J Surg Pathol 9:177, 1985.)

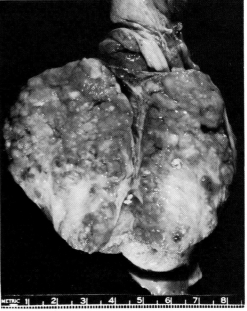

Fig. 4-3. Malignant Leydig's cell tumor. The tumor replaces the entire testis and was brown with foci of hemorrhage and necrosis in the fresh state. (Kim I, Young RH, Scully RE: Leydig cell tumor of the testis. A clinicopathological analysis of 40 cases and review of the literature. Am J Surg Pathol 9:177, 1985.)

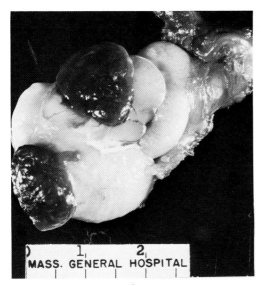

Fig. 4-2. Leydig cell tumor. A well-circumscribed tumor, which was greenish-brown, from a boy with isosexual pseudoprecocity. (Engel LL, Lanman G, Scully RE, Villee DB: Studies on an interstitial cell tumor of the testis: formation of cortisol -14_C from acetate -1 -14_C1. J Clin Endocrinol Metab 26:381, 1966 © Endocrine Society.)

nor degree; the mitotic rate varies greatly, but is low in most cases. Occasional tumors, however, appear highly malignant cytologically, with a considerable mitotic rate (Fig. 4-8). The ultrastructural features of Leydig cell tumors are discussed in Chapter 7.

Leydig cell tumors must be distinguished from the nodular Leydig cell hyperplasia or condensation that may be seen in atrophic testes, including those from patients with Klinefelter's syndrome. In these cases, Leydig cells do not displace the tubules completely but surround them; the sclerotic tubules may be difficult to identify on low-power examination, especially in patients with Klinefelter's syndrome. Leydig cell tumors, in contrast, almost always replace the seminiferous tubules. The clinical features associated with Klinefelter's syndrome may also be helpful diagnosti-

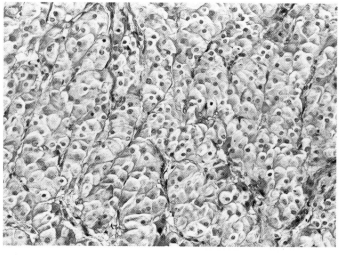

Fig. 4-4. Leydig cell tumor. The neoplastic cells contain abundant, peripherally vacuolated cytoplasm and round nuclei. H & E. × 246. (Kim I, Young RH, Scully RE: Leydig cell tumor of the testis. A clinicopathological analysis of 40 cases and review of the literature. Am J Surg Pathol 9:177, 1985.)

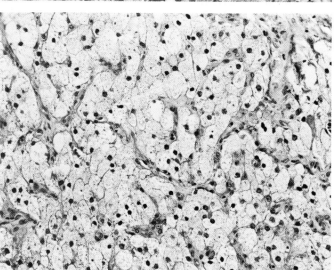

Fig. 4-5. Leydig cell tumor. The neoplastic cells contain abundant spongy, lipid-rich cytoplasm and small nuclei. H & E. × 400. (Kim I, Young RH, Scully RE: Leydig cell tumor of the testis. A clinicopathological analysis of 40 cases and review of the literature. Am J Surg Pathol 9:177, 1985.)

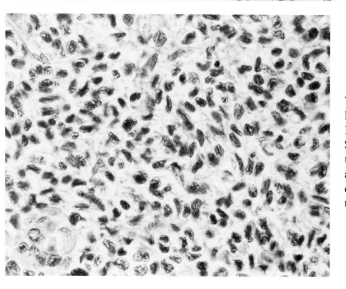

Fig. 4-6. Leydig cell tumor. The nuclei of the neoplastic cells have prominent grooves. H & E. × 640. (Kim I, Young RH, Scully RE: Leydig cell tumor of the testis. A clinicopathological analysis of 40 cases and review of the literature. Am J Surg Pathol 9:177, 1985.)

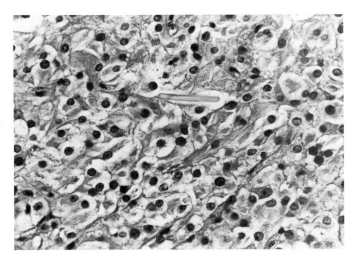

Fig. 4-7. Leydig cell tumor. Reinke crystalloid is seen in the center. H & E. × 600. (Courtesy of A. Talerman, M.D.)

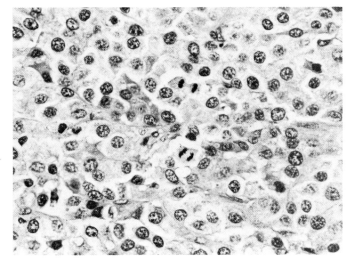

Fig. 4-8. Malignant Leydig cell tumor. The neoplastic cells exhibit nuclear hyperchromatism; several mitotic figures are visible. H & E. × 640. (Kim I, Young RH, Scully RE: Leydig cell tumor of the testis. A clinicopathological analysis of 40 cases and review of the literature. Am J Surg Pathol 9:177, 1985.)

cally. It should be remembered that, as mentioned above, a rare patient with Klinefelter's syndrome has developed a true Leydig cell tumor.

The differentiation of Leydig cell tumors from other sex cord-stromal tumors is generally not difficult because foci of epithelial differentiation are typically present in the latter. The rare Leydig cell tumors that contain cells with nuclear grooves (Fig. 4-6) however, may resemble granulosa cell tumors. Likewise, a pseudotubular or trabecular pattern in a Leydig cell tumor may suggest the diagnosis of a Sertoli cell tumor. In such cases the presence

of typical foci of Leydig cell neoplasia elsewhere is diagnostic. Leydig cell tumors may also be confused with malignant lymphomas or plasmacytomas, particularly when their cells contain less cytoplasm and are more atypical than in the usual case. Features of lymphomas and plasmacytoma that are helpful in the differential diagnosis include: a higher frequency of bilaterality, the common presence of invasion of the epididymis and spermatic cord, characteristic intertubular infiltration of the tumor cells, invasion of the tubules in one-third of the cases, and characteristic cytologic features of the neoplastic cells. A final category of tumors that may be mistaken rarely for a Leydig cell tumor is metastatic carcinoma, particularly of prostatic origin. In such cases other areas characteristic of prostatic adenocarcinoma can usually be identified; immunocytochemical staining for prostate-specific acid phosphatase and prostate-specific antigen is almost always diagnostic.

Malacoplakia may be confused with a Leydig cell tumor on both gross and microscopic examination. It results in the formation of a generally homogenous, yellow or brown mass; the finding of an abscess, which is present in most cases is an important clue to the diagnosis. On low-power examination, the testicular parenchyma is replaced by epithelioid cells with abundant granular cytoplasm (von Hansemann's cells), which superficially resemble Leydig cells, but these cells occupy tubules as well as the interstitium and are typically admixed with other inflammatory cells. In addition, many of the von Hansemann's cells contain in their cytoplasm round to oval, basophilic, calcific inclusions (Michaelis-Gutmann bodies), small structures thought to be phagolysosomes containing remnants of gram-negative bacteria. In two cases of which we are aware, malacoplakia was initially misdiagnosed as a Leydig cell tumor.

Approximately 11 percent of the Leydig cell tumors encountered to date have been clinically malignant; follow-up, however, has been of variable duration and short in many of the cases.[14] Metastases have appeared as long as 8 years postoperatively and in the series of Kim and her associates[14] occurred an average of 16 months postoperatively. Therefore, a higher proportion of reported tumors would probably have proved malignant had longer follow-up been available at the time of publication. The average age of the patients with malignant tumors has been higher than that of those with benign tumors (63 years for the former in contrast to 40 years for Leydig cell tumors in general).[14] No patients with clinically malignant tumors have presented with

endocrine manifestations, although elevated levels of various hormones or their metabolites have been recorded in many of them. None of the tumors in prepubertal patients have recurred or metastasized. Only one patient with a malignant tumor was alive at the time of last follow-up, 4 years after presentation; all the others died 2 months to 9 years (average, 34 months) postoperatively.[14] In the series of Kim et al., the survival from the initial operation to death ranged from 10 to 31 months (average, 22 months). The most common sites of metastasis have been retroperitoneal and inguinal lymph nodes (68 percent), liver (45 percent), lungs (45 percent), and bone (27 percent). Mediastinal lymph nodes, cervical lymph nodes, the kidneys, pleura, adrenal glands, and other abdominal viscera have been involved in occasional cases.

Although no single histologic criterion has proved reliable to distinguish benign from malignant Leydig cell tumors, the latter have generally been larger than the former, and have had infiltrative margins, invaded lymphatics or blood vessels, contained foci of necrosis, and had a mitotic rate of more than 3 per 10 high-power fields and significant nuclear atypicality much more often than the former.[14] All five clinically malignant tumors in the series of 40 cases reported by Kim et al.[14] had four or more of the above features; in contrast, 12 of the 14 tumors that appeared to be benign on the basis of follow-up data of 2 or more years' duration had none of these features; one benign tumor had only one and the final tumor had three features.[14]

The primary treatment of a Leydig cell tumor is inguinal orchiectomy. If the gross or histologic features indicate a likelihood of malignancy, a retroperitoneal lymphadenectomy should be considered.[14] In one case in which this procedure disclosed a microscopic focus of tumor in a lymph node, the patient was alive and well when last seen 4 years later.[14] The treatment by chemotherapy of Leydig cell tumors that have spread outside the testis has been unsatisfactory up to the present time.

TUMORS OF ADRENOCORTICAL TYPE

Testicular "tumors," which are typically bilateral, usually synchronously, develop in a significant proportion of male patients with untreated or inadequately treated adrenogenital syndrome (AGS).[36-43] Although these "tumors" may not belong, strictly speaking, in the category of sex cord stromal tumors, they resemble Leydig cell tumors microscopically, and they may even be of Leydig cell origin. They should be distinguished, however, from Leydig cell tumors because of differences in prognosis and therapy.

Testicular "tumors" of the adrenogenital syndrome (TTAGS), which occur most often in patients with the salt-losing form of this disorder (21-hydroxylase deficiency), may become evident in childhood or in adult life. Clinical clues to the diagnosis include the established presence of the syndrome in the patient, a family history of it, and bilateral testicular enlargement, which is rare in cases of Leydig cell tumor. Laboratory examination reveals the typical findings of AGS: an increase of adrenocorticotropic hormone (ACTH), androstenedione, and 17-hydroxy-progesterone levels in the plasma and 17-ketosteroid and pregnanetriol levels in the urine. A high level of urinary 17-ketosteroids in the apparent absence of metastatic disease after the excision of a testicular tumor resembling a Leydig cell tumor also suggests the possibility of an underlying AGS. Other characteristic features of the TTAGS are their enlargement and increased hormonal secretion after the administration of ACTH, and a decline in their size and hormone output after suppression of the elevated ACTH level by the administration of corticosteroids.

The testicular "tumor" of the AGS may attain a diameter as large as 10 cm. It appears to originate in the hilar region and subsequently extends peripherally into the parenchyma; sectioning reveals dark brown, lobulated tissue traversed by fibrous septa (Fig.

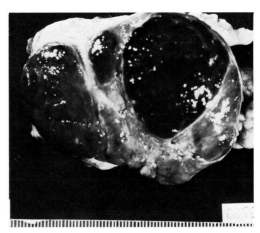

Fig. 4-9. Testicular "tumor" of the adrenogenital syndrome. The tumor is well circumscribed, lobulated, and dark brown.

4-9). Microscopic examination discloses large cells resembling Leydig cells with abundant eosinophilic cytoplasm (Fig. 4-10), which typically contains a large amount of lipochrome pigment (Fig. 4-11), but lacks crystalloids of Reinke (Fig. 4-7). The "tumor" tissue has been demonstrated to secrete cortisol and to function like hyperplastic adrenal glands. The nature of the "tumor" cells remains in doubt. Some authors contend that they are derived from adrenocortical rests, others, that they are Leydig cells that have been "captured" by ACTH, and still others, that they originate from testicular stromal cells capable of differentiating into either Leydig or adrenocortical cells, depending on the type of tropic stimulation.[43]

In an ultrastructural study, Chakraborty et al.[43] described three types of cells within a TTAGS: "giant" cells with abundant smooth endoplasmic reticulum, lamellar and tubular cristae, and numerous lysosomes and lipid droplets, (ultrastructural features shared by normal Leydig and adrenocortical cells); small cells characterized by prominent Golgi regions but otherwise relatively devoid of organelles; and modified smooth muscle cells. Crystalloids of Reinke were not identified. The "tumor" was demonstrated to produce cortisol

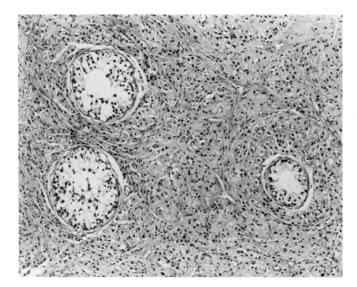

Fig. 4-10. Testicular "tumor" of the adrenogenital syndrome. Cells with abundant cytoplasm that was eosinophilic and small nuclei infiltrate between the seminiferous tubules. H & E. × 80.

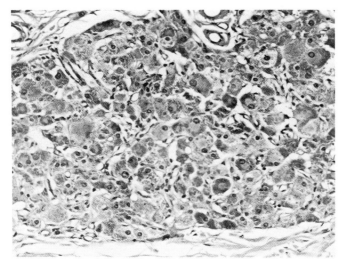

Fig. 4-11. Testicular "tumor" of the adrenogenital syndrome. The cells are large and contain abundant lipochrome pigment. H & E. × 200.

and testosterone in vitro after treatment with HCG and ACTH. The authors postulated that the "giant" cells demonstrated by electron microscopic examination were responsible for the steroid secretion.

Although TTAGS may not be true neoplasms in view of their dependence on ACTH and the lack of evidence of a malignant behavior in the cases reported to date, they are "tumors" in a clinical sense and are difficult to differentiate from Leydig cell tumors on microscopic examination. Since they respond to suppression by hormones that reduce the

ACTH levels, their presence does not warrant orchiectomy except for cosmetic reasons.

A few patients with Nelson's syndrome (development of an ACTH-secreting pituitary tumor, typically accompanied by cutaneous hyperpigmentation, after bilateral adrenalectomy for Cushing's disease) have had testicular "tumors," paratesticular "tumors," or both that have resembled those associated with AGS.[44-46] These "tumors" have been demonstrated to produce corticosteroids, including cortisol, as well as androgens.

Although they closely resemble Leydig cell

tumors, the testicular "tumors" of the AGS differ from the former in several respects. They are typically dark brown, whereas Leydig cell tumors are more often yellow or yellow–tan. Seminiferous tubules may be present within a TTAGS (Fig. 4-9) but are found only rarely within a Leydig cell tumor. The cells of the former tend to be larger and to have more abundant cytoplasm than those of the latter and contain lipochrome pigment more frequently and in greater amounts; the presence of this pigment is responsible for the dark color of the lesion on gross examination; crystalloids of Reinke have not been identified within the cells of the TTAGS. Of the eight bilateral "Leydig cell tumors" reported in the literature, one was later proven to be from a patient with AGS,[47, 48] and another was highly suggestive of this disorder.[49] The patient with the latter tumor had sexual precocity, bilateral testicular tumors, and high urinary 17-ketosteroid levels, which did not decrease after removal of both testes.

SERTOLI CELL TUMORS

Although pure Sertoli cell tumors are often indistinguishable from those that contain other cell types as well, if one relies on the descriptions and illustrations of cases in the literature, several forms of Sertoli cell tumor can be identified as specific subtypes within the sex cord-stromal category. The resemblance of some of these tumors to the lipid-rich estrogenic Sertoli cell tumor of the canine testis[50] led to the initial recognition of estrogenic Sertoli cell tumors of the human testis by Teilum.[51, 52] Two neoplasms in this category have been encountered in boys with the Peutz-Jeghers syndrome.[53, 54] This occurrence is interesting in view of the frequency of sex cord tumors with annular tubules, which appear to contain Sertoli cells,[55] in the ovaries of patients with this syndrome.[56, 57]

On gross examination, pure Sertoli cell tumors are typically well-circumscribed, some-

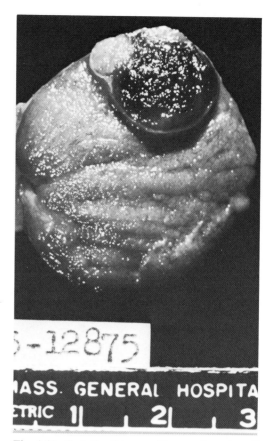

Fig. 4-12. Sertoli cell tumor. The neoplasm is well circumscribed, lobulated, and predominantly hemorrhagic. (Marshall FF, Kerr WS Jr, Kliman B, Scully RE: Sex cordstromal (gonadal stromal) tumors of the testis: a report of 5 cases. J Urol 117:180, 1977.)

times lobulated, yellow, tan, or white masses; foci of hemorrhage are occasionally present (Fig. 4-12). Microscopic examination reveals tubules that are usually solid, but occasionally hollow (Figs. 4-13 to 4-16), and cords (Fig. 4-17), nests, and masses of cells compatible with Sertoli cells, lying within a fibrous stroma. The tumor cells may contain abundant intracytoplasmic lipid (Fig. 4-16). The microscopic appearance may simulate that of certain ovarian Sertoli cell tumors,[51, 52, 58] but we have not seen a testicular neoplasm that resembled closely the well-differentiated Ser-

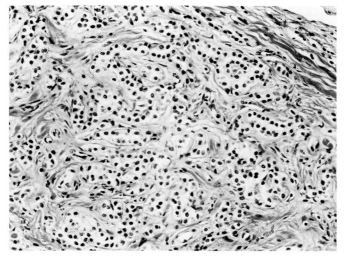

Fig. 4-13. Sertoli cell tumor. Network of solid, poorly formed tubules containing cells with pale cytoplasm and small round nuclei. H & E. × 200.

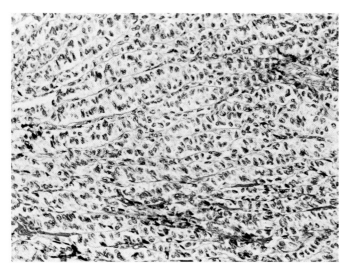

Fig. 4-14. Sertoli cell tumor. Closely packed solid tubules composed of cells with pale cytoplasm are aligned in parallel array. H & E. × 200.

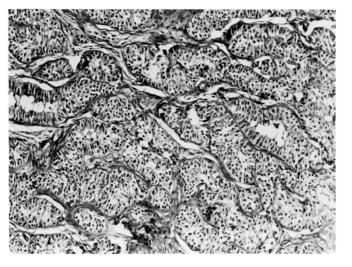

Fig. 4-15. Sertoli cell tumor. The tumor is composed of well-formed tubules, most of which are solid, but a few of which exhibit early lumen formation. H & E. × 125.

Fig. 4-16. Sertoli cell tumor. Closely packed solid tubules merging with a solid area in which many cells contain large vacuoles composed of lipid. The tumor resembles the Sertoli's cell tumor of the canine testis. H & E. × 156. (Marshall FF, Kerr WS Jr, Kliman B, Scully RE: Sex cord-stromal (gonadal stromal) tumors of the testis: a report of 5 cases. J Urol 117:180, 1977 The Williams & Wilkins Co., Baltimore.)

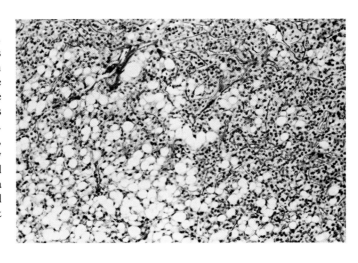

Fig. 4-17. Sertoli cell tumor. The cells are arranged in anastomosing cords in a fibrous stroma. H & E. × 125.

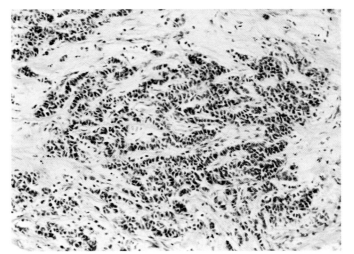

toli cell tumor composed of hollow tubules (Pick's tubular adenoma) that is a common form of this tumor in the ovary. The majority of testicular Sertoli cell tumors are probably benign, but at least six clinically malignant tumors interpreted as being composed exclusively of Sertoli cells have been reported,[59-63] including one from an 8-year-old boy[59] (Table 4-2). Malignant Sertoli cell tumors have most frequently metastasized to lymph nodes, including retroperitoneal, inguinal, paraaortic, lumbar, and supraclavicular sites; however, skin and pulmonary involvement was reported in one case.[61]

Sertoli cell tumors must be distinguished from focal nonneoplastic aggregates of small tubules that are lined by immature Sertoli cells and, in occasional cases, scattered spermatogonia as well.[64] Occasionally, small hyaline bodies resembling Call-Exner bodies or laminated calcified bodies are found within the tubules (Fig. 4-18). These lesions are usually of microscopic size, but are occasionally visible grossly as white nodules; they are encountered much more often in cryptorchid than in scrotal testes. In a large autopsy study of apparently normal descended testes from male patients 15 to 39 years of age, however, Hedinger et al.[65] found these lesions in 22 percent of the cases; approximately two-thirds of them

Table 4-2. Malignant Sex Cord-Stromal Tumors (Excluding Leydig Cell Tumors)

Study	Age (yr)	Type of Tumor	Size (cm)	Site of Metastases	Outcome
Rosvoll & Woodard[59]	8	Sertoli cell	10 x 7 x 6	Retroperitoneal lymph nodes	Alive; 5 yrs
Talerman[60]	79	Sertoli cell	7 x 5 x 4.5	Right inguinal lymph node; paraaortic lymph nodes enlarged	DOD[a]; 3 mo
Talerman[60]	29	Sertoli cell	15 x 12 x 4	Right lumbar lymph nodes	Alive; 6 yrs
Koppikar & Sirsat[62]	33	Sertoli cell	8 x 7 x 6.2	Left supraclavicular lymph node; enlarged paraaortic lymph node	Alive; 2 yrs, 3 mo
Hansen[63]	42	Sertoli cell	4 x 3.5 x 3	Inguinal, left iliac, and bilateral paraaortic lymph nodes	Alive; 1 yr
Morin & Loening[61]	60	Sertoli cell	3 x 3 x 2	Skin and lung	DOD; 3 yrs, 3 mo
Proppe & Scully[66]	44	Large-cell calcifying Sertoli cell	Not reported	Paraaortic and supraclavicular lymph nodes; bone	DOD; 16 mo
Mostofi et al.[6]	41	Granulosa cell	10.5 x 7.5 x 5	Cervical lymph node and widespread metastases	DOD; 5 mo
Nagy et al.[91]	35	Sex cord-stromal, mixed cell type	6 x 4 x 3	Clinical evidence of metastases	DOD; 1 yr, 2 mo
Nagy et al.[91]	62	Sex cord-stromal, mixed cell type	Not reported	Enlarged abdominal lymph nodes	DOD; 10 mo
Hopkins & Parry[90]	63	Sex cord-stromal, mixed cell type	8 x 5 x 4	Bone, adrenal, lungs	DOD; 5 yrs
Campbell & Middleton[88]	16	Sex cord-stromal, unclassified	15 x 10 x 8	Retroperitoneal lymph nodes	Alive; 6 mo
Herrera et al.[87]	20	Sex cord-stromal, unclassified	8.5 x 7.7 x 6.5	Left retroperitoneum	Alive; 2 yr, 3 mo
Eble et al.[89]	34	Sex cord-stromal, mixed cell type	2	Retroperitoneum	DOD; 13 mo
Collins & Symington[92]	27	Sex cord-stromal, mixed cell type	Not reported	Retroperitoneal and mediastinal lymph nodes, liver, lung, brain, bone	DOD; 3 mo

[a] DOD, dead of disease.

were bilateral. They were most common in patients 15 to 19 years of age, in whom they were present in nearly 50 percent of the cases. Although these lesions have sometimes been referred to as tubular adenomas or Sertoli cell adenomas, they have a limited growth potential and are presently regarded as hyperplastic nodules rather than neoplasms.

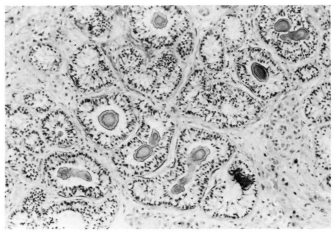

Fig. 4-18. Hyperplastic Sertoli cell nodule. A cryptorchid contains an aggregate of small tubules lined by immature Sertoli cells. Laminated microcalcifications are present within lumens. H & E. × 125.

LARGE-CELL CALCIFYING SERTOLI CELL TUMOR

In 1980 Proppe and Scully[66] reported 10 cases of an unusual subtype of testicular Sertoli cell tumor, for which they proposed the term "large-cell calcifying Sertoli cell tumor" (LCCSCT). Two cases of this type of neoplasm had been identified in the earlier literature[67, 68] and five additional examples have been reported subsequently.[69-73]

The age of the 17 patients with this neoplasm ranged from 5 to 44 years, with an average of 16 years. Four patients were in the first decade, ten in the second, two in the third, and one in the fifth decade. The only clinical manifestation in 10 of the cases was the presence of a testicular mass, but in 7 cases various other disorders were present as well. One 9-year-old boy, who also had a pituitary adenoma, was sexually precocious at the age of 2 years. Another patient, who had bilateral adrenocortical hyperplasia, had been sexually precocious at the age of 3 years, 8 years before his testicular tumor was discovered. A 16-year-old boy had a pituitary adenoma associated with gigantism and intermittent marked elevation of the plasma cortisol level. These three patients all had "steroid cell tumors" of the testis of Leydig cell or possibly adrenocortical rest cell origin in addition to their LCCSCT. Another patient presented because

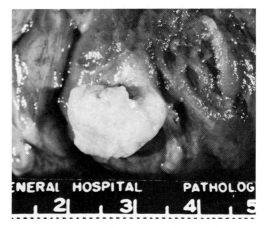

Fig. 4-19. Large-cell calcifying Sertoli cell tumor. The cut surface of the testis shows a circumscribed nodule which was gray-white, firm, and gritty.

of gynecomastia and had elevated plasma estrogen levels. Two brothers, one of whom had bilateral adrenocortical nodular hyperplasia, died as a result of cardiac myxomas. In a final case, in which examination of the testes revealed intratubular LCCSCT, the patient was a phenotypic female with the complete form of the androgen-insensitivity syndrome.

The tumors, which were unilateral in 11 of the 17 cases, ranged in size from microscopic to 4 cm in diameter in 16 of the cases; in the 17th case the tumor "had replaced the entire testis." Most of the tumors were firm, yellow to tan, and apparently well-circumscribed (Fig. 4-19). Microscopic examination,

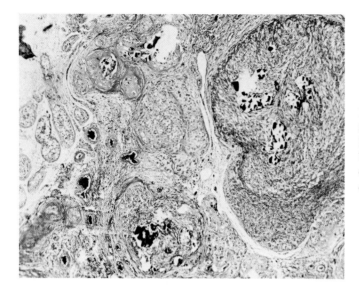

Fig. 4-20. Large-cell calcifying Sertoli cell tumor. Irregular islands of tumor cells separated by fibrous stroma. Multiple foci of calcification are present. H & E. × 40.

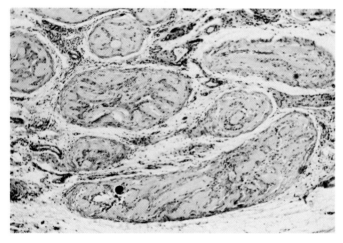

Fig. 4-21. Large-cell calcifying Sertoli cell tumor. Foci of intratubular growth with hyalinization have coalesced; a small focus of calcification is present. H & E. × 64.

however, revealed that the margin was ill-defined in most of the cases (Fig. 4-20). The neoplastic cells, which were large and contained abundant eosinophilic cytoplasm, were arranged in diffuse sheets or within nests (Fig. 4-20), trabeculae, cords, small clusters, or solid tubules. The stroma ranged from loose, myxoid connective tissue to dense collagenous tissue. Foci of intratubular tumor were found in approximately half of the cases (Fig. 4-21). A characteristic feature was the presence of calcification, which was usually conspicuous and sometimes massive, with the formation of large, basophilic, laminated nodules (Fig.

4-22). The neoplastic cells were usually rounded (Fig. 4-22), but occasionally cuboidal or columnar and rarely spindle-shaped. In most of the cases, the cytoplasm was eosinophilic and had a ground-glass or finely granular texture, but occasionally it appeared amphophilic and slightly vacuolated. The nuclei were round or oval and contained finely stippled chromatin and one or two small nucleoli. Mitotic figures were rare in most of the tumors, but in the only one that was associated with a malignant behavior four mitotic figures were identified per 10 high-power fields; in that case, metastases were present in a left

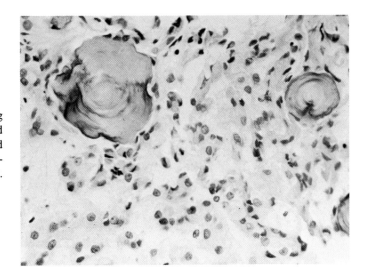

Fig. 4-22. Large-cell calcifying Sertoli cell tumor. Laminated calcific bodies are surrounded by large tumor cells with abundant cytoplasm. H & E. × 350.

supraclavicular lymph node and in a cervical vertebral body.[66] Intracytoplasmic lipid was present in the two cases investigated for this material.

Ultrastructural studies have supported the Sertoli cell origin of the LCCSCT. These studies have demonstrated solid tubular structures surrounded by basal lamina and hollow clusters of epithelial cells with pseudolumens lined by basal lamina,[67] and intracellular microfilaments in moderate to large numbers.[69, 71, 72] Only Waxman et al.[73] have identified Charcot-Bottcher filaments, which are thought to be specific inclusions of Sertoli cells, in the cytoplasm of the neoplastic cells.

The large-cell calcifying Sertoli cell tumor may be misinterpreted as a Leydig cell tumor because it is composed of cells that typically contain abundant eosinophilic cytoplasm. A number of features, however, facilitate its diagnosis: its unusual clinical associations, its multifocality and bilaterality, the presence of intratubular growth and calcification. Intratubular growth has not been recorded in Leydig cell tumors and calcification has been encountered in them only very rarely.[74] Moreover, although abundant smooth endoplasmic reticulum, lipid, and lipochrome have been reported within the neoplastic cells of the LCCSCT on ultrastructural examination,

crystalloids of Reinke, paracrystalline inclusions, or membranous whorls, all of which are characteristic of Leydig cell tumors, have not been identified.

GRANULOSA CELL TUMORS

ADULT-TYPE

Granulosa cell tumors (GCTs) of the histologic types typically encountered in the ovaries of adult patients are very rare in the testis, with only five examples in the literature.[4, 6, 75-77] Three additional cases have been encountered in a review of 90 testicular sex cord-stromal tumors from the consultation files of one of us (RES). The age range of the eight patients was 21–73 years. Four of the reported tumors were associated with gynecomastia;[6, 75, 76] no hormonal assays were recorded in four of the cases, but one of the patients[75] had a urinary level of estrogen that was said to be approximately twice normal. Clinical evidence of feminization was specifically denied in two of the three unreported cases, but there was no mention of the presence or absence of endocrine effects in the third case. The youngest patient had a complex clinical history, with associated congeni-

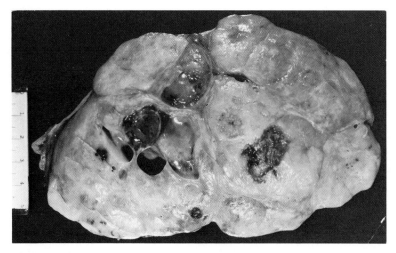

Fig. 4-23. Granulosa cell tumor, adult type. The sectioned surface, which was yellow, is divided into lobules by fibrous septa. Areas of necrosis and hemorrhage are present. (Case Records of Massachusetts General Hospital, Case 41471. N Engl J Med 253:926, 1955.)

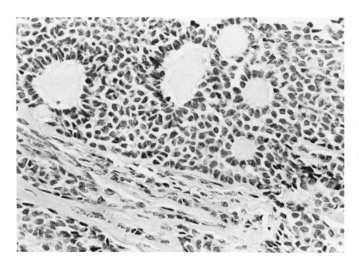

Fig. 4-24. Granulosa cell tumor, adult type. A nest of granulosa cells contains Call-Exner bodies. H & E. × 200.

tal anomalies of the urinary tract and generalized osteitis fibrosa.[76]

The tumors ranged from 5 to 13 cm in diameter. Most of them were homogeneous, yellow to yellow-gray, firm, and lobulated (Fig. 4-23). The microscopic patterns were mainly microfollicular with structures resembling Call-Exner bodies (Fig. 4-24) and diffuse (Fig. 4-25). The granulosa cells resembled those seen in ovarian GCTs, typically having angular nuclei containing grooves (Fig. 4-25). A fibro-

thecomatous stromal component was prominent in one case.[75] One patient died of metastatic tumor 5 months postoperatively; this patient had widespread metastases, including to the cervical lymph nodes.[6]

JUVENILE-TYPE

Granulosa cell tumors that correspond histologically to the juvenile granulosa cell tumor of the ovary[78] are the most common form of

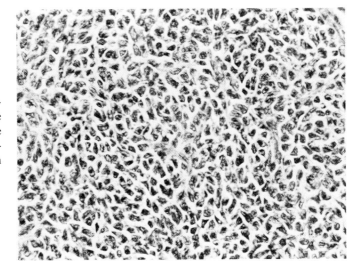

Fig. 4-25. Granulosa cell tumor, adult type. The cells are growing in a diffuse pattern; the cytoplasm is scanty and the nuclei are angular and contain grooves. H & E. × 200.

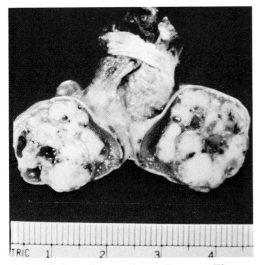

Fig. 4-26. Juvenile granulosa cell tumor. The sectioned surface of the testis is largely replaced by a predominantly solid, lobulated tumor; several cysts are visible (Lawrence WD, Young RH, Scully RE: Juvenile granulosa cell tumor of the infantile testis. A report of fourteen cases. Am J Surg Pathol 9:87, 1985.)

sex cord-stromal tumor of the infantile testis, and account for approximately three-quarters of the cases. Of the 14 tumors of this type in our reported series of cases,[79] one was found at autopsy in an abdominal testis of an infant of 30 weeks' gestational age, seven were dis-

covered during the first few days of life, and the remainder were detected in infants from 3 weeks to 4½ months of age. We have recently seen an additional example in a child 21 months of age. In 11 cases in our series, enlargement of the testis was the presenting manifestation, in one case an abdominal mass that proved to be a multicystic retroperitoneal tumor on surgical exploration was palpable, one tumor was found in the inguinal canal during a herniorrhaphy, and a final tumor was detected in a descended testis that had undergone torsion.

The 14 tumors ranged from 0.8 to 5 cm in diameter. Most of them formed thin-walled cysts that contained viscid or gelatinous fluid, but a prominent solid, nodular component was also present in one-half of them (Fig. 4-26). Microscopic examination revealed follicular (Fig. 4-27) and solid patterns (Fig. 4-28). The follicles varied in size and shape (Fig. 4-29), but were most often large and round to oval (Fig. 4-26); typically they contained watery fluid, which was basophilic or eosinophilic and usually mucicarminophilic. The solid component was in the form of sheets, nodules, and irregular clusters. Hyalinization was often extensive, and in some cases intercellular basophilic mucinous fluid was conspicuous within the cellular areas. The granulosa cells lining

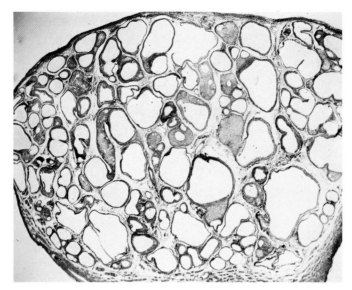

Fig. 4-27. Juvenile granulosa cell tumor. The tumor has a predominantly follicular pattern. A small rim of compressed testis is seen at the bottom of the photograph. H & E. × 10. (Lawrence WD, Young RH, Scully RE: Juvenile granulosa cell tumor of the infantile testis. A report of fourteen cases. Am J Surg Pathol 9:87, 1985.)

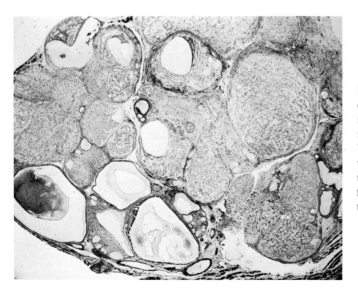

Fig. 4-28. Juvenile granulosa cell tumor. The tumor has solid nodular and follicular components. H & E. × 10. (Lawrence WD, Young RH, Scully RE: Juvenile granulosa cell tumor of the infantile testis. A report of fourteen cases. Am J Surg Pathol 9:87, 1985.)

the follicles and in the solid areas had moderate to large amounts of pale to eosinophilic cytoplasm and hyperchromatic, round to oval nuclei, some of which contained nucleoli. The number of mitotic figures varied, but was often high (Fig. 4-30), ranging up to 24 per 10 high-power fields. Follow-up evaluation was documented in only four patients, none of whom had a recurrence.

It is unclear why the juvenile granulosa cell tumor is the most common form of sex cord-stromal tumor of the testis in infants, whereas the Leydig cell tumor, Sertoli cell tumor, and sex cord-stromal tumors of unclassified or mixed cell types are much more frequent in older patients. In view of the very young age of almost all the patients with this neoplasm, most of these neoplasms must have arisen in utero, which suggests that the hormonal milieu of pregnancy had a role in their development. Rare juvenile granulosa cell tumors of the ovary have also originated prenatally.[80, 81]

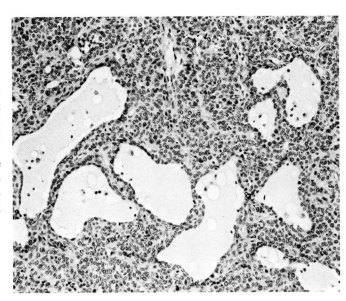

Fig. 4-29. Juvenile granulosa cell tumor. Follicles of varying sizes and shapes are separated by immature granulosa cells. H & E. × 160. (Lawrence WD, Young RH, Scully RE: Juvenile granulosa cell tumor of the infantile testis. A report of fourteen cases. Am J Surg Pathol 9:87, 1985.)

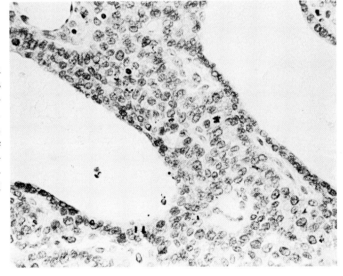

Fig. 4-30. Juvenile granulosa cell tumor. The granulosa cells have immature nuclei and several mitotic figures are visible. H & E. × 400. (Lawrence WD, Young RH, Scully RE: Juvenile granulosa cell tumor of the infantile testis. A report of fourteen cases. Am J Surg Pathol 9:87, 1985.)

SEX CORD-STROMAL TUMORS OF MIXED AND UNCLASSIFIED (INCOMPLETELY DIFFERENTIATED) CELL TYPES

In evaluating cases reported in the literature it is not always possible to differentiate pure Sertoli cell tumors from those in the mixed and unclassified categories and even from granulosa cell tumors. Therefore, the tumors that will be discussed under this heading may include a few unrecognized examples of Sertoli cell tumors and granulosa cell tumors. Unquestionable or very probable examples of pure Sertoli cell tumor and granulosa cell tumor, however, have been eliminated from the neoplasms reviewed in this section.

Sex cord-stromal tumors of mixed or not otherwise specified cell types occur within a wide age range; the youngest patients have

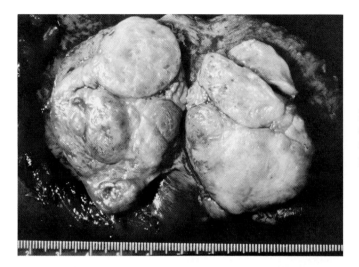

Fig. 4-31. Sex cord-stromal tumor, unclassified. A lobulated mass almost completely replaces the testis.

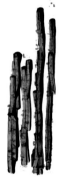

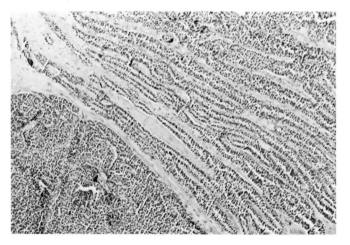

Fig. 4-32. Sex cord-stromal tumor of mixed cell types. A diffuse pattern of cells of sex-cord type lies adjacent to an array of elongated tubules. Elsewhere areas of granulosa cell tumor with Call-Exner bodies were present (lower left). H & E. × 100.

been newborn and the oldest over 80 years of age.[6, 82-92] Almost half of the patients have been children and approximately one-third are infants less than 1 year of age (although, as indicated in the previous section, our experience suggests that the great majority of the infantile cases are examples of juvenile granulosa cell tumor). The most common clinical symptom of these tumors is painless testicular enlargement usually of several months' to 5 years' duration; in one case, however, the tumor had been present for 30 years before diagnosis.[51] A review by Gabrilove et al.[85] of 50 patients with these tumors revealed that at least seven (14 percent) had gynecomastia. The frequency of gynecomastia was higher in

association with clinically malignant tumors than with benign tumors (four of four vs. three of seven, respectively).

On gross examination the tumors vary widely in size from tiny nodules to large masses that have replaced the testis. Most of the tumors are well-circumscribed and are composed of white to yellow, often lobulated tissue (Fig. 4-31), traversed by grayish-white fibrous septa. Cysts are present in some cases; hemorrhage and necrosis are uncommon.

Microscopic examination reveals a spectrum of patterns, ranging from predominantly epithelial to predominantly stromal (Fig. 4-32 to 4-34). Considerable histologic variation may be encountered within a single specimen.

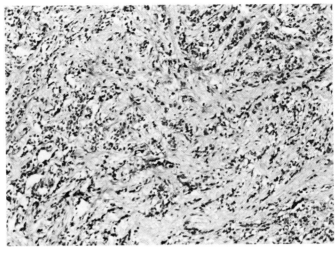

Fig. 4-33. Sex cord-stromal tumor, unclassified. Irregular aggregates of tumor cells of sex cord type are embedded in a fibrous stroma. H & E. × 125.

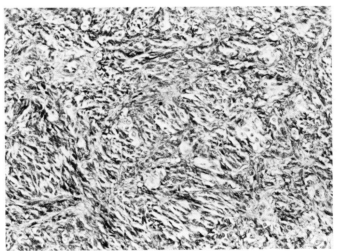

Fig. 4-34. Sex cord-stromal tumor, unclassified. Clusters of large cells with pale cytoplasm are scattered in a background of spindle cells. H & E. × 200.

The better-differentiated tumors typically contain well-formed solid or hollow tubules composed of or lined by cells resembling Sertoli cells. These cells may be columnar or polyhedral; the cytoplasm varies from scanty to abundant, and may be eosinophilic, amphophilic, or vacuolated and lipid-laden; the nuclei are round to oval and often vesicular, and sometimes contain single small nucleoli; mitotic figures are generally rare or absent. The less well differentiated tumors are composed of varying proportions of epithelial and stromal cells, which exhibit varying degrees of pleomorphism and mitotic activity. Diffuse and sarcomatoid patterns are frequent, and in some areas it may be difficult or impossible to differentiate the epithelial and stromal components. Islands and masses of cells resembling granulosa cells may also be present in both well- and poorly differentiated tumors.

The tumors resemble to varying extents neoplasms composed of similar cell types occurring in the ovary, but are more difficult to subclassify because differentiation is more often in the direction of both testicular and ovarian cell types. Also, tubular differentiation is more frequently encountered in the testicular tumors than in their ovarian counterparts.

Kurman and his associates[93] have demonstrated by immunocytochemical techniques the presence of estradiol, progesterone, and testosterone in the four major cell types of sex cord-stromal tumors of the testis and ovary as well as in the spindle cells that resemble fibroblasts in routine sections. The only sex cord-stromal tumor of the testis included in their investigation was interpreted as an undifferentiated Sertoli–Leydig cell tumor, and contained both testosterone and estradiol within its cells. Subsequently, Kurman[94] stated that one cannot be certain on the basis of light microscopic immunocytochemistry whether a positive intracellular reaction indicates synthesis, binding, or storage of a demonstrated hormone. He also noted that the same reactions seen in the neoplastic cells of these gonadal tumors are demonstrable in cells that are targets of steroid hormones, such as those of the breast and endometrium in the case of estradiol. He concluded that, at the present time, the diagnosis of a sex cord-stromal tumor is not warranted on the basis of immunocytochemical demonstration of a steroid hormone content alone.

The literature contains only rare ultrastructural studies of testicular sex cord-stromal tumors. In one report of a poorly differentiated neoplasm in this category,[95] foci corresponding to tubular structures contained cells with smooth endoplasmic reticulum, large membrane-bound inclusions, and 50-Å filaments; neither crystalloids of Reinke nor lamellar bodies were identified. Stromal cells surrounding the tubules were considered by the authors to have features suggestive of myofibroblasts. In less well differentiated foci without tubule formation, the neoplastic cells had more primitive features; organelles were sparse and basement membranes were absent or only partially surrounded the cells. Goellner and Myers[96] also found incomplete basement membranes around tumor nests and frequent pinocytosis at cell membranes; they also noted extensive interdigitations of the cell membrane and numerous desmosomes. Greco et al.[97] studied two sex cord-stromal tumors of the testis, both of which were composed exclusively of stromal elements. The cells contained numerous intracytoplasmic myofilaments similar to those seen in the contractile peritubular cells of the normal testis. Similar findings were reported by Evans and Glick.[98] These workers postulated that tumors of this type may arise from intertubular mesenchymal cells, which have the potential for differentiation into cells with contractile elements. The great morphologic heterogeneity of sex cord-stromal tumors apparent on light microscopic examination indicates that large numbers of cases must be studied with the electron microscope before the full range of their ultrastructural characteristics is elucidated.

Most testicular sex cord-stromal tumors of mixed or not otherwise specified cell types have been benign. In the review by Gabrilove et al.[85] of reported cases including these tumors, 82 percent of all the patients for whom follow-up results of 1 year or more were available had a benign course. Thirty-eight percent of the tumors occurred in children 10 years of age or younger; none of these tumors was malignant. If one considers only tumors from patients 10 years of age or older who were evaluated for 1 year or more, however, 29 percent exhibited a malignant behavior.

Five of the patients with clinically malignant sex cord-stromal tumors (excluding Leydig cell tumors) in the review of Eble et al.[89] had tumors of the mixed or unclassified type (Table 4-2). Three of them died from 3 months to 5 years after orchiectomy. Two were still alive with metastases, one of them 27 months after excision of a retroperitoneal recurrence of tumor 15 years following orchiectomy. The malignant tumors of the mixed or unclassified type have metastasized to retroperitoneal, abdominal, and mediastinal lymph nodes, as well as to the liver, lungs, brain, and bone.

MANAGEMENT

Sex cord-stromal tumors are treated by inguinal orchiectomy. If the clinical or pathologic features suggest the possibility of malignant behavior, lymphadenectomy should be performed because of the high frequency of lymph node spread in the clinically malignant cases. The age of the patient is an important consideration in this regard, since no malignant tumors have been reported to date in infants and children under 8 years of age. The pathologic features that should be evaluated in attempting to assess the prognosis of the tumor are: its size, invasive properties including vascular invasion, nuclear atypia, and mitotic activity. The average largest diameter of the reported malignant tumors (7.75 cm) has been almost twice as large as that of the benign tumors (4.25 cm); however, three malignant tumors that were 4 cm or less in greatest diameter have metastasized, indicating that size alone is not entirely reliable as a prognostic criterion. While data do not exist at the present to establish the aforementioned microscopic features as having prognostic significance, it appears reasonable to take them into account in assessing the desirability of lymph node dissection, in view of their demonstrated importance in cases of Leydig cell tumors. Computed tomography may be helpful in detecting lymph node involvement. It is to be hoped that authors reporting these tumors in the future will describe pathologic features of possible prognostic importance in detail so that more accurate information will be available. Whether radiation therapy or chemotherapy will prove useful in the management of residual or recurrent tumor is not known at the present time.

REFERENCES

1. Mostofi FK, Sobin LH: International histological classification of tumours, No. 16, Histological typing of tumours of the testis. World Health Organization, Geneva, 1977
2. Serov SF, Scully RE, Sobin LH: International histological classification of tumours No. 9. Histological typing of ovarian tumours. World Health Organization, Geneva, 1973
3. Teilum G: Homologous tumors in the ovary and testis. Contribution to classification of the gonadal tumors. Acta Obstet Gynecol Scand 24:480, 1944
4. Laskowski J: Feminizing tumors of testis. General review with case report of granulosa cell tumor of testis. Endokrynol Pol 3:337, 1952
5. Teilum G: Classification of testicular and ovarian androblastoma and Sertoli cell tumours. A survey of comparative studies with consideration of histogenesis, endocrinology, and embryological theories. Cancer 11:769, 1958
6. Mostofi FK, Theiss EA, Ashley DJB: Tumors of specialized gonadal stroma in human male subjects. Cancer 12:944, 1959
7. Symington T, Cameron KM: Endocrine and genetic lesions. In: Pugh RCB (ed): Pathology of the Testis. Blackwell Scientific Publications, Oxford, 1976
8. Mostofi FK, Price EB Jr: Tumors of the male genital system. In Atlas of Tumor Pathology, Second series, Fascicle 8. Armed Forces Institute of Pathology, Washington, D.C., 1973
9. Collins DH, Pugh RCB: The pathology of testicular tumors. Br J Urol 36 (suppl):1, 1964
10. Dixon FJ, Moore RA: Tumors of the male sex organs. In Atlas of Tumor Pathology, Section 8, Fascicle 31b and 32. Armed Forces Institute of Pathology, Washington, D.C., 1952
11. Friedman NB, Moore RA: Tumors of the testis: a report of 922 cases. Milit Surg 99:573, 1946
12. Pugh RCB: Testicular tumours—introduction. In Pugh RCB (ed): Pathology of the Testis. Blackwell Scientific Publication, Oxford, 1976
13. Scully RE, Parham AR: Testicular tumours, II. Interstitial cell and miscellaneous neoplasms. Arch Pathol 46:229, 1949
14. Kim I, Young RH, Scully RE: Leydig cell tumors of the testis. A clinicopathological analysis of 40 cases and review of the literature. Am J Surg Pathol 9:177, 1985
15. Caldamone AA, Altebarmakian V, Frank IN, Linke CA: Leydig cell tumor of testis. Urology 14:39, 1979
16. Klippel KF, Jonas U, Hohenfellner R, Walther D: Interstitial cell tumor of testis: a delicate problem. Urology 14:79, 1979.
17. Sohval AR, Churg J, Gabrilove JL et al: Ultrastructure of feminizing testicular Leydig cell tumors. Ultrastruct Pathol 4:335, 1982
18. Symington T, Cameron KM: Endocrine and genetic lesions. In Pugh RCB (ed): Pathology

of the Testis. Blackwell Scientific Publications, Oxford, 1976

19. Largiader F: Maligner tumor der Leydigschen Zwischenzellen des Hodens. Frankfurt Z Pathol 70:630, 1960

20. Weber HFJ: Hodentumor verursacht Gynakomastie. Wien Med Wchnschr 98:261, 1948

21. Johnstone G: Prepubertal gynecomastia in association with an interstitial-cell tumour of the testis. Br J Urol 39:211, 1967

22. Jolly H: Sexual Precocity. Charles C Thomas et al: Springfield, IL, 1955

23. Jungck EC, Thrash AM, Ohlmacher AP et al: Sexual precocity due to interstitial cell tumor of the testis: Report of 2 cases. J Clin Endocrinol Metab 17:291, 1957

24. Kay S, Fu YS, Koontz WW, Chen ATL: Interstitial-cell tumor of the testis. Tissue culture and ultrastructural studies. Am J Clin Pathol 63:366, 1975

25. Staubitz WJ, Oberkircher OJ, Blick MS: Precocious puberty in a case of bilateral interstitial cell tumor of testes. J Urol 69:562, 1953

26. Yuval E, Eidelman A, Beer SI, Vure E: Local excision of a virilizing Leydig-cell tumour of the testis. Br J Urol 46:237, 1974

27. Akdas A, Remzi D, Finci R: Bilateral interstitial cell tumour of testes. Br J Urol 55:123, 1983

28. Arduino LJ, Glucksman MA: Interstitial cell tumor of the testis associated with Klinefelter's syndrome: a case report. J Urol 89:246, 1963

29. Dodge OG, Jackson AW, Muldal S: Breast cancer and interstitial cell tumor in a patient with Klinefelter's syndrome. Cancer 24:1027, 1969

30. Fox H, Reeve NL: Endocrine effects of testicular neoplasms. Invest Cell Pathol 2:63, 1979

31. Wilson BE, Netzloff ML: Primary testicular abnormalities causing precocious puberty. Leydig cell tumor, Leydig cell hyperplasia and adrenal rest tumor. Ann Clin Lab Sci 13:315, 1983

32. Boulanger P, Somma M, Chevalier S et al: Elevated secretion of androstenedione in a patient with a Leydig cell tumour. Acta Endocrinol 107:104, 1984

33. Gabrilove JL, Nicolis GL, Mitty HA, Sohval AR: Feminizing interstitial cell tumor of the testis. Personal observations and a review of the literature. Cancer 35:1184, 1975

34. Bercovici P, Nahoul K, Tater D et al: Hormonal profile of Leydig cell tumors with gynecomastia. J Clin Endocrinol Metab 59:625, 1984

35. Perez C, Novoa J, Alcaniz J et al: Leydig cell tumour of the testis with gynaecomastia and elevated oestrogen, progesterone and prolactin levels: case report. Clin Endocrinol 13:409, 1980

36. Fore WW, Bledsoe T, Weber DM et al: Cortisol production by testicular tumors in adrenogenital syndrome. Arch Intern Med 130:59, 1972

37. Burke EF, Gilbert E, Uehling DT: Adrenal rest tumors of the testis. J Urol 109:649, 1973

38. Newell ME, Pippe BM, Ehrlich RM: Testis tumors associated with congenital adrenal hyperplasia: a continuing diagnostic and therapeutic dilemma. J Urol 117:256, 1977

39. Kirkland RT, Kirkland JL, Keenan BS et al: Bilateral testicular tumors in congenital adrenal hyperplasia. J Clin Endocrinol Metab 44:369, 1977

40. Kadair RG, Block MB, Katz FH, Hofeldt FD: "Masked" 21-hydroxylase deficiency of the adrenal presenting with gynecomastia and bilateral testicular masses. Am J Med 62:278, 1977

41. Franco-Saenz R, Antonipillai I, Tan SY et al: Cortisol production by testicular tumors in a patient with congenital adrenal hyperplasia (21-hydroxylase deficiency). J Clin Endocrinol Metab 53:85, 1981

42. Chrousos GP, Loriaux DL, Sherins RJ, Cutler GB Jr: Unilateral testicular enlargement resulting from inapparent 21-hydroxylase deficiency. J Urol 126:127, 1981

43. Chakraborty J, Franco-Saenz R, Kropp K: Electron microscopic study of testicular tumor in congenital adrenal hyperplasia. Hum Pathol 14:151, 1983

44. Hamwi GJ, Gwinup G, Mostow JH, Besch PK: Activation of testicular adrenal rest tissue by prolonged excessive ACTH production. J Clin Endocrinol Metab 23:861, 1963

45. Krieger DT, Samojlik E, Bardin CW: Cortisol and androgen secretion in a case of Nelson's syndrome with paratesticular tumors: response to cyproheptadine therapy. J Clin Endocrinol Metab 47:837, 1978

46. Johnson RE, Scheithauer B: Massive hyperplasia of testicular adrenal rests in a patient with Nelson's syndrome. Am J Clin Pathol 77:501, 1982

47. Garvey FK, Daniel TB: Bilateral interstial cell tumor of the testicle. J Urol 66:713, 1951

48. Miller EC, Murray HL: Congenital adrenocortical hyperplasia: case previously reported as "bilateral interstitial cell tumor of the testicle." J Clin Endocrinol Metab 22:655, 1962

49. Staubitz WJ, Oberkircher OJ, Blick MS. Precocious puberty in a case of bilateral interstitial cell tumor of testes. J Urol 69:562, 1953

50. Scully RE, Coffin DL: Canine testicular tumors with special reference to their histogenesis, comparative morphology and endocrinology. Cancer 5:592, 1952

51. Teilum G: Arrhenoblastoma–androblastoma; homologous ovarian and testicular tumors; II, including so-called "luteomas" and "adrenal tumors" of ovary and interstitial cell tumors of testis. Acta Pathol Microbiol Scand 23:252, 1946

52. Teilum G: Estrogen producing Sertoli-cell tumors (androblastoma tubulare lipoides of the human testis and ovary). Homologous ovarian and testicular tumors, III. J Clin Endocrinol 9:301, 1949

53. Cantu JM, Rivera H, Ocampo-Campos R et al: Peutz-Jeghers syndrome with feminizing Sertoli cell tumor. Cancer 46:223, 1980

54. Dubois RS, Hoffman WH, Krishnan TH et al: Feminizing sex cord tumor with annular tubules in a boy with Peutz-Jeghers syndrome. J Pediatr 101:568, 1982

55. Tavassoli FA, Norris HJ. Sertoli tumors of the ovary. A clinicopathologic study of 28 cases with ultrastructural observations. Cancer 46:2281, 1980

56. Scully RE: Sex cord tumor with annular tubules. A distinctive ovarian tumor of the Peutz-Jeghers syndrome. Cancer 25:1107, 1970

57. Young RH, Welch WR, Dickersin GR, Scully RE: Ovarian sex cord tumor with annular tubules. Review of 74 cases including 27 with Peutz-Jeghers syndrome and four with adenoma malignum of the cervix. Cancer 50:1384, 1982

58. Young RH, Scully RE: Ovarian Sertoli cell tumors: a report of 10 cases. Int J Gynecol Pathol 2:349, 1984

59. Rosvoll R, Woodard JR: Malignant Sertoli cell tumor of the testis. Cancer 22:8, 1968

60. Talerman A: Malignant Sertoli cell tumor of the testis. Cancer 28:446, 1971

61. Morin LJ, Loening S: Malignant androblastoma (Sertoli cell tumor of the testis). A case report with a review of the literature. J Urol 114:476, 1975.

62. Koppikar DD, Sirsat MV: A malignant Sertoli cell tumor of the testis. Br J Urol 45:213, 1973

63. Hansen GVO: Malignant testicular androblastoma with gynecomastia. Dan Med Bull 22:33, 1975

64. Halley JBW: The growth of Sertoli cell tumors: a possible index of differential gonadotropin activity in the male. J Urol 90(2):220, 1963

65. Hedinger CE, Huber R, Weber E: Frequency of so-called hypoplastic or dysgenetic zones in scrotal and otherwise normal human testes. Virchows Arch Pathol Anat 342:165, 1967

66. Proppe KH, Scully RE: Large-cell calcifying Sertoli cell tumor of the testis. Am J Clin Pathol 74:607, 1980

67. Fligiel Z, Kaneko M, Leiter E: Bilateral Sertoli cell tumor of testis with feminizing and masculinizing activity occurring in a child. Cancer 38:1853, 1976

68. Lange J, Leger MH, Etcheverry M: Androblastoma testiculaire: observation d'une forme bilaterale chez l'enfant. J Urol Med Chir 66:259, 1960

69. Proppe KH, Dickersin GR: Large-cell calcifying Sertoli cell tumor of the testis: light microscopic and ultrastructural study. Hum Pathol 13:1109, 1982

70. Rosenzweig JL, Lawrence DA, Vogel DL et al: Adrenocorticotropin-independent hypercortisolemia and testicular tumors in a patient with a pituitary tumor and gigantism. J Clin Endocrinol Metab 55:421, 1982

71. Perez-Atayde AR, Nunez AE, Carroll WL et al: Large-cell calcifying Sertoli cell tumor of the testis. An ultrastructural, immunocytochemical, and biochemical study. Cancer 51:2287, 1983

72. Horn T, Jao W, Keh PC: Large-cell calcifying Sertoli cell tumor of the testis: a case report with ultrastructural study. Ultrastruct Pathol 4:359, 1983

73. Waxman M, Damjanov I, Khapra A, Landal SJ: Large cell calcifying Sertoli tumor of testis. Light microscopic and ultrastructural study. Cancer 54:1574, 1984

74. Minkowitz S, Solway H, Soscia JL: Ossifying interstitial cell tumor of the testis. J Urol 94:592, 1965

75. Case Records of The Massachusetts General Hospital (Case 41471). N Engl J Med 253:926, 1955

76. Cohen J, Diamond I: Leontiasis ossea, slipped epiphyses, and granulosa cell tumor of testis with renal disease; report of case with autopsy findings. Arch Pathol 56:488, 1953

77. Melicow MM: Classification of tumors of testis; clinical and pathological study based on 105 primary and 13 secondary cases in adults, and 3 primary and 4 secondary cases in children. J Urol 73:547, 1955

78. Young RH, Dickersin GR, Scully RE: Juvenile granulosa cell tumor of the ovary. A clinicopathologic analysis of 125 cases. Am J Surg Pathol 8:575, 1984

79. Lawrence WD, Young RH, Scully RE: Juvenile granulosa cell tumor of the infantile testis. A report of fourteen cases. Am J Surg Pathol 9:87, 1985

80. Roth LM, Nicholas TR, Ehrlich CE: Juvenile granulosa cell tumor. A clinicopathologic study of three cases with ultrastructural observations. Cancer 44:2194, 1979

81. Pysher TJ, Hitch DC, Krous HF: Bilateral juvenile granulosa cell tumors in a 4-month old dysmorphic infant. A clinical, histologic and ultrastructural study. Am J Surg Pathol 5:789, 1981

82. Culp DA, Frazier RG, Butler JJ: Sertoli cell tumor in infant. J Urol 76:162, 1956

83. Batsakis JG: Tumors of the testis in infancy and childhood. Arch Pathol 72:41, 1961

84. Holtz F, Abell MR: Testicular neoplasms in infant children. II. Tumors of nongerm origin. Cancer 16:982, 1963

85. Gabrilove JL, Freiberg EK, Leiter E, Nicolis GL: Feminizing and nonfeminizing Sertoli cell tumors. J Urol 124(6):757, 1980

86. Fuglsang F, Ohlsen AS: Androblastoma predominantly feminizing. With report of case. Acta Chir Scand 112:405, 1957

87. Herrera LD, Wilk H, Wills JS, Lopez GE: Malignant (androblastoma) Sertoli cell tumor of testes. Urology 18(3):287, 1981

88. Campbell CM, Middleton AW Jr: Malignant gonadal stromal tumor: case report and review of the literature. J Urol 125:257, 1981

89. Eble JN, Hull MT, Warfel KA, Donohue JP: Malignant sex cord-stromal tumor of testis. J Urol 131:546, 1984

90. Hopkins GB, Parry HD: Metastasizing Sertoli-cell tumor (androblastoma). Cancer 23:463, 1969

91. Nagy L, Thurzo R, Pinter J: Zur pathologie der androblastoma. Zentralbl Allg Pathol 105:215, 1964

92. Collins DH, Symington T: Sertoli cell tumor. Br J Urol 36:52, 1964

93. Kurman RJ, Andrade D, Goebelsmann U, Taylor CR: An immunohistological study of steroid localization in Sertoli–Leydig tumor of the ovary and testis. Cancer 42:1772, 1978

94. Kurman RJ: Contributions of immunocytochemistry to gynecological pathology. Clin Obstet Gynaecol 11:5, 1984

95. Wiederhold MD, Gonzalez-Crussi F, Ou DW, Yokoyama MM: Ultrastructure of an undifferentiated Sertoli cell tumor of the testicle. Urol Int 37:297, 1982

96. Goellner JR, Myers RP: Sertoli cell tumor. Case report with ultrastructural findings. Mayo Clin Proc 50:459, 1975

97. Greco MA, Feiner HD, Theil KS, Mufarrij AA: Testicular stromal tumor with myofilaments: ultrastructural comparison with normal gonadal stroma. Hum Pathol 15(3):238, 1984

98. Evans HL, Glick AD: Unusual gonadal stromal tumor of the testis. Case report with ultrastructural observations. Arch Pathol Lab Med 101:317, 1977

5

Miscellaneous Neoplasms and Nonneoplastic Lesions

Robert H. Young and Robert E. Scully

This chapter will discuss the neoplasms and nonneoplastic lesions listed in categories V through IX of the World Health Organization (WHO) classification of testicular tumors (Table 5-1).[1] These categories include several entities that arise most commonly or exclusively in the testicular tunics or the epididymis. A number of additional lesions not included in the WHO classification will also be discussed.

TUMORS AND PSEUDOTUMORS OF THE RETE

The very rare carcinomas that appear to arise from the rete testis have been the subject of a recent review by Nochomovitz and Orenstein,[2] who added 1 case to 21 collected from the literature. Two-thirds of these tumors occurred in men over 50 years of age and none was encountered in patients under the age of 30 years. Approximately one-quarter of the tumors were associated with a hydrocele.

Carcinomas of the rete are usually solid, but may contain cysts. Microscopic examination reveals tubular, papillary, and solid patterns. The tubules are typically elongated, compressed, and slitlike. The papillae, which may project into cysts, may be small and cellular, superficially resembling glomeruli, or large with fibrous or hyalinized cores. The stroma, which is often prominent, may be extensively hyalinized. The neoplastic cells are typically small and cuboidal with scanty cytoplasm; nuclear stratification and at least moderate nuclear pleomorphism and mitotic activity are usually present. The ultrastructural features of the tumor reported by Nochomovitz and Orenstein[2] (groups of cells surrounded by a basal lamina and containing lumens lined by numerous microvilli, complicated interdigitations of the cell membranes, desmosomes, and cytoplasm rich in ribosomes, rough endoplasmic reticulum, and mitochondria) were similar to those of the normal rete testis. Another ultrastructural study[3] also documented resemblances to the normal rete.

Three criteria should be fulfilled before a diagnosis of carcinoma of the rete is made: a predominant location in the region of the rete; an adenocarcinomatous pattern consistent with an origin from rete epithelium; and absence of evidence of a primary carcinoma elsewhere. Metastatic adenocarcinomas, particularly from the lung and prostate gland, may simulate adenocarcinoma of the rete and a careful clinical investigation to exclude such tumors is indicated before making the latter diagnosis. Immunocytochemical staining for prostatic-specific acid phosphatase and prostatic-specific antigen should be helpful in confirming the diagnosis of metastatic carcinoma of prostatic origin in problem cases. Additional support for the diagnosis of carcinoma of the rete is the recognition of a transition between the tumor and uninvolved rete.

Almost half the patients with carcinoma of the rete have died as a result of tumor spread, usually within 2 years; follow-up study of most of the other patients has been unavailable or

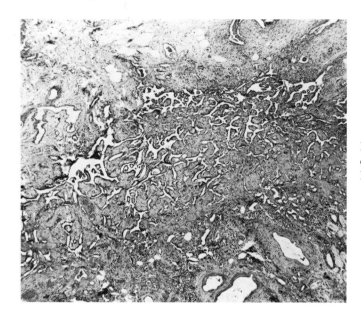

Fig. 5-1. Relative prominence of rete in atrophic testis. H & E. × 31.

Table 5-1. WHO Classification of Tumors of
the Testis: Categories V–IX

V. Lymphoid and Hematopoietic tumors

VI. Secondary tumors

VII. Tumors of collecting ducts, rete, epididymis, spermatic cord, capsule, supporting structures, and appendices
  A. Adenomatoid tumor
  B. Mesothelioma
  C. Adenoma
  D. Carcinoma
  E. Melanotic neuroectodermal tumor
  F. Brenner tumor
  G. Soft tissue tumors
    1. Embryonal Rhabdomyosarcoma
    2. Others

VIII. Unclassified tumors

IX. Tumor-like lesions
  A. Epidermal (epidermoid) cyst
  B. Nonspecific orchitis
  C. Nonspecific granulomatous orchitis
  D. Specific Orchitis
  E. Malacoplakia
  F. Fibromatous periorchitis
  G. Sperm granuloma
  H. Lipogranuloma
  I. Adrenal rests
  J. Others

of short duration. Many of those who died had advanced disease at the time of presentation. The tumor metastasizes to lymph nodes, lung, skin, liver, and bones in decreasing order of frequency[4]; recurrence in the skin has occurred in seven cases.[2] Inguinal orchiectomy is indicated as initial management; the frequent presence of lymph node metastases suggests that a lymphadenectomy should also be performed.

Acceptable adenomas of the rete testis have not been reported to the best of our knowledge; occasionally, however, a relatively prominent rete in an atrophic testis (Fig. 5-1) has been misinterpreted as an adenoma or even an adenocarcinoma.

ADENOMATOID TUMOR

In males this neoplasm (Figs. 5-2 to 5-5), which is also seen in the fallopian tube, uterus, and, rarely, the ovarian hilus of female patients, is typically located in the epididymis (Fig. 5-2), but may also arise in the spermatic cord or testicular tunics[5-12] (Fig. 5-3). Occasionally, the testicular parenchyma is involved by local extension[12] (Fig. 5-5). The adenomatoid tumor is the most common tumor of the

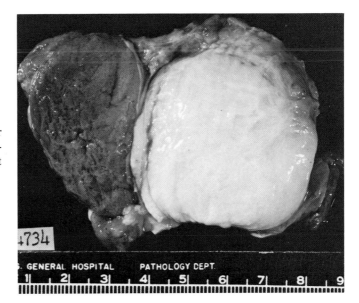

Fig. 5-2. Adenomatoid tumor of epididymis. A well-circumscribed white mass is adjacent to the testis.

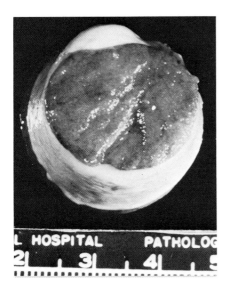

Fig. 5-3. Adenomatoid tumor of tunica albuginea.

epididymis, where it usually occurs at the lower pole[6, 7]; it has been reported in all age groups but is most common from the third through fifth decades.[8-11] The tumor is almost always unilateral and solitary and rarely exceeds 5 cm in diameter. Although typically round or oval and well-demarcated (Fig. 5-2), the tumor may be plaque-like (Fig. 5-3) and have an ill-defined margin.[12] It is composed of solid, tan to gray–white glistening tissue. Microscopic examination reveals a network of tubules, which are round, oval or slit-like (Figs. 5-4, 5-5) and range from very small to cystic; small cords and clusters of cells are characteristically seen as well. The neoplastic cells lining the tubules vary from flat to columnar and have abundant dense cytoplasm or contain large intracytoplasmic vacuoles. The stroma, which is often prominent, is usually fibrous and sometimes hyalinized; it may contain smooth muscle, which rarely predominates.[1] Lymphoid aggregates may be prominent throughout the tumor or at its periphery (Fig. 5-4). Nogales et al.[13] have reported an adenomatoid tumor of the tunica vaginalis that was admixed with a Brenner tumor. The infiltrative borders of some adenomatoid tumors (Fig. 5-5) may suggest malignancy, and rare examples have disquieting cytologic features as well. Two neoplasms interpreted as malignant adenomatoid tumors have been reported,[14, 15] but this diagnosis is not convincing in the absence of clear transitions to easily recognizable benign forms of the tumor.

The histogenesis of adenomatoid tumors in patients of both sexes has been investigated by light-microscopic, electron-microscopic,

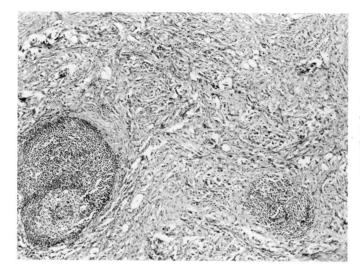

Fig. 5-4. Adenomatoid tumor of epididymis. Small spaces lined by flattened cells in a fibrous stroma. Two lymphoid follicles are present. H & E. × 79.

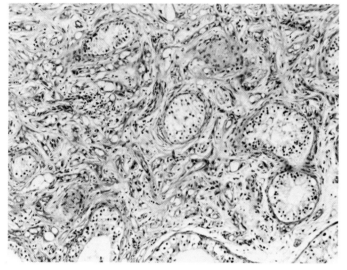

Fig. 5-5. Adenomatoid tumor invading between seminiferous tubules. H & E. × 125.

and immunocytochemical techniques[16-26]; the findings of most studies, including the demonstration of direct continuity with a benign papillary mesothelioma in one case,[18] ultrastructural similarities of the neoplastic cells to mesothelial cells,[19, 20] the demonstration of cytokeratin[22, 23] and mesothelium-specific antigen[25] in the tumor cells, and the absence of carcinoembryonic antigen within them,[23] favor a mesothelial origin. A vascular origin for several of the tumors has been suggested by the ultrastructural finding of Weibel-Palade bodies and a multilayered basal lamina in one

study,[21] and the demonstration of factor VIII in the cytoplasm of the neoplastic cells in another.[24] Staining for this substance has been negative, however, in the experience of other investigators.[22, 23] The authors of a recent study suggested that these tumors result from a reactive process and may have either vascular and mesothelial characteristics or purely mesothelial features, depending on the stage of evolution of the lesion.[26] Why these tumors are almost entirely restricted to the genital organs remains a mystery. Local excision is the treatment of choice.

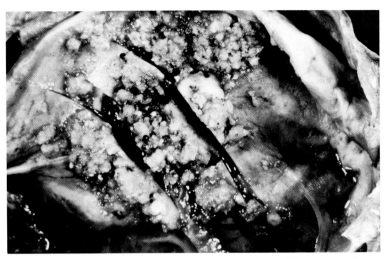

Fig. 5-6. Malignant mesothelioma of tunica vaginalis. Papillary, tumor tissue covers a large portion of the tunica.

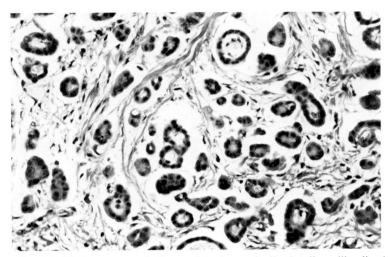

Fig. 5-7. Malignant mesothelioma of tunica vaginalis. Small papillae lined by cells resembling mesothelial cells. H & E. × 256.

MALIGNANT MESOTHELIOMA

Twenty-four malignant mesotheliomas of the tunica vaginalis have been reported.[27-34] Clinical attention is often drawn to these tumors by the presence of a hydrocele, which may recur repeatedly after tapping; a mass or ill-defined firmness may be palpated preoperatively but the diagnosis of a neoplasm is often not apparent until surgery is performed. In one case the tumor was diagnosed preoperatively by cytologic examination of hydrocele fluid.[30] In six of the reported cases,[34] and in an additional unreported case in our files, the patient had been exposed to asbestos.

On gross examination, tumor tissue may coat the tunica vaginalis or form multiple nodules on its surface (Fig. 5-6). Microscopic ex-

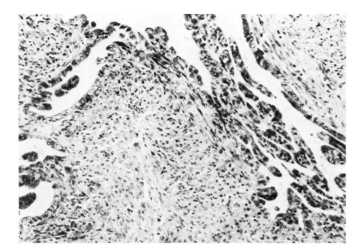

Fig. 5-8. Malignant mesothelioma of tunica vaginalis. Biphasic pattern. H & E. × 300.

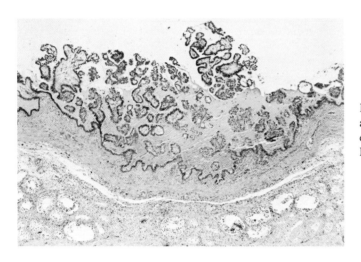

Fig. 5-9. Serous papillary cystadenoma of testis. Abundant extracellular mucin is present. H & E. × 31.

amination reveals papillary (Fig. 5-7), tubular, diffuse, and, less commonly, biphasic[32] (Fig. 5-8) or fibrous[29] patterns similar to those encountered in malignant mesotheliomas of the peritoneum and pleura. The neoplastic cells are typically cuboidal with moderate amounts of eosinophilic cytoplasm in well-differentiated tumors (Fig. 5-7), but may have highly malignant features in other cases. The ultrastructural findings, including the presence of microvilli, glycogen, tonofilaments, desmosomes, and the perinuclear location of mitochondria, have been compatible with a tumor of mesothelial type.[29-31, 33]

The initial surgical treatment should be an inguinal orchiectomy or a more radical surgical procedure if the tumor has spread beyond the testis.[30] Three of the seven patients who have had a subsequent diagnostic laparotomy have had lymph node metastases, suggesting that a lymphadenectomy should be included in the primary surgical approach. The tumor may also spread extensively to the peritoneum and metastasize to the lungs. Both radiation therapy and chemotherapy have proved beneficial in treating inoperable disease in small numbers of cases. Follow-up data are included in 23 of the reported cases. Thirteen of the patients had a relapse from 6 weeks to 10 years (mean, 20 months) after diagnosis. Ten

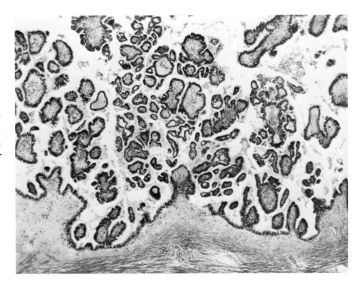

Fig. 5-10. Serous papillary cystadenoma of borderline malignancy. Numerous papillae are covered by proliferating cells of serous type. H & E. × 50.

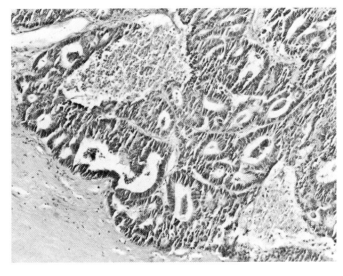

Fig. 5-11. Endometrioid adenoacanthoma. Tubular glands resembling those of the typical endometrial adenocarcinoma. Squamous differentiation is not evident in this field. H & E. × 125.

patients were disease-free from 6 weeks to 15 years postoperatively but only three of them had been evaluated for more than 18 months.[34]

MULLERIAN-TYPE TUMORS

One of us (RES) has seen in consultation several testicular tumors with microscopic features similar to those of ovarian tumors of surface epithelial type. These tumors have included one serous surface papilloma of borderline malignancy, one intra testicular serous papillary cystadenoma of borderline malignancy (Figs. 5-9, 5-10), and one tumor that replaced the testicular parenchyma and had the appearance of an endometrioid adenoacanthoma (Fig. 5-11). Reported examples of mullerian-type tumors include an additional serous cystadenoma of borderline malignancy[35] a paratesticular mucinous cystadenoma[36] and two testicular[37, 38] and one paratesticular Brenner tumor[39] (Fig. 5-12). We have also seen a paratesticular mass composed of tissue resembling endometrium and myometrium (Fig. 5-13) that lay adjacent to the tail of the

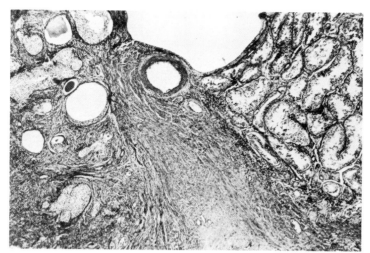

Fig. 5-12. Paratesticular Brenner tumor. H & E. × 60.

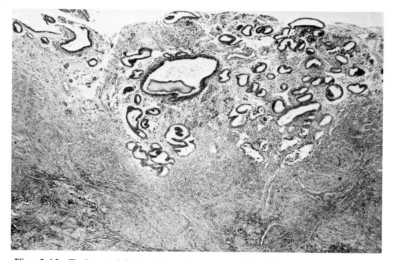

Fig. 5-13. Endometrial glands and stroma with adjacent smooth muscle in a patient treated with estrogens for carcinoma of the prostate. H & E. × 64.

epididymis. It had been removed from an 82-year-old man who had been receiving diethylstilbestrol treatment for carcinoma of the prostate gland.

MISCELLANEOUS TUMORS OF SOFT TISSUE TYPE

Benign and malignant soft tissue tumors are very rare in the testis, but somewhat more common in the epididymis and spermatic cord. We have seen one fibroma (Fig. 5-14) and two hemangiomas of the testis[40] (Fig. 5-15), and rare examples of fibroma, lipoma, leiomyoma, neurofibroma, and hemangioma have been reported.[40-44] We have examined in consultation one rhabdomyosarcoma confined to the testis of a child, and most of the reported malignant tumors of soft tissue type have also been rhabdomyosarcomas.[45] Rare intratesticular sarcomas of other types have been recorded in the literature.[46]

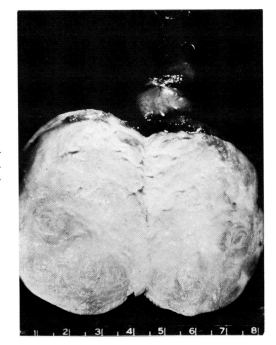

Fig. 5-14. Fibroma of the testis. Lobulated, tan–white tissue has replaced the testicular parenchyma. Microscopic examination showed relatively acellular dense fibrous tissue.

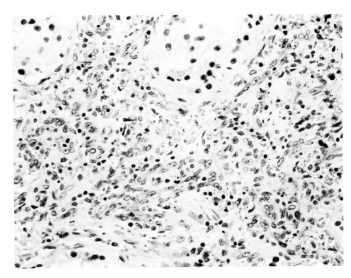

Fig. 5-15. Hemangioma of testis. Small compressed vessels separate the seminiferous tubules. H & E. × 256.

LYMPHOMA

Although malignant lymphomas account for only 5 percent of all testicular neoplasms, they account for about 50 percent in men over 60 years of age.[47-51] Approximately 75 percent of these tumors are detected after the age of 50 years. Lymphoma is the most common form of tumor that involves both testes, with the frequency of bilaterality ranging from 6 to 38 percent of the cases.[52-54] The bilateral involvement is much more often metachronous than synchronous.[51, 53] Gross examination of a testis involved by lymphoma reveals replacement of part or all of the parenchyma by a firm or soft, fleshy, homogeneous mass,

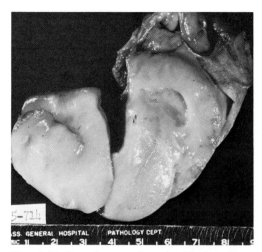

Fig. 5-16. Lymphoma of testis. Fleshy tissue, which was cream-colored, replaces the testicular parenchyma and has spread to the epididymis.

which may be cream-colored, tan, or slightly pink (Fig. 5-16); lobulation is occasionally conspicuous; necrosis is uncommon. The gross appearance closely resembles that of a seminoma. A helpful clue to the differential diagnosis is the spread of lymphoma to the epididymis (Fig. 5-16) or spermatic cord in up to 50 percent of the cases,[54] in contrast to only approximately 8 percent in cases of seminoma.[9]

Low-power microscopic examination provides a diagnostic clue in the form of predominant intertubular infiltration of the neoplastic cells (Fig. 5-17), a finding that is not conspicuous in most other types of testicular neoplasia. In one-third of the cases, the lymphoma cells also invade the tubules (Fig. 5-18), effacing their normal cellular population to varying extents. Involvement of tubules is typically confined to those within the tumor. Microscopic evidence of epididymal involvement occurs in up to 80 percent of the cases, and involvement of the spermatic cord, somewhat less frequently.[54]

Between 70 and 90 percent of testicular lymphomas are of the diffuse, large-cell, or "histiocytic" type, but almost all forms,[52-61] including rare examples of Hodgkin's lym-

phoma,[62, 63] have been reported. Turner and his co-workers[59] have found that subdivision of testicular lymphomas into the subtypes in the Working Formulation disclosed a far better prognosis for those tumors in the intermediate-grade than in the high-grade group.

Testicular lymphomas must be differentiated from typical seminomas, spermatocytic seminomas, embryonal carcinomas, and several forms of orchitis, including viral orchitis, granulomatous orchitis, and malacoplakia, all of which can resemble lymphomas on gross examination. Although characteristic patterns of growth are helpful in the differential diagnosis (Fig. 5-17), the essential criteria for distinguishing these lesions are the morphologic features and staining characteristics of their cells. Lymphoma cells are unlike those of typical seminomas, which have prominent cell membranes, an abundant content of clear, glycogen-rich cytoplasm, and rounded but flattened central nuclei with one or a few prominent nucleoli. The cells of spermatocytic seminomas have mostly spherical, dark nuclei of unequal size and glycogen-free cytoplasm, and those of embryonal carcinoma are anaplastic, often contain clear cytoplasm, and grow in a variety of distinctive epithelial patterns; embryonal carcinoma cells also stain positively for cytokeratin.[64] The various forms of orchitis have distinctive features, which will be discussed below. Rarely, a testis involved by chronic epididymoorchitis may have histologic features simulating those of a malignant lymphoma and the designation "pseudolymphoma" has been applied to these cases.[51, 65]

The overall survival rate for patients with lymphoma presenting in the testis is 15 to 30 percent at 2 years,[53, 54] but more than 50 percent if the tumor appears to be confined to the testis on the basis of careful staging.[52, 59] The importance of staging is emphasized by the finding in one series[59] of confinement of extratesticular spread to the spleen in three of six patients who underwent a staging laparotomy. Other sites of involvement by the lymphoma have been varied but there is relatively frequent involvement of Waldeyer's

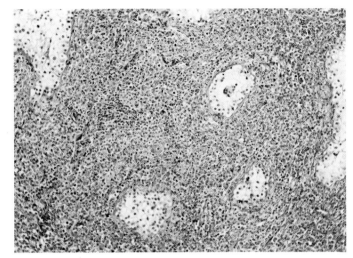

Fig. 5-17. Lymphoma of testis. Large lymphoid cells separate the seminiferous tubules. H & E. × 100.

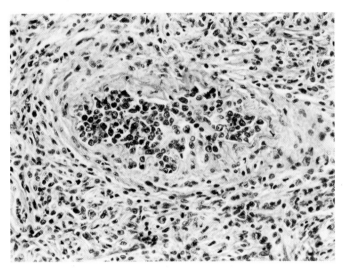

Fig. 5-18. Lymphoma of testis. Seminiferous tubules invaded by large lymphoid cells. H & E. × 313.

ring[52, 56, 58, 60] and central nervous system involvement was present in almost one-third of the cases in one large series.[59] Orchiectomy alone is inadequate therapy for testicular lymphoma, and should be supplemented by chemotherapy or radiation therapy.[56, 58-61]

PLASMACYTOMA AND MULTIPLE MYELOMA

The testis is involved in approximately 2 percent of patients with multiple myeloma, but the involvement is usually apparent only at autopsy.[66-71] The first example of testicular myeloma in the English-language literature was reported by Ulrich,[72] who described the case of a 55-year-old man with multiple myeloma in whom a testicular tumor was the only extraosseous manifestation of the disease. Sporadic reports of testicular involvement in cases of clinically evident multiple myeloma, as well as testicular enlargement that preceded recognition of the disease, have appeared subsequently.[73-78] Cases of solitary plasmacytoma of the testis and testicular plasmacytoma associated with similar tumors of other organs (Fig. 5-19) have also been reported,[51, 79-81] but

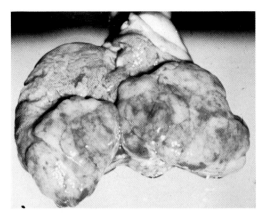

Fig. 5-19. Plasmacytoma of testis. A lobulated, fleshy mass replaces the lower pole of the testis. Patient had plasmacytoma of nasopharynx 3 years previously and plasmacytoma of contralateral epididymis 8 years later. He was alive and well 26 years after orchiectomy.

follow-up in most of these cases has been short, and multiple myeloma may subsequently have become evident in some of them. No case has been reported in which long-term follow-up has established cure of a testicular plasmacytoma by orchiectomy. Testicular involvement has been bilateral in approximately 30 percent of the patients, including those with multiple myeloma and those with plasmacytoma; the bilateral involvement is typically metachronous. On microscopic examination a predominantly interstitial growth pattern is encountered, but intratubular extension of the neoplastic cells may also occur.[77]

LEUKEMIC INFILTRATION

Microscopic involvement of the testis has been found at autopsy in 64 percent of 140 patients with acute leukemia, and 22 percent of 76 patients with chronic leukemia.[82] The testis was enlarged in 7 percent of the patients; the enlargement was invariably bilateral and usually asymmetrical. Testicular swelling had been evident during life in only 4.5 percent of the patients. In another autopsy series restricted to children, 62 percent of the patients

with acute leukemia had microscopic testicular involvement.[83] Only very rarely is testicular enlargement the presenting manifestation of leukemia.[84]

Recent interest in involvement of the testis by leukemia has been focused on the role of this organ as a sanctuary for leukemic cells during clinical "remission,"[85-95] and most testicular specimens containing leukemic infiltrates that the pathologist sees are biopsy specimens, usually from children, that have been obtained to determine the presence or absence of involvement (Fig. 5-20). Approximately 16 percent of patients with acute lymphocytic leukemia have relapses initially in the form of testicular infiltration.[87, 88] The affected patient usually has testicular swelling, which, although unilateral on clinical examination in most cases, is usually proven to be bilateral if a biopsy of the contralateral testis is also performed.[86] Testicular relapse is frequently a harbinger of systemic relapse[87, 88] and is considered an indication for radiation therapy to the testis, central nervous system chemoprophylaxis, and systemic chemotherapy.[95] On microscopic examination, the pattern of leukemic infiltration is similar to that of lymphoma (Fig. 5-20), with tubular invasion in some of the cases.[88]

METASTATIC TUMORS

Unlike the ovary, which is a common site of metastasis, the testis is rarely involved by tumor originating elsewhere. Because of the decreased incidence of testicular germ cell tumors and the increased incidence of cancer of other organs in men over the age of 50 years, metastatic tumors account for a much higher percentage of testicular neoplasms in this age group than in younger men. In their recent review, Haupt et al.[96] found that the mean age of patients with tumors metastatic to the testis was 55 years.

In a prospective autopsy study, in which both testes were sliced thinly and examined carefully, Tiltman[97] found testicular metas-

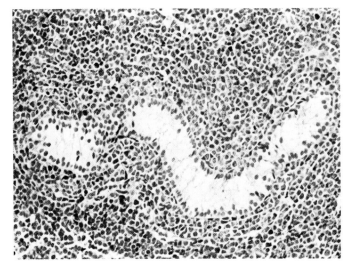

Fig. 5-20. Acute lymphoid leukemia. Infiltrate of leukemic cells surrounds the seminiferous tubules. H & E. × 313.

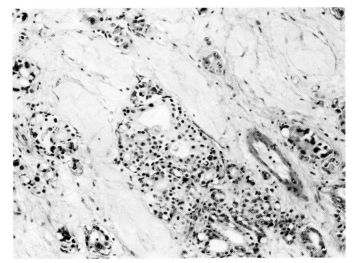

Fig. 5-21. Carcinoma of prostate metastatic to testis. Adenocarcinomatous glands invading among seminiferous tubules, which are hyalinized and atrophic. H & E. × 160.

tases in only 6 of 248 (2.4 percent) men with malignant tumors. The primary tumors were carcinoma of the prostate (two cases), malignant melanoma of the skin (two cases), carcinoma of the lung, and mesothelioma of the pleura (one case each). Other autopsy studies have been retrospective and included patients dying of all causes, which eliminates the possibility of accurately determining the frequency of testicular metastases in cancer patients.

Testicular metastases are bilateral in 15 percent of the cases. Prostatic (Figs. 5-21–5-23) and pulmonary carcinomas are the most common primary tumors, with the former ac-

counting for about one-third and the latter about one-fifth of the cases in the literature.[96-102] The high frequency of prostatic cancer is due partly to the occasional finding of occult metastases in patients who have undergone therapeutic orchiectomy.[102] The next most frequent primary tumors have been malignant melanomas of the skin and carcinomas of the colon, kidney, stomach, and pancreas.[96] Metastatic melanoma has been reported to be manifested by melanospermia in one case.[103] Isolated examples or only a few examples of metastatic carcinomas of the urinary bladder, ureter, biliary tract, salivary gland, and thy-

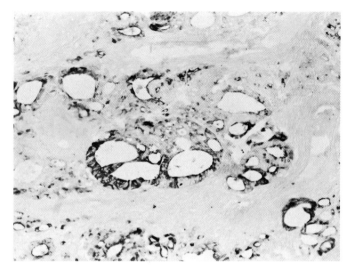

Fig. 5-22. Carcinoma of prostate metastatic to testis. The tumor cells stain positively for prostate-specific antigen. Immunoperoxidase technique. × 125. Same case as Figure 5-21.

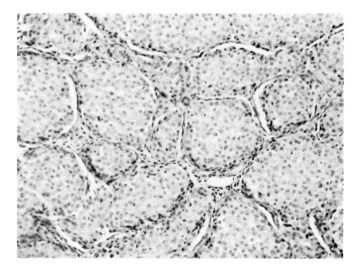

Fig. 5-23. Carcinoma of prostate metastatic to testis. The lack of glandular differentiation and the presence of moderate to abundant amounts of eosinophilic cytoplasm impart a superficial resemblance to a Leydig cell tumor. H & E. × 160.

roid gland have been reported, as well as cases of pleural mesothelioma, carcinoid tumor, retinoblastoma, neuroblastoma, and "fibroliposarcoma."[96-101] We have also seen single cases of urethral carcinoma and angiosarcoma that metastasized to the testis.

Of the almost 130 examples of metastases to the testis in the literature, the testicular tumor was the initial manifestation of the disease in only 10 patients.[96, 104] The primary tumors in eight of these cases were in the prostate gland (three cases), kidney (two cases), pancreas (one case), stomach (one case), and colon (one case).[96] In one case the tumor was

a carcinoid, probably of gastrointestinal origin,[105] and in another the primary site was never determined.[96] We have examined in consultation an additional unpublished case in which a metastastic tumor from the prostate gland was the presenting manifestation of the disease (Figs. 5-21, 5-22).

On gross examination a testis involved by a metastasis usually shows single or multiple nodules but diffuse effacement of the entire parenchyma is occasionally seen.[98] The presence of multiple nodules should suggest the possibility of metastasis, particularly in a patient over 50 years of age, but differentiation between a primary and metastatic tumor depends on microscopic examination. Although metastatic tumors occasionally resemble primary testicular neoplasms microscopically (Fig. 5-23), identification of the tumor as metastatic is almost always established not only by awareness of the presence of a primary tumor elsewhere, but also by the distinctive features of the individual neoplasm, lymphatic and blood vessel invasion, which is often present, and a predominant localization of the tumor in the interstitial tissue. Metastatic tumors, however, may also invade and fill the seminiferous tubules.[97] Special stains, particularly for mucin, and immunoperoxidase studies (Fig. 5-22) may also be helpful in establishing or confirming the nature of a metastatic lesion.

CYSTS

Epidermoid cysts, which account for approximately 1 percent of testicular enlargements, occur at all ages, but are most common during the second to fourth decades.[106-108] They average 2 cm in diameter, are round to oval, and composed of laminated cheesy material surrounded by a fibrous wall (Fig. 5-24). Microscopic examination shows that at least part of the cyst wall is lined by keratinizing squamous epithelium (Fig. 5-25); the lining may be denuded over large areas with ulceration and foreign body giant cell reaction. It is important to sample epidermoid cysts, which are not considered true neoplasms, extensively to exclude an association with small foci of invasive or in situ germ cell neoplasia or scars, the presence of which warrant the diagnosis of teratoma, a tumor with a metastatic potential. Orchiectomy for epidermoid cysts results in 100 percent survival.

Other types of testicular cyst are extremely rare; they include parenchymal cysts of undetermined origin, lined by cuboidal or flattened epithelium,[109-111] and cysts arising from the mesothelium of the tunica albuginea.[112] True hermaphrodites, who are phenotypic males in

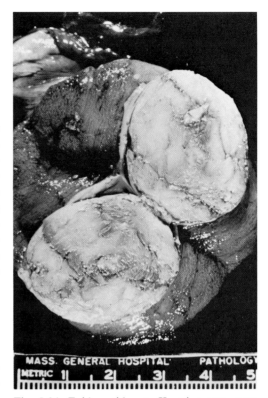

MASS. GENERAL HOSPITAL   PATHOLOGY
METRIC 1| 2| 3| 4| 5|

Fig. 5-24. Epidermoid cyst. Keratinaceous material fills the cyst.

a minority of the cases, may have ovotestes or, very rarely, an ovary in the scrotum.[113] The ovarian tissue often contains cystic follicles and corpora lutea, and on occasion, the patient presents with pain and a mass in the scrotum, which may simulate a testicular tumor. The diagnosis should be suspected because of the almost invariable presence of hypospadias, gynecomastia, and other stigmata of true hermaphroditism, including an abnormal karyotype, usually 46XX.

CYSTIC DYSPLASIA

This lesion, which occurs rarely in infants and children, is characterized by the presence of multiple anastomosing cysts of varying sizes and shapes, separated by fibrous septa.[114-116] The term "cystic dysplasia" was proposed by Leissring and Oppenheimer[114]; only five cases

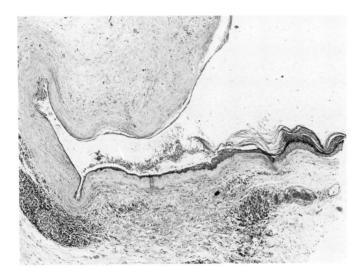

Fig. 5-25. Epidermoid cyst. Keratinizing squamous epithelium lines the cyst. H & E. × 50.

have been described. Two patients were newborns; the others were 4, 9, and 10 years of age. Two patients had ipsilateral renal agenesis and one had bilateral renal dysplasia. Gross examination has revealed a multicystic mass replacing most of the testis. The lesion was bilateral in the two newborns, but unilateral in the older children. The process begins in the region of the rete and extends into the parenchyma, which may be compressed to form a thin rim at the periphery. The cysts are lined by a single layer of flat or cuboidal epithelial cells, which have been shown by ultrastructural studies to be similar to those of the rete testis.[116]

ORCHITIS

Numerous agents may be responsible for orchitis,[117, 118] which will be discussed under the following headings: bacterial, viral, granulomatous, and malacoplakia.

BACTERIAL ORCHITIS

The bacteria that have been reported to cause orchitis have been enumerated by Mikuz and Damjanov[117]: *Escherichia coli, Neisseria gonorrheae, Aerobacter aerogenes, Pseudomonas, Klebsiella, Streptococcus, Staphylococcus,* *Pneumococcus, Hemophilus, Brucella, and Salmonella.* In most cases, orchitis is a complication of epididymitis or a urinary tract infection, but it may also result from bloodborne dissemination. The pathologist only occasionally examines testes involved by bacterial infection because the diagnosis is usually obvious clinically and curative treatment is instituted. When an orchiectomy is performed, the gross appearance varies, depending on the relative extents of epididymal and testicular involvement and the chronicity of the process. The testis may contain abscesses or be fibrotic and adherent to adjacent tissues. Rarely, a neoplasm may be suggested in the chronic stage of the disease.[119] Microscopic examination discloses acute and chronic inflammation, abscess formation, granulation tissue, and fibrosis, depending on the duration of the process. In some cases, there is focal infarction, which may be the result of venous occlusion.[120] Orchitis associated with tuberculosis, leprosy, and syphilis is discussed in the section on granulomatous orchitis.

VIRAL ORCHITIS

The most familiar form of viral orchitis is that caused by the mumps virus[121-124] (Fig. 5-26), but a wide variety of other viruses have

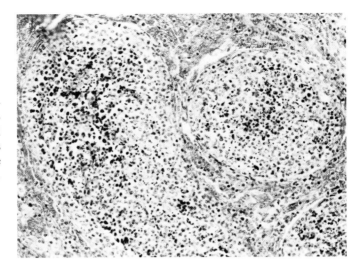

Fig. 5-26. Mumps orchitis. Numerous inflammatory cells, including many neutrophils, fill the lumens of the seminiferous tubules. Interstitial hemorrhage is also present. H & E. × 200.

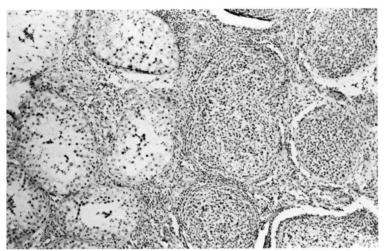

Fig. 5-27. Viral orchitis. Some of the tubules are normal whereas others are filled with an inflammatory infiltrate. H & E. × 156.

also been implicated,[125, 126] most often the Coxsackie B virus.[127] The testis is involved in 14 to 36 percent of adults with mumps, but in well under 1 percent of children with this disease.[121-124] Testicular involvement is accompanied by epididymitis in 85 percent of the cases, and bilateral testicular involvement is present in almost 20 percent of the cases.[121] On clinical examination the testis is swollen and tender. Incision of the tunica albuginea reveals edema and, in some cases, hemorrhage. Microscopic examination discloses interstitial edema early in the course, followed by vascu-

lar dilatation and interstitial lymphocytic infiltration.[123] Interstitial hemorrhage occurs subsequently, accompanied by polymorphonuclear leukocytic infiltration of the seminiferous tubules and degeneration of the germinal epithelium (Fig. 5-26). Healing results in patchy hyalinization of tubules and interstitial fibrosis, with intervening areas of normal testis. In 13 percent of the cases bilateral involvement is sufficiently extensive to result in infertility.[121, 122]

The microscopic features of other forms of viral orchitis (Fig. 5-27) have been investigated much less extensively, but appear to resemble those of mumps orchitis. In the rare cases in which mumps orchitis precedes parotitis or is the sole evidence of the infection, or in those cases in which orchitis is the exclusive or major manifestation of another viral illness, the gross and microscopic findings may be confused with those of a malignant tumor, particularly a seminoma or lymphoma. Careful examination of the cellular infiltrate, however, enables one to make the correct diagnosis.

GRANULOMATOUS ORCHITIS

Infectious

Granulomatous inflammation of the testis may be encountered in a variety of infectious diseases, including tuberculosis, leprosy, syphilis, and fungal infections. In one large series, approximately one-third of the patients with genitourinary tuberculosis presented because of involvement of the epididymis or testis.[128] Although tuberculous epididymo-orchitis has decreased greatly in frequency in Western countries, it is not exceedingly rare, as evidenced by the occurrence of 20 cases over a decade in a single hospital in Great Britain.[129] The epididymis is the primary site of the disease; the testis is usually affected only in the late stages of the disease.[128, 132] This sequence of involvement, the 30 percent frequency of bilaterality, and the 50 percent frequency of an abscess or sinus tract are important clues to the infectious nature of the process, which is unlikely to be mistaken for a neoplasm.

Involvement of the testis is very common in patients with lepromatous leprosy, but rare in those with other forms of the disease.[133-137] Leprosy, in contrast to tuberculosis, involves the testis more commonly than the epididymis. Both testes are usually affected; they are typically normal or decreased in size, but occasionally enlarged. Rarely, a patient with lepromatous leprosy presents because of testi-

cular involvement.[137] The microscopic findings have been classified into three stages: vascular, characterized by thickening of vessel walls and a perivascular inflammatory infiltrate; interstitial, with progressive obliterative endarteritis and interstitial fibrosis; and obliterative, with loss of the normal architecture and replacement of the parenchyma by fibrous tissue.[133] Lepra bacilli can usually be identified readily during the first two stages.

The testis may be involved in congenital syphilis and in the tertiary stage of acquired syphilis.[118, 138] In congenital syphilis, bilateral painless testicular enlargement is usually present, and microscopic examination shows interstitial inflammation, endarteritis, and fibrosis. A similar appearance may also characterize involvement by tertiary syphilis, but in the latter, gummas of varying sizes may also be encountered (Figs. 5-28, 5-29).

On very rare occasions fungal and parasitic diseases involve the testis.[118, 139] Sarcoidosis may affect the epididymis and rarely the testis,[140-143] and in at least one case[142] testicular enlargement suggested a neoplasm, resulting in an orchiectomy.

Idiopathic

Idiopathic granulomatous orchitis is one of the more common forms of nonneoplastic testicular enlargement.[144-150] In the experience of the Armed Forces Institute of Pathology,[9] 120 of 6,000 testicular masses (0.2 percent), and in another series[48] 12 of 597 testicular masses (0.2 percent) were caused by this lesion, which usually occurs during the fifth or sixth decade.[144] It follows a urinary tract infection with gram-negative bacilli in about two-thirds of the cases, and is characterized by testicular enlargement, sometimes associated with pain or tenderness, which may disappear, leaving a painless mass.[144] The contralateral testis is also affected, usually metachronously, in occasional cases.[144, 147] Rarely there is a sinus tract between the testis and the scrotum.[147] Although granulomatous orchitis

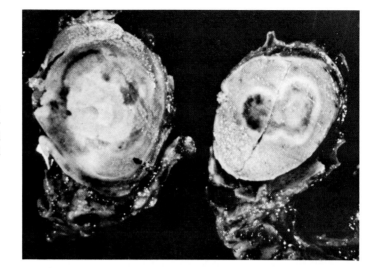

Fig. 5-28. Gumma of testis. The testis is extensively involved by a circumscribed zone of necrosis surrounded by a fibrous capsule.

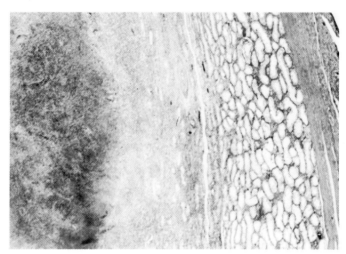

Fig. 5-29. Gumma of testis. Sharply circumscribed granuloma with central necrosis lies adjacent to testicular tissue. H & E. × 20.

may be indistinguishable from a neoplasm in some cases, in others the history of symptoms consistent with a "flu-like" illness, the sudden onset of testicular swelling, and associated pain or tenderness suggest a nonneoplastic process.[144]

Gross examination reveals replacement of the testicular parenchyma by homogeneous, sometimes lobulated, tan–yellow, grey, or white tissue (Fig. 5-30). The process is usually diffuse but a localized, well-circumscribed nodule is sometimes seen. The epididymis and spermatic cord are involved in about half the cases and an exudate is often present on the tunica. Microscopic examination shows prominent invasion of the seminiferous tubules by an inflammatory infiltrate, in which epithelioid histiocytes predominate (Fig. 5-31); Langhans type giant cells are seen in one-third of the cases. The interstitial tissue typically contains numerous chronic inflammatory cells (Fig. 5-31), including eosinophils in most of the cases. The primarily intratubular location of the granulomatous process is helpful in differentiating the lesion from granulomatous orchitis of infectious origin and from the very rare cases of sarcoidosis involving the testis, in both of which the granulomas are predomi-

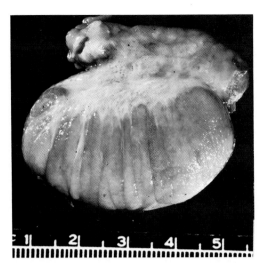

Fig. 5-30. Granulomatous orchitis. The testicular tissue has a homogeneous, bulging, lobulated appearance.

nantly interstitial. Also, necrosis within the granulomas may be seen in the infectious lesions, but not in idiopathic granulomatous orchitis. Identification of organisms by smear or culture is the most effective way to diagnose specific forms of granulomatous orchitis. It must be emphasized, however, that remnants of sperm may give positive results on acid-fast staining in cases of idiopathic granulomatous orchitis.[144]

MALACOPLAKIA

Although encountered most frequently in the urinary bladder, malacoplakia has been reported in a wide variety of other locations, including the testis.[151-154] In a recent review, McClure[154] summarized the findings in 37 reported cases in which the testis, epididymis, or both were involved. The testis was affected alone in about 60 percent of the cases, and the epididymis alone on rare occasions. Testicular malacoplakia has been reported in patients at every age except the first two decades. The symptoms are nonspecific; occasionally, there is a history of a prior urinary tract infection. The involved testis, which has been the right testis in three-quarters of the cases, is usually enlarged and may be difficult to remove because of fibrous adhesions to surrounding tissues. Bilateral involvement has not been reported.

Sectioning of the testis shows replacement of all or a portion of it by yellow, tan, or brown tissue, which is often divided into lobules by streaks of fibrous tissue (Fig. 5-32); the consistency is usually soft, but may be firm if a significant degree of fibrosis is present. The frequent finding of one or more abscesses (Fig. 5-32) is gross evidence that the process is not neoplastic. Another clue is the presence of reactive inflammatory changes in the tunica albuginea and involvement of the epididymis, which may become firm and fibrotic. Culture of an abscess usually yields *Escherichia coli,* but other organisms, such as *Proteus,* are occasionally recovered. Microscopic examination reveals replacement of the tubules and interstitial tissue by large histiocytic cells with abundant granular eosinophilic cytoplasm (von Hansemann's cells) (Fig. 5-33), some of which contain solid and targetoid basophilic inclusions of varying sizes (Michaelis-Gutmann bodies) (Fig. 5-34). Acute and chronic inflammatory cells, granulation tissue, and fibrosis are also present and may obscure the characteristic features of the process, especially if Michaelis-Gutmann bodies are inconspicuous. These structures are accentuated by von Kossa's, periodic acid-Schiff (PAS), and iron stains, which show positive findings in almost all the cases. The PAS stain also demonstrates retention of the underlying tubular architecture and accentuates the granules in the cytoplasm of the von Hansemann cells. Ultrastructural studies have shown that the Michaelis-Gutmann bodies are phagolysosomes that have ingested the breakdown products of bacteria.[155-157]

SCLEROSING LIPOGRANULOMA

A distinctive granulomatous reaction to exogenous lipids may be encountered in the male genitalia, usually outside, but occasionally also

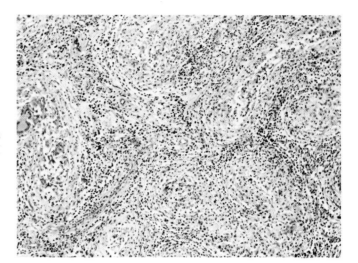

Fig. 5-31. Granulomatous orchitis. Epithelioid histiocytes have invaded the seminiferous tubules, which are obscured. H & E. × 125.

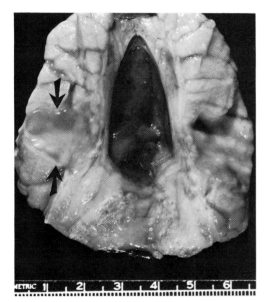

Fig. 5-32. Malacoplakia of testis. The testis has been bisected in such a fashion that congested tunica vaginalis appears in the center of the picture. Lobulated tissue, which was yellow–tan, has replaced the testicular parenchyma. Note abscess (arrows).

within, the testis[158-160] (Fig. 5-35). Palpation of a hard mass may lead to orchiectomy because of the suspicion of a neoplasm. The lesion has been encountered in mentally deranged patients and draft evaders who have injected paraffin or other oily material into the genitalia to enhance their size or produce a tumorlike mass. Gross examination reveals an ill-defined, firm, oily mass and microscopic examination discloses lipid vacuoles of varying size surrounded by foreign-body giant cells (Fig. 5-35), with chronic inflammation and fibrosis, which is often extensive and may be hyaline.

FIBROMATOUS PERIORCHITIS (FIBROUS PSEUDOTUMOR, NODULAR PERIORCHITIS)

These terms describe the presence of diffuse or focal fibromatous proliferation involving the tunica vaginalis or albuginea.[161-164] In the diffuse form, the testis is surrounded by dense fibrous tissue (Fig. 5-36) and in the localized form, there may be single or disseminated nodules, which may suggest a neoplasm on clinical examination. Sectioning reveals firm white tissue and microscopic examination typically demonstrates hyalinized collagen, which may be focally calcified (Fig. 5-37); in some cases the lesion is more cellular, with inflammation and granulation tissue formation. This disorder is generally thought to be reactive; a mesothelial origin has recently been proposed for some of these lesions on the basis of ultrastructural features characteristic of mesotheliomas including microvilli, a basal lamina, rudimen-

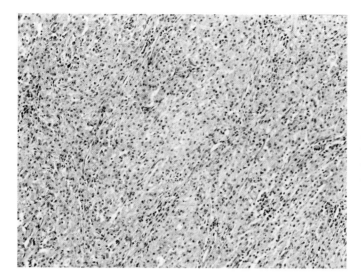

Fig. 5-33. Malacoplakia of testis. Sheets of histiocytes with abundant cytoplasm that was eosinophilic are admixed with chronic inflammatory cells. H & E. × 125.

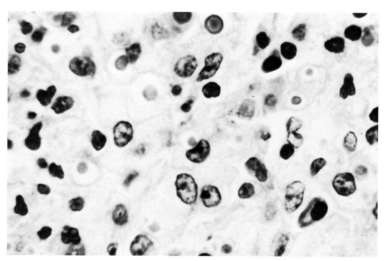

Fig. 5-34. Malacoplakia of testis. Michaelis–Gutmann bodies, most of which have a targetoid appearance. H & E. × 400.

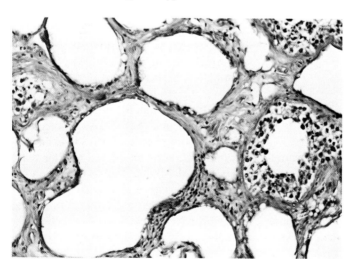

Fig. 5-35. Sclerosing lipogranuloma involving testis. Large lipid vacuoles, surrounded by flattened foreign body giant cells, are present in the interstitial tissue. H & E. × 160.

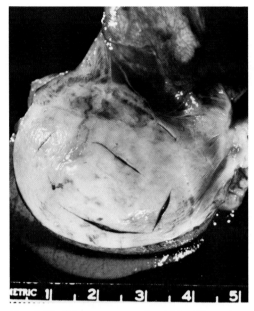

Fig. 5-36. Fibromatous periorchitis. Firm tissue, which was white, coats the tunica vaginalis.

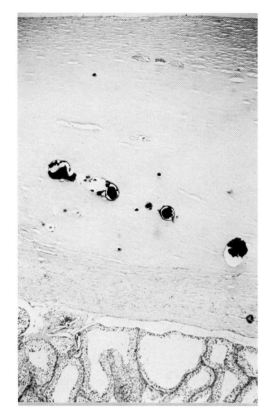

Fig. 5-37. Fibromatous periorchitis. Dense hyalinized tissue with focal calcification surrounds the testis. H & E. × 50.

tary desmosome-like attachments, tight junctions, and cytoplasmic filaments in one case.[164] Identification of the nature of the process by frozen section examination may result in avoidance of an unnecessary orchiectomy. Shafik[165] has suggested the term "constrictive albuginitis" to describe diffuse fibrosis of the tunica albuginea.

CHOLESTEROL GRANULOMA

Rarely, a granulomatous and foreign body giant cell reaction to cholesterol crystals in the tunica vaginalis produces a firm mass that may suggest a testicular or paratesticular tumor[166, 167]; in one case the lesion was considered to resemble tuberculosis on gross examination.[166] Diffuse calcification of the tunica vaginalis, visible on x-ray examination, has also been reported.[168]

MICROLITHIASIS

In this rare condition, calcified concretions are present within the seminiferous tubules (Fig. 5-38). Six cases have been reported in the literature[169-173]; testicular involvement was not documented histologically in one of them but appears to have been present on the basis of x-ray findings.[173] Four patients were children. In one of the two adult patients the lesion was found during an investigation for infertility, and we have seen an additional case of this type. The process has involved both cryptorchid and scrotal testes and has been bilateral in three cases, in all of which diffuse calcification was noted on x-ray examination. It has been suggested that microlithiasis results from calcification of the corpora-amylacea-like bodies that may be found in the semi-

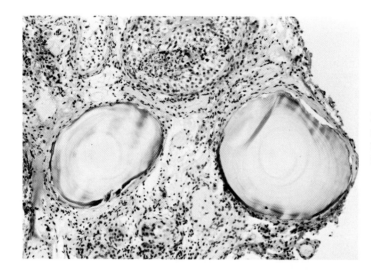

Fig. 5-38. Testicular microlithiasis. Two seminiferous tubules are replaced by calcific bodies. H & E. × 125.

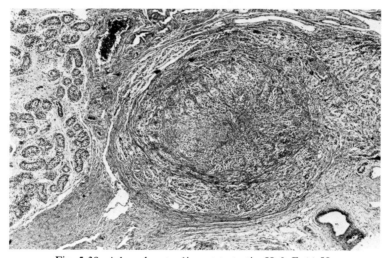

Fig. 5-39. Adrenal rest adjacent to testis. H & E. × 50.

niferous tubules of both cryptorchid and otherwise normal scrotal testes.[174, 175]

ADRENAL RESTS

Small yellow nodules of ectopic adrenocortical tissue, usually less than 1 cm in diameter, have been found in the spermatic cord, epididymis, between the epididymis and testis, in the rete, and occasionally within the tunica albuginea in approximately 10 percent of infants[176, 177] (Fig. 5-39). Their major clinical significance is in the role they may have as a source for the tumorlike masses in and adjacent to the testis that may develop in patients with the adrenogenital syndrome and Nelson's syndrome. The latter lesions are discussed in more detail in Chapter 4.

SPLENIC–GONADAL FUSION

In cases of this unusual abnormality, splenic and gonadal tissues become adherent and fuse during early intrauterine development[178-184] (Fig. 5-40). Less than 100 cases have been reported; males are affected more often than females, with a ratio of about 12:1. In males, the left testis has been involved with one possi-

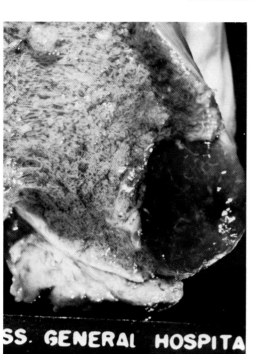

Fig. 5-40. Splenic–gonadal fusion. Nodule of splenic tissue in lower pole of testis.

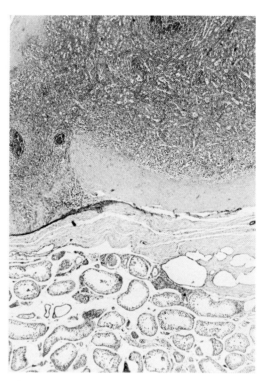

Fig. 5-41. Splenic–gonadal fusion. Splenic tissue separated from testicular tissue by band of fibrous tissue. H & E. × 50.

ble exception. This abnormality occurs in two forms, continuous and discontinuous.[179] In the continuous form a cord connects the splenic tissue attached to the testis with the spleen, while in the discontinuous form no cord is present. The cord usually arises from the upper pole of the spleen, but may also originate from the hilus or lower pole. Small aggregates of splenic tissue may be found in the cord as it traverses the peritoneal cavity, or the cord may be composed entirely of splenic tissue. The splenic tissue attached to the testis typically forms a discrete mass, which is usually small, but may be as large as 12 cm. It is almost always fused to the upper pole of the testis or the head of the epididymis, but occasionally it is attached to the lower pole and rarely it is intratesticular (Fig. 5-40). The gross and microscopic features of the lesion are similar to those of normal spleen (Fig. 5-41).

In 1956, Putschar and Manion[179] summarized the world literature on splenic–gonadal fusion, and observed that almost one-third of the patients with the continuous form had severe defects of the extremities (peromelia), sometimes associated with micrognathia. A variety of other malformations have also been reported. The coexistence of splenic–gonadal fusion and limb bud anomalies indicates that the lesion may be induced between the fifth and eighth weeks of gestation. In patients without associated congenital abnormalities the clinical presentation is in the form of a scrotal mass or an inguinal mass. The latter may be discovered during an operation for an inguinal hernia, which is present in more than one-third of the cases, or for an undescended testis, which has been present in about one-sixth of the cases. Two patients have had pain in the scrotum associated with attacks of malaria.

POLYORCHIDISM

Approximately 50 examples of this condition have been reported.[185-188] Among the patients with this disorder, from two to five testes have been present within the scrotum. Although usually discovered during childhood or early adult life, the condition has occasionally gone undetected until the seventh decade.

INFARCTS, HEMATOMAS, AND VASCULITIS

Torsion of the spermatic cord with resultant testicular infarction necessitates an orchiectomy in approximately 40 percent of cases.[189] Torsion of the testicular appendages may simulate torsion of the entire organ, but the former diagnosis is usually readily apparent on exploration.[190] Occasionally, a testicular infarct may simulate a neoplasm on clinical examination.[191]

Although testicular hemorrhage is usually a complication of a malignant neoplasm, we have seen one case in which rupture of an artery involved by arteritis led to the formation of a large hematoma (Fig. 5-42) which simulated a choriocarcinoma on gross examination. The arteritis had the microscopic features of polyarteritis nodosa, but was confined to the testis (Fig. 5-43); the patient was alive and well 14 years after orchiectomy. We have seen one other patient with long-term follow-up data, in whom necrotizing arteritis was confined to the testis.

The testes may be involved in patients with polyarteritis nodosa.[192-194] In one autopsy study 93 percent of patients with this disease were found to have one or more testicular abnormalities, including characteristic arterial lesions in 86 percent of the cases, recent infarcts in 27 percent, healed infarcts in 30 percent, hematomas in 5 percent, interstitial hemorrhage in 55 percent, and varying degrees of atrophy and tubular hyalinization in most of the cases.[192] The testes were abnormally small in 25 percent of the patients and the tunica vaginalis often exhibited blue or red

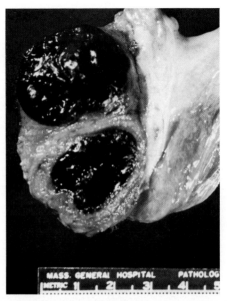

Fig. 5-42. Hematoma of testis associated with localized necrotizing vasculitis.

mottled discoloration. Despite the frequency of these morphologic abnormalities, only 9 percent of the patients had complained of testicular pain or tenderness. The authors of this study estimated that a testicular biopsy specimen should be diagnostic of polyarteritis in approximately 20 percent of patients with that disease and symptoms referable to testicular involvement based on the distribution of the arterial lesions within the testis. Testicular involvement has also been reported in cases of Henoch-Schönlein purpura[195] and in patients with juvenile rheumatoid arthritis.[196]

PAPILLARY CYSTADENOMA OF THE EPIDIDYMIS

Price[197] reviewed 20 cases of this type of tumor[197-199] in 1970, including some from the files of the Armed Forces Institute of Pathology. The tumors occurred in patients with a wide age range and were bilateral in approximately one-third of the cases; the bilateral tumors were usually associated with concomitant or subsequent evidence of von Hippel-Lindau's disease.[200] The diameter of the tumors ranged up to 5 cm; they were cys-

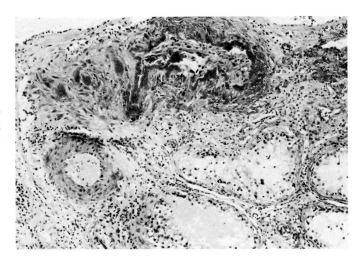

Fig. 5-43. Arteritis of testis. Extensive fibrinoid necrosis of wall of large artery. H & E. × 125. Same case as Figure 5-36.

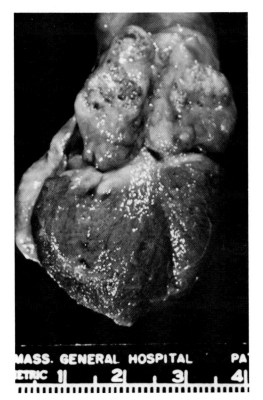

MASS. GENERAL HOSPITAL

Fig. 5-44. Papillary cystadenoma of epididymis from a patient with von Hippel-Lindau's disease. A lobulated mass, which was yellow, has replaced the epididymis.

tic, solid, or cystic and solid (Fig. 5-44). Microscopic examination discloses tubules and cysts, which may contain complex papillae (Fig. 5-45), lined by cytologically benign columnar cells; the lining cells often contain clear, glycogen-rich cytoplasm.

A small number of carcinomas of the epididymis have been reported;[201-203] we have seen one example of the papillary, clear-cell type, which may be the malignant counterpart of the papillary cystadenoma. Because of the rarity of primary carcinomas of the epididymis, the possibility of a metastatic carcinoma[204] should be considered in the differential diagnosis when a malignant epithelial tumor is encountered at this site. Benign and malignant soft tissue tumors of various types have also been reported in the epididymis, with smooth muscle tumors most commonly encountered.[205-207] Very rare teratomas of the epididymis have been reported.[208]

RETINAL ANLAGE TUMOR (MELANOTIC NEUROECTODERMAL TUMOR, MELANOTIC HAMARTOMA, MELANOTIC PROGONOMA) OF THE EPIDIDYMIS

The retinal anlage tumor occurs most often in the maxilla of young children, but four examples that arose in the epididymis have been

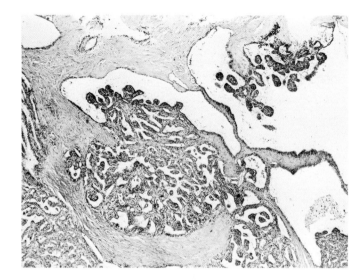

Fig. 5-45. Papillary cystadenoma of epididymis. Tubules and cysts with papillae projecting into their lumens. H & E. × 75.

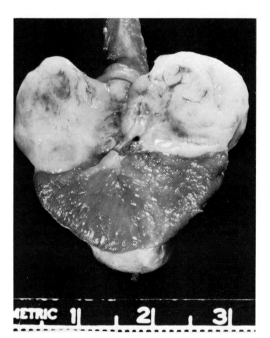

Fig. 5-46. Retinal anlage tumor of epididymis. Well-circumscribed mass that was predominantly cream-colored abuts the testis. Arrow points to an area of discoloration that was grayish-brown.

reported in detail.[209-213] Three additional tumors of this type have been seen at the Armed Forces Institute of Pathology,[9] and we have encountered an additional case at our hospital (Figs. 5-46, 5-47). Seven of the eight patients were 6 months of age or less, and one was 2 years old.[9] Seven tumors were 3 cm or less in diameter, and one was described as having "largely replaced the epididymis."[213] On gross examination, the tumors may be closely apposed to the testis, but do not invade it. Most of them have been well-circumscribed and round to oval, but the tumor reported by Johnson et al.[213] had an "irregular" margin. In that case microscopic foci of metastatic tumor were present in inguinal and retroperitoneal lymph nodes, including a lymph node from the right renal pedicle. The sectioned surfaces of the neoplasm are typically brown or black, at least focally, but may be predominantly cream-colored or gray (Fig. 5-46). Microscopic examination reveals nests, cords, and spaces composed of or lined by cells of two types: cuboidal cells, many of which contain melanin pigment in their cytoplasm; and smaller cells with round to oval, hyperchromatic nuclei and scant cytoplasm, resembling the cells of a neuroblastoma (Fig. 5-47). These cellular components are dispersed in a typically prominent fibrous stroma (Fig. 5-47). The patient from our hospital was well 3 years postoperatively; six other patients for whom follow-up data are available, including the child with lymph node metastases, were alive and well from 1 to 4 years after presentation.

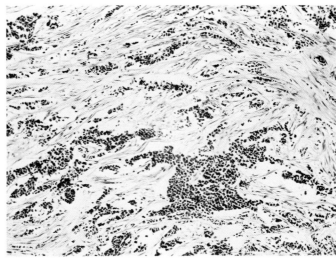

Fig. 5-47. Retinal anlage tumor of epididymis. Irregularly shaped nests of small round cells with prominent fibromatous stroma. H & E. × 156.

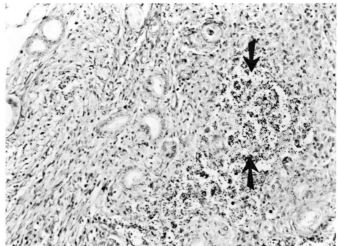

Fig. 5-48. Vasitis nodosa with sperm granuloma. Small tubules have invaded the wall of the vas. A sperm granuloma is indicated by arrows. H & E. × 156.

SPERM GRANULOMA OF EPIDIDYMIS AND VAS DEFERENS

In cases of this lesion, which almost always involves the epididymis or vas deferens[214-219] (Fig. 5-48), a granulomatous reaction to extravasated sperm produces a painful nodule, which may measure up to 4 cm in greatest dimension[217] and has occasionally been mistaken for a testicular tumor[215] and treated by orchiectomy.[220] Sperm granulomas are now seen most often in patients who have had a vasectomy[217-219] in whom they are encountered in up to 42 percent of cases.[219] In some patients the lesion may be associated with a history of trauma or inflammation.[214] Approximately 90 percent of sperm granulomas encountered after vasectomy are in the vas and 10 percent in the epididymis.[217] Those occurring in the vas are associated with vasitis nodosa (Fig. 5-48) in approximately one-third of the cases.[217]

On gross examination, sperm granulomas are typically firm but may have small, soft yellow to white foci on sectioning.[215] The microscopic appearance varies depending on the stage of the process. In the initial phase there is an infiltrate of neutrophils which is gradually replaced by epithelioid histiocytes that surround the sperm and give the most characteristic appearance of this lesion (Fig. 5-48); calcification is occasionally seen.[215, 217] In the later stages of the lesion there is progressive fibrosis and hyalinization, and lipochrome pigment may be prominent.[215]

VASITIS NODOSA

This process,[221-223] which has also been referred to by a number of other terms,[222] is characterized by an irregular proliferation of small ductlike structures within the wall, and occasionally extending to the adventitia, of the vas deferens[222] (Fig. 5-48). It is believed to develop in most cases secondary to obstruction, which results in increased intraluminal pressure and escape of sperm into the wall of the vas, with the formation of a sperm granuloma. In one study,[222] sperm granulomas were found in about half the cases of vasitis nodosa. This process is followed by penetration of the wall by ductal epithelium. The lesion is encountered most often as a complication of vasectomy but may also develop in the absence of such a history, possibly due to inflammation in some cases.[225]

Vasitis nodosa, which is occasionally bilateral,[222, 226] presents typically as a firm, fusiform nodule, usually 1 cm or less in greatest dimension, in the scrotal portion of the vas.[222] Sectioning reveals tissue that is usually white and may contain milky fluid. Low-power microscopic examination reveals a haphazard arrangement of ductules lined by cuboidal epithelium which may simulate the appearance of a low-grade adenocarcinoma. Invasion of nerves by the proliferating epithelium may enhance the resemblance to carcinoma.[224-226] The epithelial lining cells may exhibit reactive atypia but on high-power examination the cytologic features are not those of a malignant tumor. The association with a sperm granu-

loma and the presence of sperm within the lumens of the ductules in many of the cases are of additional help in establishing the benign nature of the process. This lesion is analogous to the form of endosalpingiosis[227] that develops in women after operations on the fallopian tube and the appearance of haphazardly arranged small ductules in vasitis nodosa has been compared[221, 222] to salpingitis isthmica nodosa occurring in the fallopian tube.[228]

REFERENCES

1. Mostofi FK, Sobin LH: Histologic types of tumors of the testis. International Histological Classification of Tumours, No. 16. World Health Organization, Geneva, 1977
2. Nochomovitz LE, Orenstein JM: Adenocarcinoma of the rete testis. Case report, ultrastructural observations, and clinicopathologic correlates. Am J Surg Pathol 8:625, 1984
3. Fukunaga M, Aizawa S, Furusato M et al: Papillary adenocarcinoma of the rete testis. A case report. Cancer 50:134, 1982
4. Gisser SD, Nayak S, Kaneko M, Tchertkoff V: Adenocarcinoma of the rete testis: a review of the literature and report of a case with associated asbestosis. Hum Pathol 8:219, 1977
5. Golden A, Ash JE: Adenomatoid tumors of the genital tract. Am J Pathol 21:63, 1945
6. Longo VJ, McDonald JR, Thompson GJ: Primary neoplasms of the epididymis. Special reference to adenomatoid tumors. JAMA 147:937, 1951
7. Broth G, Bullock WK, Morrow J: Epididymal tumors: I. Report of 15 new cases including review of literature. 2. Histochemical study of the so-called adenomatoid tumor. J Urol 100:530, 1968
8. Yasuma T, Saito S: Adenomatoid tumor of the male genital tract. A pathological study of eight cases and review of the literature. Acta Pathol Jpn 30:883, 1980
9. Mostofi FK, Price EB: Tumors of the male genital system. In Atlas of Tumor Pathology, second series, Fascicle 8. Armed Forces Institute of Pathology, Washington, D.C., 1973
10. Viprakasit D, Tannenbaum M, Smith AM: Adenomatoid tumor of the male genital tract. Urology 4:325, 1974

11. DeKlerk DP, Nime F: Adenomatoid tumors (mesothelioma) of testicular and paratesticular tissue. Urology 6:635, 1975

12. Miller F, Lieberman MK: Local invasion in adenomatoid tumors. Cancer 21:933, 1968

13. Nogales FF, Matill A, Ortega I, Alvares T: Mixed Brenner and adenomatoid tumor of the testis. An ultrastructural study and histogenetic considerations. Cancer 43:539, 1979

14. Fisher ER, Klieger H: Epididymal carcinoma (malignant adenomatoid tumor, mesonephric, mesodermal carcinoma of epididymis). J Urol 95:568, 1966

15. Söderström J, Liedberg CF: Malignant "adenomatoid" tumor of the epididymis. Acta Pathol Microbiol Scand 67:165, 1966

16. Jackson JR: The histogenesis of the "adenomatoid" tumor of the genital tract. Cancer 11:337, 1958

17. Sundarasivarao D: The mullerian vestiges and benign epithelial tumors of the epididymis. J Pathol Bacteriol 66:417, 1953

18. Hanrahan JB: A combined papillary mesothelioma and adenomatoid tumor of the omentum. Cancer 16:1497, 1963

19. Taxy JB, Battifora H, Oyasu R: Adenomatoid tumors: a light microscopic, histochemical, and ultrastructural study. Cancer 34:306, 1974

20. MacKay B, Bennington JL, Skoglund RW: The adenomatoid tumor: fine structural evidence for a mesothelial origin. Cancer 27:109, 1971

21. Davy CL, Tang C-K: Are all adenomatoid tumors adenomatoid mesotheliomas? Hum Pathol 12:360, 1981

22. Barwick KW, Madri JA: An immunohistochemical study of adenomatoid tumors utilizing keratin and Factor VIII antibodies. Evidence for a mesothelial origin. Lab Invest 47:276, 1982

23. Said J, Nash G, Lee M: Immunoperoxidase localization of keratin proteins, carcinoembryonic antigen, and factor VIII in adenomatoid tumors: Evidence for a mesothelial derivation. Hum Pathol 13:1106, 1982

24. Bell DA, Flotte TJ: Factor VIII related antigen in adenomatoid tumors. Implications for histogenesis. Cancer 50:932, 1982

25. Mucientes F, Govindarajan S, Burotto S: Immunoperoxidase study of adenomatoid tumor of the epididymis using anti-mesothelial cell serum. Cancer 55:363, 1985

26. Nistal M, Paniagua R, Fuentes E, Regadera J: Histogenesis of adenomatoid tumor associated to pseudofibromatous periorchitis in an infant with hydrocele. J Pathol 144:275, 1984

27. Kasdon EJ: Malignant mesothelioma of the tunica vaginalis propria testis. Report of two cases. Cancer 23:1144, 1969

28. Fligiel Z, Kaneko M: Malignant mesothelioma of the tunica vaginalis propria testis in a patient with asbestos exposure. A case report. Cancer 37:1478, 1976

29. Eimoto T, Inoue I: Malignant fibrous mesothelioma of the tunica vaginalis. A histologic and ultrastructural study. Cancer 39:2059, 1977

30. Japko L, Horta AA, Schreiber K et al: Malignant mesothelioma of the tunica vaginalis testis. Report of first case with preoperative diagnosis. Cancer 48:119, 1982

31. Mikuz G, Hopfel-Kreiner I: Papillary mesothelioma of the tunica vaginalis propria testis. Case report and ultrastructural study. Virchows Arch (Pathol Anat) 396:231, 1982

32. Chen KT, Arhelger RB, Flam MS, Hanson JH: Malignant mesothelioma of tunica vaginalis testis. Urology 20:316, 1982

33. McDonald RE, Sago AL, Novicki DE, Bagnall JW: Paratesticular mesotheliomas. J Urol 130:360, 1983

34. Antman K, Cohen S, Dimitrov NV et al: Malignant mesothelioma of the tunica vaginalis testis. J Clin Oncol 2:447, 1984

35. Hershman BR, Ross MR: Papillary cystadenoma within the testis. Am J Clin Pathol 61:724, 1974

36. Kellert E: An ovarian type pseudomucinous cystadenoma in the scrotum. Cancer 12:187, 1959

37. Goldman RL: A Brenner tumor of the testis. Cancer 26:853, 1970

38. Vechinski TO, Jaeschke WH, Vermund H: Testicular tumors. An analysis of 112 consecutive cases. Am J Roentgenol 95:495, 1965

39. Ross L. Paratesticular Brenner-like tumor. Cancer 21:722, 1968

40. Hargreaves HK, Scully RE, Richie JP: Benign hemangioendothelioma of the testis: case report with electron microscopic documentation and review of the literature. Am J Clin Pathol 77:637, 1982

41. Henline RB: The differential diagnosis and treatment of tumors of the testicle with report of a case of bilateral fibroma of the testes. J Urol 32:177, 1934

42. Collins DH, Symington T: Sertoli-cell tumor. Br J Urol 36:52, 1964

43. Honore LH, Sullivan LD: Intratesticular leiomyoma: a case report with discussion of differential diagnosis and histogenesis. J Urol 114:631, 1975

44. Livolsi V, Schiff M: Myxoid neurofibroma of the testis. J Urol 118:341, 1977

45. Ravich L, Lerman PH, Drabkin JW, Foltin E: Pure testicular rhabdomyosarcoma. J Urol 94:596, 1965

46. Matthew T, Prabhakaran K: Osteosarcoma of the testis. Arch Pathol Lab Med 105:38, 1981

47. Teppo L: Testicular cancer in Finland. Acta Pathol Microbiol Scand [A] (Suppl 238):7, 1973

48. Ferguson JD: Tumors of the testis. Br J Urol 34:407, 1962

49. Abell MR, Holtz F: Testicular and paratesticular neoplasms in patients 60 years of age and older. Cancer 21:852, 1968

50. Gowing NFC: Malignant lymphoma of the testis. Br J Urol 36:85, 1964

51. Gowing NFC: Malignant lymphoma of the testis. P. 334. In Pugh RCB (ed): Pathology of the Testis. Blackwell Scientific Publications, Oxford, 1976

52. Kiely JM, Massey BD, Harrison EG, Utz DC: Lymphoma of the testis. Cancer 26:847, 1970

53. Sussman EB, Hajdu SI, Lieberman PH, Whitmore WF: Malignant lymphoma of the testis: a clinicopathological study of 37 cases. J Urol 118:1004, 1977

54. Talerman A: Primary malignant lymphoma of the testis. J Urol 118:783, 1977

55. Jackson SM, Montessori GA: Malignant lymphoma of the testis: review of 17 cases in British Columbia with survival related to pathological subclassification. J Urol 123:881, 1980

56. Read G: Lymphomas of the testis—results of treatment 1960–77. Clin Radiol 32:687, 1981

57. Paladugu RR, Bearman RM, Rappaport H: Malignant lymphoma with primary manifestation in the gonad. A clinicopathologic study of 38 patients. Cancer 45:561, 1980

58. Duncan PR, Checa F, Gowing NFC et al: Extranodal non-Hodgkin's lymphoma presenting in the testicle. A clinical and pathologic study of 24 cases. Cancer 45:1578, 1980

59. Turner RR, Colby TV, MacKintosh FR: Testicular lymphomas: A clinicopathologic study of 35 cases. Cancer 48:2095, 1981

60. Buskirk SJ, Evans RG, Banks PM et al: Primary lymphoma of the testis. Int J Radiat Oncol Biol Phys 8:1699, 1982

61. Baldetorp LA, Brunkvall J, Cavallin-Stahl E, et al: Malignant lymphoma of the testis. Br J Urol 56:525, 1984

62. Hamlin JA, Kagan AR, Friedman NB: Lymphomas of the testicle. Cancer 29:1352, 1972

63. Sampat MB, Sirsat MV, Kamat MR: Malignant lymphoma of the testis in Indians. Br J Urol 46:569, 1974

64. Battifora H, Sheibani K, Tubbs RR et al: Antikeratin antibodies in tumor diagnosis: Distinction between seminoma and embryonal carcinoma. Cancer 54:843, 1984

65. Jass JR, Farrell MA, Ellis H: Pseudolymphoma of the testis. Br J Urol 56:102, 1984

66. Pasmantier MW, Azar HA: Extraskeletal spread in multiple plasma cell myeloma. A review of 57 autopsied cases. Cancer 23:167, 1969

67. Hayes DW, Bennett WA, Heck FJ: Extramedullary lesions in multiple myeloma—review of literature and pathologic studies. Arch Pathol 53:262, 1952

68. Gordon AJ, Churg J: Visceral involvement in multiple myeloma. NY State J Med 49:282, 1949

69. Dolin S, Dewar JP: Extramedullary plasmacytoma. Am J Pathol 32:83, 1956

70. Carson CP, Ackerman LV, Maltby JD: Plasma cell myeloma—clinical, pathologic and roentgenologic review of 90 cases. Am J Clin Pathol 25:849, 1955

71. Anderson PF: Extramedullary plasmacytomas. Acta Radiol 32:365, 1949

72. Ulrich H: Multiple myeloma. Arch Intern Med 64:994, 1939

73. Weitzner S: Metastatic plasma cell myeloma in testis—report of a case and review of the literature. Rocky Mt Med J 66:48, 1969

74. Melicow MM, Cahill GF: Plasmacytoma (multiple myeloma) of testis: a report of four cases and review of the literature. J Urol 71:103, 1951

75. Osman R, Morrow JW: Myeloma of the testicle: a case report. J Urol 96:353, 1966
76. Chica G, Johnson DE, Ayala AG: Plasmacytoma of testis presenting as primary testicular tumor. Urology 11:90, 1978
77. Levin HS, Mostofi FK: Symptomatic plasmacytoma of the testis. Cancer 25:1193, 1970
78. Kirshbaum JD: Metastatic plasma cell myeloma of the testicles. Urol Cutan Rev 51:456, 1947
79. Soumerai S, Gleason EA: Asynchromous plasmacytoma of the stomach and testis. Cancer 45:396, 1980
80. Steinberg D: Plasmacytoma of the testis. Report of a case. Cancer 36:1470, 1975
81. Oldham RK, Polmar SH: Extramedullary plasmacytomas following successful radiotherapy of Hodgkin's disease—clinical and immunologic aspects. Am J Med 54:761, 1973
82. Givler RL: Testicular involvement in leukemia and lymphoma. Cancer 23:1290, 1969
83. Reid H, Marsden HB: Gonadal infiltration in children with leukemia and lymphoma. J Clin Pathol 33:722, 1980
84. Jampol ML, Ohnysty J: Acute leukemia seen as testicular tumor. NY State J Med 67:1903, 1967
85. Nies BA, Bodey GP, Thomas LB et al: The persistence of extramedullary leukemic infiltrates during bone marrow remission of acute leukemia. Blood 26:133, 1965
86. Finkelstein JZ, Dyment PG, Hammond GD: Leukemic infiltration of the testes during bone marrow remission. Pediatrics 43:1042, 1969
87. Stoffel TJ, Nesbit ME, Levitt SH: Extramedullary involvement of the testes in childhood leukemia. Cancer 35:1203, 1975
88. Kuo T-T, Tschang T-P, Chu J-Y: Testicular relapse in childhood acute lymphocytic leukemia during bone marrow remission. Cancer 38:2604, 1976
89. Saiontz HI, Gilchrist GS, Smithson WA et al: Testicular relapse in childhood leukemia. Mayo Clin Proc 53:212, 1978
90. Eden OB, Hardisty RM, Innes EM et al: Testicular disease in acute lymphoblastic leukaemia in childhood. Br Med J 1:334, 1978
91. Nesbit ME, Robison LL, Ortega JA et al: Testicular relapse in childhood acute lymphoblastic leukemia: association with pretreatment patient characteristics and treatment. Cancer 45:2009, 1980
92. Sullivan MP, Perez CA, Herson J et al: Radiotherapy (2500 RAD) for testicular leukemia: local control and subsequent clinical events: A Southwest Oncology Group study. Cancer 46:508, 1980
93. Askin FB, Land VJ, Sullivan MP et al: Occult testicular leukemia: testicular biopsy at three years' continuous complete remission of childhood leukemia: a Southwest Oncology Group Study. Cancer 47:470, 1981
94. Klein EA, Kay R, Norris DG: Incidence and detection of testicular leukemia in children. Cleve Clin Q 51:401, 1984
95. Smith SD, Trueworthy RC, Klopovich PM, et al: Management of children with isolated testicular leukemia. Cancer 54:2854, 1984
96. Haupt HM, Mann RB, Trump DL, Abeloff MD: Metastatic carcinoma involving the testis. Clinical and pathologic distinction from primary testicular neoplasms. Cancer 54:709, 1984
97. Tiltman AJ: Metastatic tumors in the testis. Histopathology 3:31, 1979
98. Price EB, Mostofi FK: Secondary carcinoma of the testis. Cancer 10:592, 1957
99. Pienkos EJ, Jablokow VR: Secondary testicular tumors. Cancer 30:481, 1972
100. Meares EM, Ho TL: Metastatic carcinomas involving the testis: a review. J Urol 109:653, 1973
101. Hanash KA, Carney JA, Kelalis PP: Metastatic tumor to testicles: routes of metastases. J Urol 102:465, 1969
102. Weitzner S: Survival of patients with secondary carcinoma of prostate in the testis. Cancer 32:447, 1973
103. Lowell DM, Lewis EJ: Melanospermia: a hitherto undescribed entity. J Urol 95:407, 1966
104. Johnson DE, Jackson L, Ayala AG: Secondary carcinoma of the testis. South Med J 64:1128, 1971
105. Dockerty MB, Scheifley CH: Metastasizing carcinoid. Report of an unusual case with episodic cyanosis. Am J Clin Pathol 25:770, 1955
106. Price EB, Mostofi FK: Epidermoid cysts of the testis in children: a report of four cases. J Pediatr 77:676, 1970
107. Price EB: Epidermoid cysts of the testis: a clinical and pathologic analysis of 69 cases from the testicular tumor registry. J Urol 102:708, 1969

108. Shah KH, Maxted WC, Chun B: Epidermoid cysts of the testis: a report of three cases and analysis of 141 cases from the world literature. Cancer 47:577, 1981

109. Schmidt SS: Congenital simple cyst of the testis: a hitherto undescribed lesion. J Urol 96:236, 1966

110. Tosi SE, Richardson JR: Simple cyst of the testis: case report and review of the literature. J Urol 114:473, 1975

111. Takihara H, Valvo JR, Tokuhara M, Cockett ATK: Intratesticular cysts. Urology 20:80, 1982

112. Warner KE, Noyes DT, Ross JS: Cysts of the tunica albuginea testis: a report of 3 cases with a review of the literature. J Urol 132:131, 1984

113. Van Niekerk WA: True hermaphroditism. Pediat Adolesc Endocrinol 8:80, 1981

114. Leissring JC, Oppenheimer ROF: Cystic dysplasia of the testis: a unique congenital anomaly studied by microdissection. J Urol 110:362, 1973

115. Fisher JE, Jewett TC, Nelson SJ, Jockin H: Ectasia of the rete testis with ipsilateral renal agenesis. J Urol 128:1040, 1982

116. Nistal M, Regardera J, Paniagua R: Cystic dysplasia of the testis. Light and Electron Microscopic study of three cases. Arch Pathol Lab Med 108:579, 1984

117. Mikuz G, Damjanov I: Inflammation of the testis, epididymis, peritesticular membranes, and scrotum. Pathol Annu 17:101, 1982

118. Morgan AD: Inflammation and infestation of the testis and paratesticular structures. p. 79. In Pugh RCB (ed): Pathology of the Testis. Blackwell Scientific Publications, Oxford, 1976

119. Honore LH: Nonspecific peritesticular fibrosis manifested as testicular enlargement. Clinicopathological study of nine cases. Arch Surg 113:814, 1978

120. Hourihane D O'B: Infected infarcts of the testis: a study of 18 cases preceded by pyogenic epididymo-orchitis. J Clin Pathol 23:668, 1970

121. Werner CA: Mumps orchitis and testicular atrophy. I. Occurrence. Ann Intern Med 32:1066, 1950

122. Werner CA: Mumps orchitis and testicular atrophy. II. A factor in male sterility. Ann Intern Med 32:1075, 1950

123. Gall EA: The histopathology of acute mumps orchitis. Am J Pathol 23:637, 1947

124. Beard CM, Benson RC, Kelalis PP et al: The incidence and outcome of mumps orchitis in Rochester, Minnesota, 1935 to 1974. Mayo Clin Proc 52:3, 1977

125. Riggs S, Sanford JP: Viral orchitis. N Engl Med 266:990, 1962

126. Wolnisty C: Orchitis as a complication of infectious mononucleosis. N Engl J Med 266:88, 1962

127. Craighead JE, Mahoney EM, Carver DH et al: Orchitis due to Coxsackie Virus Group B, Type 5: report of a case with isolation of virus from the testis. N Engl J Med 267:498, 1962

128. Wechsler H, Westfall M, Lattimer JK: The earliest signs and symptoms in 127 male patients with genitourinary tuberculosis. J Urol 83:801, 1960

129. Ferrie BG, Rundle JSH: Tuberculous epididymo-orchitis. A review of 20 cases. Br J Urol 55:437, 1983

130. Veenema RJ, Lattimer JK: Genital tuberculosis in the male: clinical pathology and effect on fertility. J Urol 78:65, 1957

131. Christensen WI: Genitourinary tuberculosis: review of 102 cases. Medicine 53:377, 1974

132. Kahn RI, McAninch JW: Granulomatous disease of the testis. J Urol 123:868, 1980

133. Grabstald H, Swan LL: Genitourinary lesions in leprosy. With special reference to the problem of atrophy of the testes. JAMA 149:1287, 1952

134. Bernard JC, Vazquez CAJ: Visceral lesions in lepromatous leprosy. Study of sixty necropsies. Int J Leprosy 41:94, 1973

135. Watson RA, Gangai MP, Skinsnes OK: Genitourinary leprosy. Urol Int 29:312, 1974

136. El-Shiemy S, El-Hefnawi H, Abdel-Fattah A, et al: Testicular and epididymal involvement in leprosy patients, with special reference to gynecomastia. Int J Dermatol 15:52, 1976

137. Akhtar M, Ali MA, Mackey DM: Lepromatous leprosy presenting as orchitis. Am J Clin Pathol 73:712, 1980

138. Menninger WC: Congenital syphilis of the testicle. With report of twelve autopsied cases. Am J Syphilis 12:221, 1928

139. Grobert MJ, Bischoff AJ: Actinomycosis of the testicle: case report. J Urol 87:567, 1962

140. Longcope WT: Sarcoidosis or Besnier-Boeck-

Schaumann disease. JAMA 117:1321, 1941

141. Longcope WT, Frieman DG: A study of sarcoidosis. Medicine 31:1, 1952

142. Krauss L: Genital sarcoidosis. Case report and review of the literature. J Urol 80:367, 1958

143. Amenta PS, Gonick P, Katz SM: Sarcoidosis of testis and epididymis. Urology 17:616, 1981

144. Morgan AD: Inflammatory lesions simulating malignancy. Br J Urol 36(suppl):95, 1964

145. Capers TH: Granulomatous orchitis. Am J Clin Pathol 34:139, 1960

146. Spjut H, Thorpe J: Granulomatous orchitis. Am J Clin Pathol 26:136, 1956

147. Lynch VP, Eakins D, Morrison E: Granulomatous orchitis. Br J Urol 40:451, 1968

148. Fajardo LF, Dueker GE, Kosek JC: Light and electron microscopic observations on granulomatous orchitis. Invest Urol 6:158, 1968

149. Mikuz G: Ultrastructural study of two cases of granulomatous orchitis. Virchows Arch (Pathol Anat) 360:223, 1973

150. McClure J: Malakoplakia of the testis and its relationship to granulomatous orchitis. J Clin Pathol 33:670, 1980

151. Haukoul RS, Chinchinian H: Malakoplakia of the testicle. Report of a case. Am J Clin Pathol 29:473, 1958

152. Brown RC, Smith BH: Malakoplakia of the testis. Am J Clin Pathol 47:135, 1967

153. Damjanov I, Katz SM: Malakoplakia. Pathol Ann 16:103, 1981

154. McClure J: Malakoplakia. J Pathol 140:275, 1983

155. Lou TY, Teplitz C: Malakoplakia. Pathogenesis and ultrastructural morphogenesis. Hum Pathol 5:191, 1974

156. McClurg FV, D'Agostino AN, Martin JH, Race GH: Ultrastructural demonstration of intracellular bacteria in three cases of malakoplakia of the bladder. Am J Clin Pathol 60:780, 1973

157. Tamura H, Iannoti HM: Ultrastructure of Michaelis-Gutmann body. A study of testicular malakoplakia. Arch Pathol 98:409, 1974

158. Smetana HF, Bernhard W: Sclerosing lipogranuloma. Arch Pathol 50:296, 1950

159. Arduino LJ: Sclerosing lipogranuloma of male genitalia. J Urol 82:155, 1959

160. Oertel YC, Johnson FB: Sclerosing lipogranuloma of male genitalia. Review of 23 cases. Arch Pathol Lab Med. 101:321, 1977

161. Goodwin WE: Multiple, benign, fibrous tumors of tunica vaginalis testis. J Urol 56:438, 1946

162. Lewis HY, Pierce JM: Multiple fibromas of the tunica vaginalis. J Urol 87:142, 1962

163. Orlay G: Multiple fibromata of the tunica vaginalis. Review of the literature and case report. Br J Surg 49:66, 1961

164. Benisch B, Peison B, Sobel HJ, Marquet E: Fibrous mesotheliomas (pseudofibroma) of the scrotal sac: a light and ultrastructural study. Cancer 47:731, 1981

165. Shafik A: Constrictive albuginitis: report of 3 cases. J Urol 122:269, 1979

166. Lin JI, Tseng CH, Marsidi PJ, Bais VC: Cholesterol granuloma of right testis. Urology 14:522, 1979

167. Lowenthal SB, Goldstein AMB, Terry R: Cholesterol granuloma of tunica vaginalis simulating testicular tumor. Urology 18:89, 1981

168. Kokotas N, Kontogeorsos L, Kyriakidis A: Calcification of the tunica vaginalis. Br J Urol 55:128, 1983

169. Priebe CJ Jr, Garret R: Testicular calcification in a 4-year-old boy. Pediatrics 46:785, 1970

170. Weinberg AG, Curranino G, Stone IC Jr: Testicular microlithiasis. Arch Pathol 95:312, 1973

171. Schantz A, Milsten R: Testicular microlithiasis with sterility. Fertil Steril 27:801, 1976

172. Vegni-Talluri M, Bigliardi E, Vanni MG, Tota G: Testicular microliths: their origin and structure. J Urol 124:105, 1980

173. Coetzee T: Pulmonary alveolar microlithiasis with involvement of the sympathetic nervous system and gonads. Thorax 25:637, 1970

174. Sohval AR: Histopathology of cryptorchidism. A study based upon the comparative histology of retained and scrotal testes from birth to maturity. Am J Med 16:346, 1954

175. Bieger RC, Passarge E, McAdams AJ: Testicular intratubular bodies. J Clin Endocrinol 25:1340, 1965

176. Dahl EV, Bahn RC: Aberrant adrenal cortical tissue near the testis in human infants. Am J Pathol 40:587, 1962

177. Nelson AA: Accessory adrenal cortical tissue. Arch Pathol 27:955, 1939

178. Olken HG: Accessory splenic tissue within the scrotum. Report of a case. Am J Pathol 21:81, 1945

179. Putschar WG, Manion WC: Splenic–gonadal fusion. Am J Pathol 32:15, 1956

180. Watson RJ: Splenogonadal fusion. Surgery 63:853, 1968

181. Mendez R, Morrow J: Ectopic spleen simulating testicular tumor. J Urol 102:598, 1969

182. Pendse AK, Mathur PN, Sharma MM, Gupta OP: Splenic–gonadal fusion. Br J Surg 62:624, 1975

183. Halvorsen JF, Stray O: Splenogonadal fusion. Acta Pediatr Scand 67:379, 1978

184. Wick MR, Rife CC: Paratesticular accessory spleen. Mayo Clin Proc 56:455, 1981

185. Butz RE, Croushore JH: Polyorchidism. J Urol 119:289, 1978

186. Pelander WM, Luna G, Lilly JR: Polyorchidism: case report and literature review. J Urol 119:705, 1978

187. Nocks BN: Polyorchidism with normal spermatogenesis and equal sized testes: A theory of embryological development. J Urol 120:638, 1978

188. Feldman S, Drach GW: Polyorchidism discovered as testicular torsion. J Urol 130:976, 1983

189. Skoglund RW, McRoberts JW, Ragde H: Torsion of the spermatic cord: a review of the literature and an analysis of 70 new cases. J Urol 104:604, 1970

190. Skoglund RW, McRoberts JW, Ragde H: Torsion of testicular appendages: presentation of 43 new cases and a collective review. J Urol 104:598, 1970

191. Shapiro JR, Rabinovitz J, Konrad P, Tesluk H: Focal infarction of the testicle in a child simulating testicular tumor. J Urol 118:485, 1977

192. Dahl EV, Baggenstoss AH, DeWeerd JH: Testicular lesions of periarteritis nodosa with special reference to diagnosis. Am J Med 28:222, 1960

193. Nuzum JW Jr, Nuzum JW Sr: Polyarteritis nodosa. Statistical review of one hundred seventy-five cases from the literature and report of a typical case. Arch Intern Med 94:942, 1954

194. Frohnert PP, Sheps SG: Long-term follow-up study of periarteritis nodosa. Am J Med 43:8, 1967

195. Mikuz G, Hofstadter F, Hager J: Testis involvement in Schonlein-Henoch Purpura. Pathol Res Pract 165:323, 1979

196. Tangney NJ: Testicular complications in connective tissue disease. Arch Dis Child 56:651, 1981

197. Price EB: Papillary cystadenoma of the epididymis. A clinicopathologic analysis of 20 cases. Arch Pathol 91:456, 1971

198. Sherrick JC: Papillary cystadenoma of the epididymis. Cancer 9:403, 1956

199. Tsuda H, Fukushima S, Takahashi M et al: Familial bilateral papillary cystadenoma of the epididymis. Report of three cases in siblings. Cancer 37:1831, 1976

200. Melmon KL, Rosen SW: Lindau's disease. Am J Med 36:595, 1964

201. Hinman F, Gibson TE: Tumors of the epididymis, spermatic cord and testicular tunics. A review of the literature and report of three new cases. Arch Surg 8:100, 1924

202. Salm R: Papillary carcinoma of the epididymis. J Pathol 97:253, 1969

203. Brown NJ: Miscellaneous tumours of epithelial type. p. 304 In Pugh RCB (ed): Pathology of the Testis. Blackwell Scientific Publications, Oxford, 1976

204. Brotherus JV: Metastatic tumors of the epididymis and the spermatic cord. J Urol 83:171, 1960

205. Williams G, Banerjee R: Paratesticular tumors. Br J Urol 41:332, 1969

206. DeLuise VP, Draper JW, Gray GF: Smooth muscle tumors of the testicular adnexa. J Urol 115:685, 1976

207. Farrell MA, Donnelly BJ: Malignant smooth muscle tumors of the epididymis. J Urol 124:151, 1980

208. Pap S, Kiss I: Teratoma of the epididymis. Int J Urol Nephrol 5:173, 1973

209. Eaton WL, Ferguson JP: Retinoblastic teratoma of the epididymis. Case report. Cancer 9:718, 1956

210. Frank GL, Koten JW: Melanotic hamartoma ("retinal anlage tumor") of the epididymis. J Pathol Bacteriol 84:307, 1962

211. Zone RM: Retinal anlage tumor of the epididymis. A case report. J Urol 103:106, 1970

212. Cutler LS, Chaudry AP, Topazian R: Melanotic neuroectodermal tumor of infancy: an ultrastructural study, literature review, and reevaluation. Cancer 48:257, 1981

213. Johnson RE, Scheithauer BW, Dahlin DC: Melanotic neuroectodermal tumor of infancy. A review of seven cases. Cancer 52:661, 1983

214. Friedman NB, Garske GL: Inflammatory reactions involving sperm and the seminiferous tubules: extravasation, spermatic granulomas and granulomatous orchitis. J Urol 62:363, 1949

215. Glassy FJ, Mostofi FK: Spermatic granulomas of the epididymis. Am J Clin Pathol 26:1303, 1956

216. Schmidt SS: Technics and complications of elective vasectomy. The role of spermatic granulomas in spontaneous recanalization. Fertil Steril 17:467, 1966

217. Schmidt SS, Morris RR: Spermatic granuloma: the complication of vasectomy. Fertil Steril 24:941, 1973

218. Leader AJ, Axelrad SD, Frankowski R, Mumford SD: Complications of 2,711 vasectomies. J Urol 111:365, 1974

219. Silber SJ: Sperm granuloma and reversibility of vasectomy. Lancet 2:588, 1977

220. Dunner PS, Lipsit ER, Nochomovitz LE: Epididymal sperm granuloma simulating a testicular neoplasm. J Clin Ultrasound 10:353, 1982

221. Benjamin JA, Robertson TD, Cheetham JG: Vasitis nodosa: A new clinical entity simulating tuberculosis of the vas deferens. J Urol 49:575, 1943

222. Civantos F, Lubin J, Rywlin AM: Vasitis nodosa. Arch Pathol 94:355, 1972

223. Taxy JB: Vasitis nodosa. Two cases. Arch Pathol Lab Med 102:643, 1978

224. Kovi J, Agbata A: Benign neural invasion in vasitis nodosa. JAMA 228:1519, 1974

225. Goldman RL, Azzopardi JG: Benign neural invasion in vasitis nodosa. Histopathology 6:309, 1982

226. Zimmerman KG, Johnson PC, Paplanus SH: Nerve invasion by benign proliferating ductules in vasitis nodosa. Cancer 51:2066, 1983

227. Sampson JA: Postsalpingectomy endometriosis (endosalpingiosis). Am J Obstet Gynecol 20:443, 1930

228. Schenken JR, Burns EL: A study and classification of nodular lesions of the fallopian tubes. Am J Obstet Gynecol 45:624, 1943

6

Testicular and Paratesticular Tumors of Childhood

F. Gonzalez-Crussi

GENERAL CONSIDERATIONS

The incidence of testicular tumors in boys is only about 2:100,000 with less than one child per million dying of the disease each year.[1, 2] It is not likely that a number of cases sufficiently large to permit statistically valid inferences could accumulate at a single institution in a reasonably short time. For instance, in 40 years of experience at the Department of Urology of the University of Iowa, 366 testicular tumors were seen, but only 18 were in patients under 16 years of age.[3] Twelve children with testicular tumors were seen in a comparable time period at the University of California at San Francisco.[4] Up to 1958 only 160 cases of malignant testicular neoplasms in children were described,[5] (although more than 464 testicular tumors, not always histologically defined, had been reported by 1954).[6] By 1965, the number[7] of verified cases had risen to 221. Since then, increased general awareness of the problem and earlier detection have resulted in a multitude of reports, to the extent that reviewers would find it impractical to attempt to compile the entire world's literature. Nonetheless, it remains true that a testicular tumor in a child is a rare event: only 3 percent of all testicular tumors occur in children under 15 years of age.[8] There is a rapid rise with the onset of puberty, yet the incidence is only 5.9 percent within the first two decades of life.[9] Later in life the higher mortality due to testicular malignancy is unquestionable: a definite "peak" appears in early adulthood, and a second one in old age. The mortality curve for testicular malignancies is thus said to be bimodal. Epidemiologic analyses have disclosed that it is trimodal; still a "third peak," albeit a minor one, is seen in white children at about 2 years of age.[2] As will be discussed subsequently, germ cell tumors occurring in infants, and particularly yolk sac (endodermal sinus) tumor, account for the small elevation noted at this early age.

In the last few decades, a remarkable rise in the incidence of testicular tumors was noted in the United States[10] and other countries,[11] particularly in Scandinavia, although not uniformly so.[12] There was talk of a veritable "epidemic,"[13] but little information was provided on the effect that this trend may have had on children. Li and Fraumeni[2] concluded that the effect was negligible, since the rates for children did not change over a period of 35 years, during which time testicular cancer rose by nearly 50 percent in young men. These conclusions, no doubt, will require further elaboration in terms of the different populations studied. For example, a report from India disclosed an unusually high percentage of testicular tumors (17.1 percent) in children.[14] The black African population, in contrast, displays a rarity of testis cancer,[15] in a similar way to Ewing's sarcoma which occurs so rarely in blacks as to suggest that blacks may be genetically protected from this neoplasm.[16] On the other hand, the African population of Uganda, in whom testicular tumors are generally rare, has a relative excess of yolk sac tumors (orchioblastoma).[17] Does this mean that testicular tumors in children result from factors other than those determining their appearance in older patients? Clearly, much work is required before this question can be answered satisfactorily. No specific etiologic factor has yet been identified in testicular malignancy, either of adults or children. The undescended testis seems more relevant to the former, but children have developed tumors[18] as early as 6 years. This and other congenital anomalies that may occur in conjunction with testicular tumor[19, 20] suggest that genetic factors may be more important in childhood testicular cancer than is commonly assumed. The definite documentation of familial involvement appears to support this statement, although such an occurrence is very rare.[21, 23] We may state that the cause is unknown, and that risk factors such as socioeconomic status, occupation, and urban (vs. rural) residence, may be significant[24] but must be interpreted in the light of more extensive demographic investigations before they can be acknowledged as clues to the origin of testicular cancer.

GERM CELL TUMORS

The major categories of testicular germ cell tumors seen in children correspond to those represented in general classifications of testicular tumors.[25] However, seminoma, malignant teratoma ("teratocarcinoma"), and choriocarcinoma are virtually never seen in prepubertal patients. Embryonal carcinoma, as this term is understood in most classifications, does not occur in children either; the exception is the classification plan devised by Mostofi and Price,[26] in which yolk sac carcinoma is considered to be a "juvenile" or "infantile" variant of embryonal carcinoma. The confusion produced by the nonuniform use of terms may be dispelled by reference to the histogenetic concepts embodied in the classification of Dixon and Moore,[27] which forms the base for all others. Embryonal carcinoma cells are considered to be multipotential anaplastic cells, capable of giving rise to any tissue found in the body. They are, in fact, primitive embryonic cells[28] indistinguishable from those of an early blastula. If they remain in this state of undifferentiation and form a tumor, the name of such a neoplasm is embryonal carcinoma. If they differentiate into somatic tissues, the result is a teratoma; if into structures found outside the embryo, the neoplasm is either a yolk sac carcinoma or choriocarcinoma. The influences that direct embryonal carcinoma cells along one or the other lines of differentiation are largely unknown, but experimental evidence indicates that these are environmental, inductive influences, just as occur during normal embryogenesis. Obviously, the possibility of manipulating the direction of differentiation, a theoretically feasible goal, will have to await detailed answers to many fundamental questions of developmental biology. However, the accepted tenet is that embryonal carcinoma cells are the progenitor cells of choriocarcinoma, teratoma, and yolk sac tumors. Hence, the implication is that even a fully mature teratoma began as a group of embryonal carcinoma cells, which eventually attained complete differentiation. It has been suggested that the totipotentiality of germ cells lessens with age.[29] It is of considerable theoretical interest to note that before puberty, embryonal carcinoma cells in patients with testicular tumors differentiate completely along somatic lines, or as extraembryonic yolk sac structures. Three-quarters of testicular tumors occurring before puberty are germ-cell tumors, almost all of which can be classified as either yolk sac carcinoma or teratoma; the remainder are non-germ cell neoplasms of Sertoli or Leydig cell origin.[14] Seminoma is nonexistent in patients before the age of 10, and is extremely rare thereafter, until late adolescence. Accordingly, the tumor types discussed in the present chapter will be those more commonly encountered. Because of the clinical importance of malignancies arising from paratesticular connective tissues in childen, a section is devoted to these tumors. A number of other tumors may manifest as testicular masses during childhood, chief

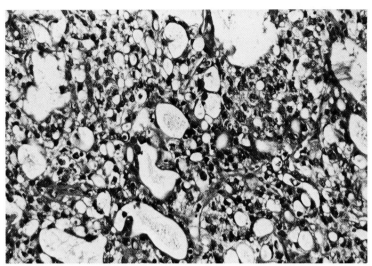

Fig. 6-1. "Honeycomb" pattern of growth, one of several histologic appearances of yolk sac tumor. H & E. × 225.

among which are lymphomas and leukemia. Discussion of this topic and of certain uncommon tumors that may affect the testicle in children is provided in Chapter 5.

YOLK SAC (ENDODERMAL SINUS) TUMOR

Yolk sac (endodermal sinus) tumor (YST, EST) has been a frequently used designation for the neoplasm defined by Teilum[31] as a primary gonadal neoplasm, but which now has been well-identified in a number of extragonadal sites.[32]

INCIDENCE AND APPEARANCE

As previously stated, this is the single most common germ cell tumor of the prepubertal testis. It corresponds to the entity that British authors referred to as orchioblastoma,[33] presumably because it was confined to infants and young children. However, the idea has prevailed that it is the same as yolk sac tumor in adults, with the difference, noted by Talerman,[34] that yolk sac tumor is found admixed with other germ cell tumors in adults, whereas in children it tends to occur in pure form. The varied microscopic patterns that this tumor may adopt have been well-described in the abundant literature on this malignancy in both gonadal and extragonadal sites.[31, 32, 34] Usually, epithelial cells are found immersed in a myxoid stroma (Fig. 6-1) but structural complexity results from the varied patterns of arrangement of the epithelial cells, which may produce interanastomotic network, "honeycombed" areas, cysts, diffuse masses, cavities and channels, and characteristic structures (PAS-positive globules, Schiller-Duval bodies) of diagnostic value (Fig. 6-2). During the last decade there has been sustained interest in identifying substances produced by tumor cells. Since it was demonstrated that the human yolk sac can produce various proteins, such as alpha-fetoprotein (AFP), alpha-1-antitrypsin (A_1AT), and transferrin,[35] it was logical to use such proteins as "markers" of diagnostic and prognostic usefulness. Implicit in much of the work published is the concept that mere production of alpha-fetoprotein is indicative of vitelline origin. This, however, is a postulate that has not been exempt from criticism. Thus, it has been pointed out that

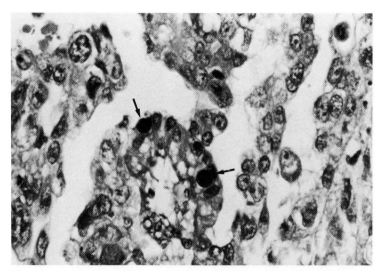

Fig. 6-2. PAS-positive, diastase-resistant "globules" (arrows) within epithelial cells of yolk sac tumor of testis. PAS with diastase digestion, × 450.

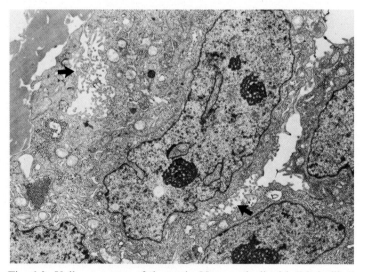

Fig. 6-3. Yolk sac tumor of the testis. Note nucleoli with "skein-like" nucleolonema, presence of microvilli (arrows), and extracellular, electron-dense deposits (upper, left side of illustration). × 17,500.

non-yolk-sac elements may be responsible for such biosynthesis,[36] which thus should not be made a criterion for classification. More important from a practical point of view has been the recent demonstration by Damjanov et al.[37] that cells from an AFP-positive yolk sac tumor may become AFP-negative, presumably as an effect of therapy. Accordingly, the search for appropriate "markers" must continue, and characterization of structural aspects by combined ultrastructural–histochemical or immunologic means is stillan appropriate endeavor for pathologists.

The ultrastructure of these tumors recapitulates, to a limited extent, that of the human yolk sac,[32] although similarities are not close.

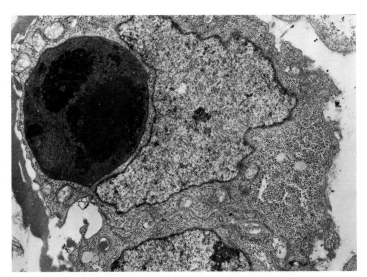

Fig. 6-4. Yolk sac tumor of testis. Large, complex secondary lysosome, abundant glycogen, and extracellular linear deposit of electron-dense substance that corresponded to material positive for PAS stain and AFP-immunostain of light microscopy. × 17,500.

Evidence of endodermal differentiation is the presence of cells with microvilli, well-developed lysosomes, and tight junctions. Other features include abundant glycogen in some cells, and prominent nucleoli with so-called skein-like nucleolonema (Figs. 6-3, 6-4). Electron-dense deposits are regularly seen in the extracellular space, often in linear configuration; such material may be seen intracellularly, and apparently corresponds topographically with areas of A_1AT and AFP-positivity. Takei and Pearl[38] observed cells with the characteristic granules of Langerhans cells in an extragonadal yolk sac tumor; to our knowledge such an observation has not been repeated. These authors proposed an interesting hypothesis of the histogenesis of germ cell tumors, in which embryonal carcinoma and yolk sac tumor are considered as two stages in a "vertical" spectrum of differentiation. Presumably, embryonal carcinoma contains a predominance of cells showing endodermal differentiation, whereas yolk sac tumor may generate germ cells (a function of the normal yolk sac) of more varied potentiality, thus explaining the presence of other elements, such as Langerhans cells, trophoblastic cells, etc. This hypothesis would also explain the mixed character of yolk sac tumor in the adult, but not the "pure" composition of this tumor in the young. It should be noted that to consider embryonal carcinoma as a more differentiated, endodermally committed type of neoplasm is contrary to the traditional view that regards embryonal carcinoma as the less differentiated, "progenitor," neoplasm from which yolk sac elements derive. Whether histiocytes with Langerhans inclusions are reactive cells of the host or tumor-derived elements is at present unknown. Obviously there is need for further work aiming to clarify the origin of these tumors.

PROGNOSIS AND THERAPY

As soon as the identity of this tumor was established, various series showed that the prognosis for children with this tumor was appreciably better than for adults with the same neoplasm,[39, 40] although the disease is potentially fatal, and certain series showed very high mortality figures for children.[41] There is no doubt that the advent of multidrug therapies has modified the prognosis of yolk sac tumor. The experience at our institution with yolk sac tumor of various anatomical sites was reported by Olsen et al.[42] From this experience it is clear that patients who would have certainly died a few years ago can now survive. We have seen dramatic regressions of large masses with the cyclic use of a six-drug regimen. Aggressive multidrug regimens are not innocuous, and may cause significant complications, but we have seen inoperable, widespread tumors disappear in complete responses brought about in a matter of weeks.

The optimal treatment for testicular yolk sac tumor of childhood continues to be debated. At issue are the specific indications for lymph node dissection, chemotherapy, and radiotherapy. It is agreed that the initial treatment should consist of orchiectomy with high ligation of the cord, and that transscrotal biopsy or orchiectomy is contraindicated. It is also agreed that a complete staging work-up is required to determine the extent of the disease. Controversy has surrounded the potential benefits and risks of extensive retroperitoneal lymph node dissection. Whereas this procedure has been hailed as both diagnostic and therapeutic, it may carry the risk of damage to the sacral plexus and consequent sexual dysfunction in later life.[43] It has been argued that if the child is under 12 months of age, the evidence does not support increased chances of survival following lymphadenectomy, even though there is no question that in children above 2 years of age the survival is much improved.[44] At our institution, 4 of 13 children with testicular yolk sac tumor had lymphatic spread, and were under 2 years of age. Therefore, extended lymph node dissection has been advocated in the treatment of young children on the grounds that it helps in staging as well as in therapy. Aggressive chemotherapeutic protocols perhaps could be reserved for those children with evidence of lymphatic spread.

TERATOMAS

Teratomas are highly prevalent in children. In the testicle, all teratomas of prepubertal children are benign. This contrasts markedly with what is observed in the adult population, in whom teratocarcinomas are about 10 times more common than benign teratomas.[33] Malignancy in a testicular teratoma may be present if the patient is in late adolescence, although the peak incidence is around 25 years of age[33]; in that case, the tumor does not differ from the adult type of neoplasm. Therefore, in this section brief consideration will be given to teratomas of the prepubertal testis, which carry an excellent prognosis.

The symptoms and signs refer to the presence of a testicular mass and are not specific. Hydroceles are very common. Associated congenital anomalies occur in more than 20 percent of children with testicular germ cell tumors (including yolk sac tumor). In Brosman's[30] review, 76 percent of testicular neoplasms in prepubertal children were yolk sac tumor, and 14 percent were benign teratomas. This differs from our experience and that of others[4, 45] who have found that the frequency of yolk sac tumor only slightly exceeds that of benign teratomas. Associated congenital anomalies include Down's syndrome (2 percent), Klinefelter's syndrome (1.5 percent), inguinal hernia (7 percent), and a number of other malformations, such as hemihypertrophy, xeroderma pigmentosum, ataxia of unknown origin, hemophilia, spina bifida, and retrocaval ureter.[46] Familial involvement, in various combinations (father and sons, siblings, etc.) has been reported; teratoma may occur in one of the involved members of the reported family, but usually the patient presents after childhood. Nonetheless, these facts favor the existence of genetic influence controlling the development of teratomas (for review, see Gilman,[46] Shinohara et al.,[47] and Damjanov[28]).

The gross appearance is typical of well-differentiated teratoma; there may be areas of

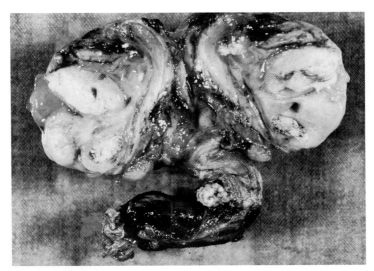

Fig. 6-5. Variegated gross appearance typical of benign teratomas of the prepubertal testis.

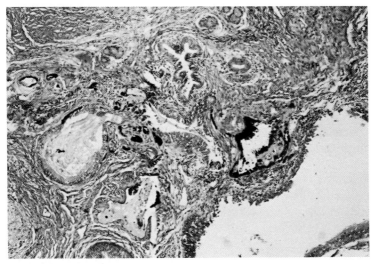

Fig. 6-6. Composite histologic structure of teratoma testis. Black structures represent melanin-producing cells. H & E. × 75.

calcification, cartilagenous plates, hairs, cystic cavities containing viscid fluid, or sebaceous material; often black deposits suggest melanin, as in retinal epithelium (Figs. 6-5, 6-6).

Whereas malignancy in testicular teratoma of the adult is related to germ cell tumor components that are part of the teratoma (embryonal carcinoma, choriocarcinoma, yolk sac tumor, and seminoma), we have yet to see such components in a testicular teratoma of a young, prepubertal child. Young children develop teratomas entirely composed of somatic tissues (although, according to theory, such tissues represent the differentiated progeny of undifferentiated cells), in which the reason for concern may be the appearance of immaturity.

We have seen examples containing abundant immature neurogenic tissues, simulating "neuroepithelioma." In spite of the relative abundance of this and other immature tissues, the course of the tumor has been invariably benign. These observations support the contention that such tissues should be designated "immature" instead of "malignant," or "suspicious of malignancy." Use of this cautious nomenclature will avoid possible misguided therapies that may be harmful in themselves. Similarly to teratomas of other sites, testicular teratomas that contain large amounts of immature somatic tissues should be identified by "histologic grading," that is, some evaluation of the amount of immature tissue present. Those showing high grade should be followed attentively. Nonetheless, the behavior of the vast majority of teratomas of the prepubertal testis justifies advocacy of conservative management by simple orchiectomy.[4]

INTERSTITIAL (LEYDIG) CELL TUMOR

Tumors of interstitial cell origin comprised only 1.6 percent of all testicular tumors referred to the British Testicular Tumor Panel,[33] and 3 percent of 6,000 testis tumors accessioned at the Armed Forces Institute of Pathology.[48] This tumor may be expected in children, since about one-fourth of all cases have involved patients between the ages of 5 and 10 years.[26] Nevertheless, the uncommon nature of this neoplasm accounts for the fact that even large pediatric oncology services see one or two cases in the course of many years. Patients from early infancy to old age may be affected.

CLINICAL MANIFESTATIONS

Precocious development of secondary sexual characteristics is manifested by all children with these tumors. In adults, the most common manifestation is simply painless enlarge-

ment of the involved testicle. Macrogenitosomia precox, premature epiphyseal closure, deepening of the voice, acne, and many other manifestations that may accompany precocious puberty are attributed to hormonal output by the tumor. Older patients may develop gynecomastia or signs of feminization (female distribution of pubic hair and gynecomastia), from days to years before seeking medical attention. Mostofi and Price[26] estimated that the average duration of these disturbances is 28 months and interpreted a long preconsultation interval as indirect evidence of slow tumor growth.

The diagnosis is often made upon demonstration of markedly elevated levels of 17-ketosteroids. A number of virilizing hormones may be identifiable. Apparently the enzyme systems present vary from tumor to tumor, and therefore the hormonal effects also vary. Certain tumor products, such as 19-hydroxyandrostenedione, may act as estrogenic precursors.[49] Androstenedione and testosterone have been identified in some cases, but no uniform secretory pattern exists, and this heterogeneity should be kept in mind when one is trying to establish the diagnosis.

PATHOLOGIC APPEARANCE

The gross appearance of the tumor is highly characteristic, and is illustrated in Figure 6-7. A well-defined, well-circumscribed nodule is seen arising within the testicular parenchyma, pushing aside the normal testicular structures. Typically, the nodule is single, mahogany brown, soft but not mucinous, and generally smaller than 5 cm in diameter.

Histologically, the tumor is constituted of lobulated sheets, cords, and/or irregular masses of large polyhedral cells with eosinophilic granular cytoplasm that may contain Reinke crystalloids (Fig. 6-8). Features of atypia may be present, but they correlate poorly with prognosis. Lipochrome pigment may be quite abundant. The uninvolved testicular parenchyma may show changes of

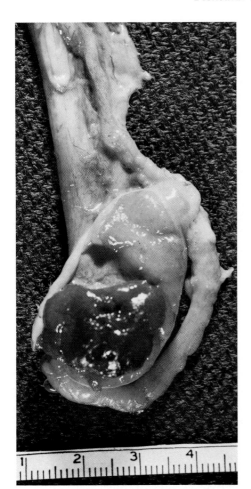

Fig. 6-7. Typical gross appearance of interstitial cell (Leydig) tumor of the testis in a prepubertal boy who showed signs of precocious masculinization. Tumor is a well-demarcated, brown nodule about 1.5 cm in greatest diameter.

spermatogenesis in areas immediately adjacent to the tumor. Therefore, the speculation is that hormonal products from the tumor diffuse locally and induce formation of spermatocytes and spermatids in neighboring seminiferous tubules.

Since the first description of the ultrastructure of this tumor by Cervos Navarro et al.,[50] the ultramicroscopic features have been well characterized. The tumor cells show abundant vesicles in the cytoplasm, very probably part of a highly developed smooth endoplasmic reticulum; characteristic membranous "whorls" are present,[51, 52] which are also found in interstitial cells of the mouse testis.[53] The tumor cells, in fact, closely reproduce the substructural morphology of normal human interstitial cells, well described by Fawcett and Burgos.[54] As is common in steroid-producing cells, the mitochondria have tubular or tubulovesicular cristae and the smooth endoplasmic reticulum shows extraordinary development; more so, perhaps, in tumors that are clearly functional, than in those that are not.[55] An elegant immunohistologic and ultrastructural study by Kurman et al.[56] localized the presence of both testosterone and estradiol within Leydig cells and Sertoli cells in Sertoli–Leydig cell tumors, but there were no boys under 15 years of age in that series. Hormones were not demonstrable, by the techniques used, in vacuolated, "light" cells positive for lipid stains, despite the fact that such cells are often assumed to be hormone-producing.

PROGNOSIS AND THERAPY

Most Leydig cell tumors are benign. Malignancy has been estimated in 10 percent of all Leydig cell tumors.[26] Since this tumor is very rare, the opportunity to see an example of malignancy in a child is exceptional. It is generally accepted that a high mitotic rate, growth in a destructive pattern, and lymphatic or vascular invasion are indications of malignancy, but that the best criterion is demonstration of metastases. Metastases usually take years to develop, and therefore the patient is often no longer a child by the time this diagnosis is made. In children, the problem is in distinguishing a tumor originating in an adrenal cell rest from a metastatic interstitial Leydig cell tumor. It is appropriate to recall that adrenal cell rests occur along the spermatic cord, or in the rete testis, but not in the testis proper, and not inside vessels. A number of subtle differences were listed by Mostofi and Price.[26] In general, lesions within the testicle should be considered Leydig cell tumors.

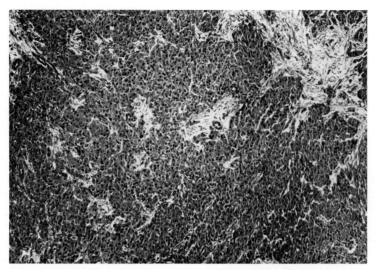

Fig. 6-8. Histologic appearance of tumor shown in Figure 6-7. Uniform composition of lobulated masses of Leydig cells which, however, did not contain demonstrable Reinke crystals H & E. × 125.

Prominent, bilateral, sometimes intratesticular nodules may be seen in children with congenital adrenal hyperplasia[57]; whether these nodules are comprised of Leydig cells or adrenal cortical cells is not always clear, but this disease should be suspected in a child with hyperadrenalism and bilateral testicular nodules. The presence crystalloids of Reinke identifies the cells as Leydig cells, but the crystalloids often cannot be found. Conservative surgical treatment is adequate for most cases of Leydig cell tumors in children. Malignancy, fortunately an extremely rare event, poses a problem for the oncologist because of the limited experience available.

SERTOLI CELL TUMOR

Although tumors of gonadal stroma are quite rare, when present they are apt to be found in infants and children. Tumors of gonadal stroma form 19 percent of testicular tumors in this age group[26] but only 3 to 4 percent of all testicular tumors referred to the Armed Forces Institute of Pathology.[58] Many authors reporting isolated observations were im-

pressed by a certain morphologic aspect, and each one devised a term that best described the observed pattern. The result was terminologic confusion which became considerably lessened in 1959, when Mostofi et al.[59] introduced the term "specialized gonadal stromal tumor." Nonetheless, the term Sertoli cell tumor has remained current and seems to describe adequately the gonadal stromal neoplasm most commonly encountered in children. Therefore, we have adhered to current use.

CLINICAL MANIFESTATIONS

Sertoli cell tumors may occur in patients of all ages, from the newborn period to old age. Of 23 Sertoli cell tumors in children reviewed by Weitzner and Groppe[60] 16 were less than 1 year of age, including 6 newborns.

A hormonal effect may be detected in children with Sertoli cell tumor; gynecomastia is noted in less than 20 percent of cases[58, 61] and may regress after surgical removal of the tumor. Elevated gonadotropin levels have been demonstrated in at least two instances and masculinization in one; the latter was a re-

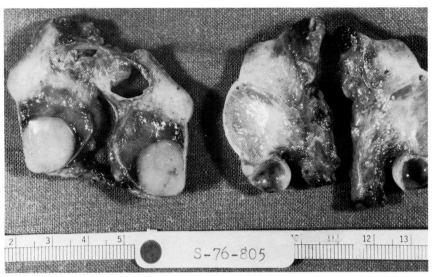

Fig. 6-9. Solid and cystic gross appearance of multifocal Sertoli-cell nodules ("adenomas") in an infant who had the androgen-insensitivity syndrome.

markable case with bilateral gonadal stromal tumors in which both neoplastic Sertoli cells and hyperplastic Leydig cells were present.[62] Most of these tumors have been unilateral[3, 60, 63-69] but a distinctive variant has been recognized (see below) with a tendency to bilaterality. The rare bilateral cases[62, 70] may belong in this category. When no endocrinologic effect is manifested, Sertoli cell tumor is indistinguishable from germ-cell neoplasms. Accordingly, inguinal orchiectomy is performed and the diagnosis is established only after histologic examination of the removed specimen. This tumor has shown a preference for the left gonad in most reported series.[26, 60]

PATHOLOGIC APPEARANCE

A cystic character may be prominent, thus leading to the mistaken preoperative diagnosis of teratoma; the cysts are assumed to arise from distended tubules[64] (Fig. 6-9).

Histologically, a wide range of appearances is reported. The best differentiated variety is distinctly tubular and difficult to distinguish from the normal prepubertal testis, in which the seminiferous tubules are lined predominantly by Sertoli cells,[71] implying a benign nature; these tumors of the best differentiated variety occupy an intermediate position between hyperplasias[72] and tumor, but their expansile nature and occasional encapsulation would seem to justify the term "adenoma." An epithelial character is usually discernible, whether it forms tubules or not. In children an epithelial component is usually present. When the tumor cells form sheets and grow in a destructive way (Figs. 6-10 to 6-12), the possibility of malignancy becomes an important consideration. This is discussed below.

The ultrastructure of well-differentiated cells (Sertoli cell adenoma) is comparable to that of normal Sertoli cells,[71, 73] as shown by the presence of abundant smooth endoplasmic reticulum, lipid droplets, smooth plasmalemma, irregular nuclear envelope, and many mitochondria. Observations on the ultrastructure of Sertoli–Leydig cell tumors of the ovary reveal many similarities, thus supporting the histogenetic unity of these neoplasms in male and female gonads.[74-76] Ramzy and Bos[75] gave a tabular comparison of the ultrastructural features of normal and neoplastic (ovarian)

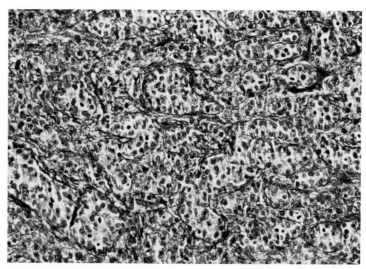

Fig. 6-10. Well-differentiated Sertoli-cell tumor with predominantly tubular arrangement. Wilder's reticulin. × 325.

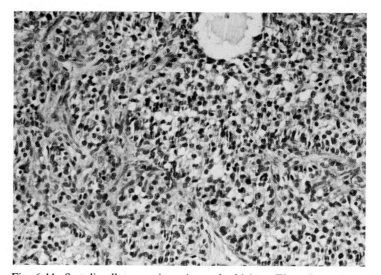

Fig. 6-11. Sertoli cell tumor in a 4-month-old boy. There is tendency to form solid cell masses, losing the tubular configuration H & E. × 225.

Sertoli cells, noting only minor differences, such as the absence of Charcot-Böttcher crystalloids from tumor cells of the testis.

A particular variant known as "large-cell calcifying Sertoli cell tumor" (LCCSCT) has been identified recently and 12 cases are now on record.[58] Patients with this tumor may have a complex clinical history. Involvement of siblings and association with cardiac myxoma and pituitary adenoma have been reported. Only one of the reported patients had gynecomastia, but five had other endocrine disorders, such as isosexual and heterosexual precocity, and some had testicular nodules of steroid-producing cells similar to those seen in adrenogenital syndrome.

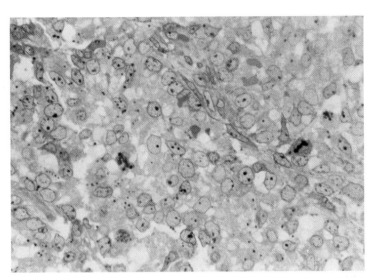

Fig. 6-12. Sertoli cell tumor; same case as in Figure 6-11. Area of high cellularity, solid growth, and abundant mitotic activity. In spite of these features the course was benign. Toluidine blue stain after epoxy embedding. × 450.

Histologically, the LCCSCT variant showed proliferation of cells in diffuse masses, cords, and tubules. Growth within seminiferous tubules was prominent in some cases. Calcification was a constant feature, from minimal to massive, inside and outside tubules (Figs. 6-13, 6-14). The tumor cells varied in size, from 12 to 35 μm in diameter, but usually were large, cuboidal, or columnar. The ultrastructure of LCCSCT was recently reported by Perez-Atayde et al.[77] as showing cells similar to normal Sertoli cells, others comparable to those in azoospermic human testis, and still others showing features displayed by cells of the common type of Sertoli cell tumors. About half the tumor cells were stained with antibodies to testosterone and estradiol by the immunoperoxidase technique; follicle-stimulating hormone (FSH) receptors were not demonstrated.

Malignant Sertoli cell tumors in children are extremely rare, but Rosvoll and Woodard[78] documented metastases to retroperitoneal lymph nodes in an 8-year-old boy, and pointed out that the criteria for diagnosis of malignancy were not defined. Talerman[79] systematically dealt with this problem, and suggested that features of concern include: lack of gross demarcation, scanty tubular formation, high mitotic activity, necrosis, invasion of epididymis, growth in solid cellular sheets, and invasion of the capsule. Lymphatic or vascular invasion was considered diagnostic of malignancy. With rare exceptions, all malignant Sertoli cell tumors of the testicle have been reported in adult patients.[80] The devastating effects of injudicious radiotherapy and chemotherapy in a growing child seem too high a risk to allow one to advocate prophylactic use of such therapies. Therefore, the conservative guidelines that have been advocated for testicular tumors of children in general[4] are applicable to Sertoli cell tumors. Inguinal orchiectomy with high ligation of the spermatic cord has been adequate therapy for most children with this disease. Strong presumption of malignancy may make further measures imperative, but the available experience is insufficient to advocate a standard form of treatment in such rare cases.

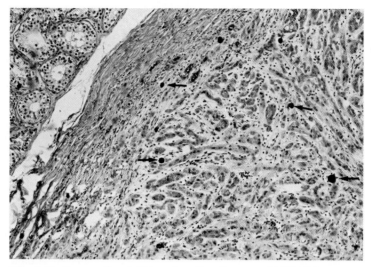

Fig. 6-13. Large-cell calcifying Sertoli cell tumor (LCCSCT) appears as an encapsulated mass containing abundant calcific spherules (arrows). H & E. × 225. (Case published by Perez-Atayde AR, Nunez AE, Carroll WL, et al: Large-cell calcifying Sertoli-cell tumor of the testis. An ultrastructural, immunocytochemical and biochemical study. Cancer 51:2287, 1983.)

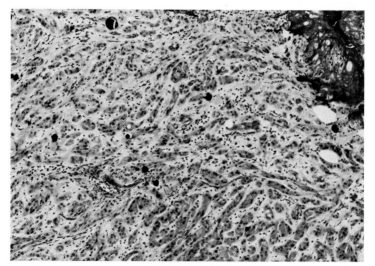

Fig. 6-14. Detail of LCCSCT shows tubular and cordlike cell proliferation; rounded and massive, irregular calcific deposits (right upper corner of illustration). Slide courtesy of Dr. Perez-Atayde. Same case as Figure 6-13. H & E. × 225.

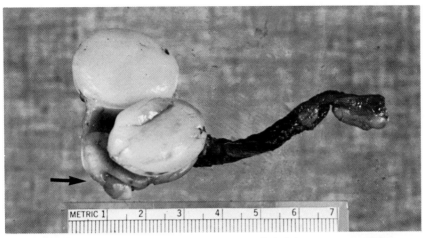

Fig. 6-15. The nodular, whitish mass is an embryonal rhabdomyosarcoma. The arrow points to the testicle, largely outside the view in the photograph.

PARATESTICULAR TUMORS

CLINICAL MANIFESTATIONS

Childhood malignancies arising from paratesticular structures, such as tunica vaginalis, spermatic cord, and connective tissue of the testicular coverings, are virtually always rhabdomyosarcomas. The chief clinical manifestation is a mass, often without any other symptoms; dull aching pain, tenderness, and a dragging sensation may be present, but the paucity of manifestations is often the cause of delay in diagnosis.[81] Other signs, such as redness of the overlying skin, localized edema, and fever simulate an orchiepididymitis, and confusion with an inflammatory condition is the direct cause of late referral to the oncologist.[82] The lesion may or may not transilluminate. The presence of a hydrocele may further contribute to the masking of a sarcoma. Whatever the reason for the delay in diagnosis, lateness in instituting treatment is common. It is warranted to assume that this time lag may be partly responsible for the observation that the tumor has spread beyond its site of origin in many cases, by the time treatment is started. Close to half the patients with genitourinary rhabdomyosarcoma (of both sexes) have tumors in clinical stage III and IV when first diagnosed.[83]

PATHOLOGIC APPEARANCE

The experienced surgeon who has exposed the tumor by the recommended inguinal incision can usually recognize the tumor grossly. The tumor is usually a lobulated, smooth, grey-white, glistening mass that may appear to displace the testicle without replacing it (Fig. 6-15). The site of origin may often be traced to the spermatic cord, the tunica vaginalis parietalis, the visceral sheet of the tunica vaginalis, or the connective tissue around the epididymis.

The most common histologic type of rhabdomyosarcoma in children, regardless of locations is the embryonal type.[84-87] This predominance is clearly apparent in paratesticular rhabdomyosarcoma; close to 90 percent of such sarcomas are embryonal. Despite persistent difficulties that hamper the histologic classification of rhabdomyosarcomas, such as the presence of different microscopic patterns in the same tumor, most paratesticular lesions can be classified into one of the traditional

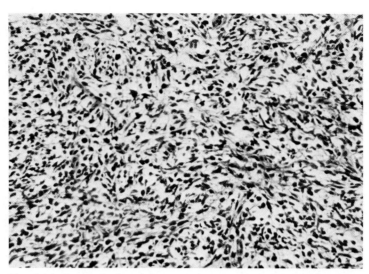

Fig. 6-16. Paratesticular embryonal rhabdomyosarcoma features small and elongated mesenchymal cells within a myxoid stroma. Cytoplasmic striations are not seen in the majority of cases. H & E. × 225.

histologic groups (embryonal, alveolar, pleomorphic, or poorly differentiated).[88] Reviews of the pathologic appearance of childhood rhabdomyosarcoma have appeared,[83, 84, 89] making it unnecessary to recapitulate the many details that help the pathologist to arrive at a diagnosis. Suffice it to state that the widespread use of techniques such as electronmicroscopy and immunocytochemistry are having an impact on our present understanding of the structure, and therefore the classification, of these tumors. Thus, demonstration of the presence of desmin has been reported as a helpful adjunct in the diagnosis of poorly differentiated rhabdomyosarcomas, that "marks" cells in alveolar and nonalveolar arrangement.[90] Accordingly, as greater sophistication in diagnostic techniques is achieved it will become possible to confirm the diagnosis of uncommon variants with greater ease, and to rule out, or be certain of, the skeletal muscle derivation of tumor cells currently considered of uncertain histogenesis (Figs. 6-16 to 6-21).

Excluding the "botryoid" type, which is most prevalent in girls and is considered to be a variant of embryonal rhabdomyosarcoma, the second most common form of genitourinary sarcoma in children is an "undifferentiated" sarcoma, often thought to be rhabdomyosarcoma merely on circumstantial evidence, such as site of origin and response to therapy comparable to that of embryonal rhabdomyosarcoma.[83, 84] Next in frequency is alveolar rhabdomyosarcoma. Whereas two decades ago this tumor was believed to be exceptional in a paratesticular location, it is now apparent that most large series will include a few examples primary in this anatomical site. Considering that about 90 percent of the cases correspond to the embryonal histologic type, it is still true that all other variants are uncommon. In particular, the pleomorphic type, common in adults, is extremely rare in children regardless of anatomical location. Because of the scarcity of case observations, there is not enough experience to evaluate the influence of histologic type on the ultimate prognosis. At present, all are treated alike. When rhabdomyosarcomas of all sites are studied, alveolar rhabdomyosarcoma emerges as a particularly aggressive variant; more treatment failures, more advanced disease at presentation, and less survivals among those who pres-

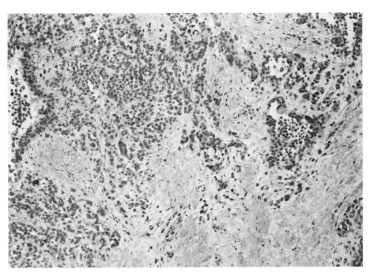

Fig. 6-17. Paratesticular alveolar rhabdomyosarcoma in a 5-year-old-boy. In addition to alveolar arrangement, there are masses of cells showing noncohesive "solid" growth, that is, undifferentiated areas. Biebrich Scarlet–acid fuchsin–hematoxylin after methacrylate embedding, × 160.

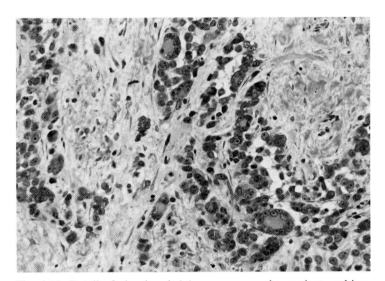

Fig. 6-18. Detail of alveolar rhabdomyosarcoma shows giant multinucleated cells, an important diagnostic feature of this tumor. Biebrich scarlet–acid fuchsin–hematoxylin after methacrylate embedding, × 450.

ent as Group I have been reported for patients with alveolar rhabdomyosarcoma.[83] However, the site of the primary is an important prognostic determinant for rhabdomyosarcoma of childhood,[91] and one should be careful not to extrapolate freely from observations pertaining to the behavior of rhabdomyosarcoma of the limbs or the trunk. Clearly, some time will have to pass before coordinated interinstitutional studies accumulate sufficient experience to be able to evaluate better the correlation of histologic findings and prognosis.

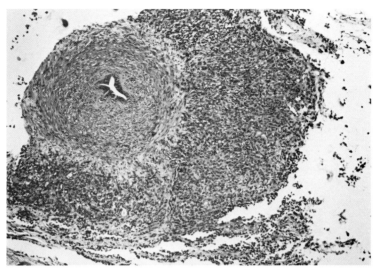

Fig. 6-19. Paratesticular rhabdomyosarcoma of "undifferentiated" type encircling vas deferens H & E. × 110.

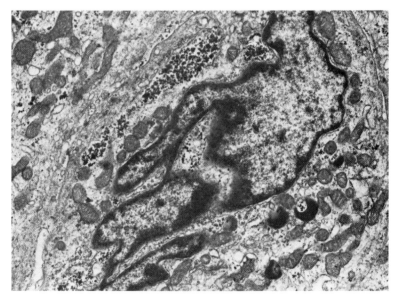

Fig. 6-20. Ultrastructure of poorly differentiated cell from a solid area of alveolar rhabdomyosarcoma. Note convoluted nucleus with lamina fibrosa, intracytoplasmic glycogen granules, and mitochondria of dense matrix. Cells were desmin-positive on light microscopic immunostain. × 20,000.

PROGNOSIS AND THERAPY

Of 20 patients with paratesticular rhabdomyosarcoma initially reported by the Intergroup Rhabdomyosarcoma Study (IRS), 15 had adequate study of the retroperitoneal lymph nodes either by retroperitoneal node dissection or biopsy; 6 of 15 (40 percent) had nodal involvement by tumor.[87, 91] In all except one, gross disease could be excised surgically.

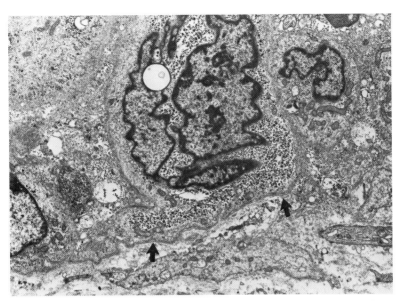

Fig. 6-21. Paratesticular alveolar rhabdomyosarcoma. Tumor cells lining alveolar spaces show formation of a distinct, but discontinuous, basement lamina (*arrows*) at site of abutment against fibrous stromal trabeculae. Despite epithelial-like arrangement and close intercellular contact, no cell-to-cell junctional devices are seen × 13,000.

The disease-free rate with combined forms of therapy was 89 percent at a median of 23 months from diagnosis (range, 8–43 months). Venous invasion was seen in only 15 percent (3 of 20) of the cases. Thus, patients with paratesticular rhabdomyosarcoma are at high risk of developing retroperitoneal lymph node metastases (40 percent); inguinal lymph node metastases were present in 2 of 13 patients (15 percent). Therefore, it is generally recommended that radical orchiectomy be followed by examination of the retroperitoneal lymph nodes. It is not known why genitourinary rhabdomyosarcoma shows such a high propensity to disseminate to lymph nodes. Rhabdomyosarcomas of certain sites, such as the orbit, rarely metastasize to lymph nodes, even though the histologic type is the same.

In another report from the IRS, 58 children with genitourinary rhabdomyosarcoma (including girls with lesions of vagina, uterus, and urinary bladder) were studied, and the frequency[92] of lymph node metastases was 26 percent. The recommendation was not to radiate lymph-node-bearing areas routinely, but only when lymph node metastases were proved to be present, because high radiation dosages are known to be necessary to ablate tumor cells, and these may exceed the maximum tolerated by some normal tissues, such as the bowel.[92] Furthermore, radiation must be given to relatively large fields, in view of the ability of rhabdomyosarcoma to extend along fascial planes. Fortunately, it has been shown that radiation need not necessarily reach the very high doses (5,000–6,000 rad) initially recommended, when maintenance chemotherapy is administered concurrently.[93]

Before the early 1960s surgery and radiation therapy were used either alone or in combination for the treatment of childhood rhabdomyosarcoma and the results were most unrewarding. Gradually, chemotherapy came into prominence when it was found that several antitumor drugs were effective in controlling occult disease following surgery and radiotherapy.[94] It then became customary to administer these drugs (actinomycin D, vincristine, cyclophophamide) prophylactically, that is, before the patient manifested any evidence of recurrence, or mestastases. The efficacy of these agents was evident; it also became possible successfully to treat patients with inoperable or metastatic rhabdomyosarcoma. Success was claimed in up to 58 percent of cases that formerly would have been considered unsalvageable.[95] Today's results, as mentioned before, are even more highly encouraging. It is thus appropriate to conclude that substantial progress has been made in the therapy of childhood rhabdomyosarcoma, particularly in the last two decades. However, complications of present-day therapies are still a major disadvantage. Radiation causes skeletal maldevelopment, fibrosis of soft tissues, and, in some cases, induces a secondary malignant tumor. Chemotherapy, despite its most gratifying results, induces serious hematologic complications; in 1975 it was reported to cause death in about 2 percent of children treated for rhabdomyosarcoma. Surgery, as is well known, is subject to the irreversible complications brought about by ablation of tissues. Surgery for paratesticular rhabdomyosarcoma included excision of lymph nodes, urinary diversions, and other procedures whose attending mortality and morbidity are well known. The goal of current protocols is, therefore, to use each treatment modality in combination with others to reduce the rate of complications of each without sacrificing antitumor efficacy. Trials of new chemotherapeutic agents, and new combinations of agents may help to achieve this goal with greater success than has been possible previously.

REFERENCES

1. Javadpour N, Bergman S: Recent advances in testicular cancer. Current Probl Surg 15:39, 1978
2. Li FP, Fraumeni JF Jr: Testicular cancers in children: epidemiologic characteristics. J Natl Cancer Inst 48:1575, 1972
3. Boatman DL, Culp DA, Wilson VB: Testicular neoplasms in children. J Urol 109:315, 1973
4. Marshall S, Lyon RP, Scott MP: A conservative approach to testicular tumors in children: 12 cases and their management. J Urol 129:350, 1983
5. Anderson RE, Huston C: Tumors of the testicle in childhood. Am J Surg 95:445, 1958
6. Phelan JT, Woolner LB, Hayles AB: Testicular tumors in infants and children. Surg Gynecol Obstet 105:569, 1957
7. Houser, R, Izant R, Persky L: Testicular tumors in children. Am J Surg 110:876, 1965
8. Scully RE, Parham AR: Testicular tumors: seminoma and teratoma. Arch Pathol 45:581, 1948
9. Sauer HR, Watson, EM, Burke, EM: Tumors of the testicle. Surg Gynecol Obstet 86:591, 1948
10. Grumet RF, MacMahon B: Trends in mortality from neoplasms of the testis. Cancer 11:790, 1958
11. Clemmesen J: A doubling of morbidity from testis carcinoma in Copenhagen. 1943–1962. Acta Pathol Microbiol Scand 72:348, 1968
12. Teppo L: Malignant testicular tumors in Finland. Acta Pathol Microbiol Scand 75:18, 1969
13. Editorial: An epidemic of testicular cancer? Lancet 2:164, 1968
14. Bhargavan MK, Reddy DG: Tumors of the testis. II Tumors of the testis in children. Cancer 19:1655, 1966
15. Tiltman AF: The racial incidence of testicular tumors. South Afr Med J 43:97, 1969
16. Fraumeni JF Jr, Glass AG: Rarity of Ewing's sarcoma among U.S. Negro children. Lancet 1:366, 1970
17. Templeton AC: Testicular neoplasms in Ugandan Africans. Afr J Med Sci 3:157, 1972
18. DeCenzo JM, Leadbetter GW: Early orchiopexy and testis tumors. Urology 5:365, 1975
19. Batata MA, Whitemore WF Jr, Chu FCH, et al: Cryptorchidism and testicular cancer. J Urol 124:382, 1980
20. Campbell HE: Incidence of malignant growth of the undescended testicle. A reply and reevaluation. J Urol 81:663, 1959
21. DiBella NJ: Familial gonadal neoplasms. N Engl J Med 309:1389, 1983
22. Thomson WO, Sinclair DM: Familial teratomas of testis. Br J Urol 49:322, 1977
23. Lapes M, Iozzi L, Ziegenfus WD et al: Familial testicular cancer in a father (bilateral semi-

noma–embryonal cell carcinoma) and son (teratocarcinoma). Cancer 39:2317, 1977

24. Muir CS, Nectoux J: Epidemiology of cancer of the testis and penis. Natl Cancer Inst Monogr 53:157, 1979

25. Nochomowitz LE, Rosai J: Current concepts on the histogenesis, pathology and immunochemistry of germ cell tumors of the testis. Pathol Annu 13(1):327, 1978

26. Mostofi FK, Price EB Jr: Tumors of the male genital system. In Atlas of Tumor Pathology, 2nd series, fascicle 8. Armed Forces Institute of Pathology, Washington, DC, 1973

27. Dixon FJ, Moore RA: Tumors of the male sex organs. In Atlas of Tumor Pathology, section 8, fascicles 31b, 32. Armed Forces Institute of Pathology, Washington, DC, 1952

28. Damjanov I: Pathology of human teratomas. p. 23. In Damjanov I, Knowles BB, Solter D (eds): The Human Teratomas. Humana Press, Clifton, New Jersey, 1983

29. Brawn PN: The origin of germ cell tumors of the testis. Cancer 51:1610, 1983

30. Brosman SA: Testicular tumors in prepubertal children. Urology 13:581, 1979

31. Teilum G: Endodermal sinus tumors of the ovary and testis. Comparative morphogenesis of so-called mesonephroma ovarii (Schiller) and extraembryonic (yolk sac-allantoic) structures of the rat placenta. Cancer 12:1092, 1959

32. Gonzalez-Crussi F: The human yolk sac and yolk sac (endodermal sinus) tumors. Perspect Pediatr Pathol 5:179, 1979

33. Pugh RCB (ed): Pathology of the Testis. Blackwell, Oxford, 1976

34. Talerman A: Endodermal sinus (yolk sac) tumor elements in testicular germ-cell tumors in adults: comparison of prospective and retrospective studies. Cancer 46:1213, 1980

35. Gitlin D, Perricelli A: Synthesis of serum albumin, prealbumin, α-foetoprotein, α-1 antitrypsin and transferrin by the human yolk sac. Nature 228:995, 1970

36. Parkinson C, Beilby JOW: Testicular germ cell tumors: should current classification be revised? Invest Cell Pathol 3:135, 1980

37. Damjanov I, Amenta PS, Zarghami F: Transformation of an AFP-positive yolk sac carcinoma into an AFP-negative neoplasm. Evidence for in vivo cloning of the human parietal yolk sac carcinoma. Cancer 53:1902, 1984

38. Takei Y, Pearl GS: Ultrastructural study of intracranial yolk sac tumor: with special reference to the oncologic phylogeny of germ cell tumors. Cancer 48:2038, 1981

39. Ross MM, Morrow JW: Yolk sac carcinoma of the testis. J Urol 108:109, 1972

40. Young PG, Mount BM, Foote FW Jr, Whitmore WF Jr: Embryonal adenocarcinoma in the prepubertal testis—a clinicopathologic study of 18 cases. Cancer 26:1065, 1970

41. Roth LM, Panganiban WG: Gonadal and extragonadal yolk sac carcinomas. A clinicopathologic study of 14 cases. Cancer 37:812, 1976

42. Olsen MM, Raffensperger JG, Gonzalez-Crussi F, et al: Endodermal sinus tumor: a clinical and pathological correlation. J Pediatr Surg 17:832, 1982

43. Smith AM, Raghunatha NR, Shelor WC: Clinical dilemma in management of yolk sac childhood tumor of testis. Urology 14:88, 1979

44. Reaman GH, Cohen LF: Less frequently encountered malignant neoplasms in the young. p. 707. In Levine A (ed): Cancer in the Young. Masson, New York, 1981

45. Karamehmedovic O, Woodtli W, Pluss HJ: Testicular tumors in childhood. J Pediatr Surg 10:109, 1975

46. Gilman PA: Epidemiology of human teratomas. p. 81. In Damjanov I, Knowles BB, Solter D (eds): The Human Teratomas. Clinical Biology. Humana Press, Clifton, NJ, 1983

47. Shinohara M, Komatsu H, Yokoyama M: Familial testicular teratomas in 2 children: familial report and review of the literature. J Urol 123:552, 1980

48. Turner JH: The testis. p. 309. In Bloodworth JMB Jr (ed): Endocrine Pathology. General and Surgical, 2nd ed. Williams & Wilkins, Baltimore, 1982

49. Ances IG, Connor TB, Gallaher EP et al: Case of feminizing interstitial-cell tumor of the testicle. Clinical and biochemical evaluation. J Clin Endocrinol 33:452, 1971

50. Cervos Navarro J, Tonutti E, Bayer JM: Elektronmikroskopische untersuchung eines androgen bildenden Leydigzell tumors. Endokrinologie 47:25, 1964

51. Kay S, Fu Y, Koontz WW, Chen ATL: Interstitial cell tumor of the testis. Tissue culture and ultrastructural studies. Am J Clin Pathol 63:366, 1975

52. Beals TF, Pierce GB, Schroeder CF: The ultra-

structure human testicular tumors. I. Interstitial cell tumors. J Urol 92:64, 1965

53. Carr I, Carr J: Membranous whorls in the testicular interstital cells. Anat Rec 144:143, 1962

54. Fawcett DW, Burgos MH: Studies on the fine structure of the mammalian testis. II. The human interstitial tissue. Am J Anat 107:245, 1960

55. Roth LM, Spurlock BO, Sternberg WH et al: Fine structure of transplantable Leydig cell tumors of the rat. Am J Pathol 60:137, 1970

56. Kurman RJ, Andrade G, Goebelsmann U, Taylor CJ: An immunohistologic study of steroid localization in Sertoli–Leydig tumors of the ovary and testis. Cancer 42:1772, 1978

57. Burke EF, Gilbert E, Uehling DT: Adrenal rest tumors of the testes. J Urol 109:649, 1973

58. Proppe KH, Scully RE: Large-cell calcifying Sertoli cell tumor of the testis. Am J Clin Pathol 74:607, 1980

59. Mostofi FK, Theiss EA, Ashley DJB: Tumors of specialized gonadal stroma in human male patients. Androblastoma, Sertoli-cell tumor, granulosa-theca cell tumor of the testis and gonadal stromal tumor. Cancer 12:944, 1959

60. Weitzner S, Gropp A: Sertoli cell tumor of testis in childhood. Am J Dis Child 128:541, 1974

61. Hopkins GB, Parry HD: Metastasizing Sertoli-cell tumor (androblastoma). Cancer 23:463, 1969

62. Fligiel Z, Kaneko M, Leiter E: Bilateral Sertoli-cell tumor of testes with feminizing and masculinizing activity occurring in a child. Cancer 38:1853, 1976

63. Batsakis JG: Tumors of testis in infancy and childhood. Arch Pathol 72:27, 1961

64. Collins DH, Symington T: Sertoli-cell tumor. Br J Urol 36: suppl 52, 1964

65. Culp DA, Frazier RG, Butler JJ: Sertoli cell tumor in an infant. J Urol 76:162, 1956

66. Holtz F, Abell MR: Testicular neoplasms in infants and children. II. Tumors of non-germ cell origin. Cancer 16:982, 1963

67. Giebnink GS, Ruymann FB: Testicular tumors in childhood. Am J Dis Child 127:433, 1974

68. Gonder MJ, Fadell, EJ: Gonadal stromal tumor in an infant. J Urol 84:357, 1960

69. Woodside JR and Borden TA: Sertoli cell tumor (gonadal stromal tumor) in an infant. J Pediatr Surg 14:138, 1979

70. Lange J, Leger MH, Etcheverry M: Androblas-

tome testiculaire: observation d'une forme bilaterale chez l'enfant. J Urol Med Chir 66:259, 1960

71. Able ME, Lee JC: Ultrastructure of a Sertoli-cell adenoma of the testis. Cancer 23:481, 1969

72. Stalker AL, Hendry WT: Hyperplasia and neoplasia of the Sertoli cell. J Pathol Bacteriol 64:161, 1952

73. Goellner JR, Myers RP: Sertoli-cell tumor. Case report with ultrastructure findings. Mayo Clin Proc 50:459, 1975

74. Murad TM, Mancini R, George J: Ultrastructure of a virilizing ovarian Sertoli–Leydig cell tumor with familial incidence. Cancer 31:1440, 1973

75. Ramzy I, Bos C: Sertoli-cell tumors of the ovary. Light and ultrastructural study with histogenetic considerations. Cancer 38:2447, 1976

76. Roth LM, Cleary RE, Rosenfield RL: Sertoli–Leydig cell tumor of the ovary, with an associated mucinous cystadenoma: an ultrastructural and endocrine study. Lab Invest 31:648, 1974

77. Perez-Atayde AR, Nunez AE, Carroll WL et al: Large-cell calcifying Sertoli-cell tumor of the testis. An ultrastructural, immunocytochemical and biochemical study. Cancer 51:2287, 1983

78. Rosvoll RV, Woodard JR: Malignant Sertoli cell tumor of the testis. Cancer 22:8, 1968

79. Talerman A: Malignant Sertoli-cell tumor of the testis. Cancer 28:446, 1971

80. Koppikar DD, Sirsat MV: A malignant Sertoli cell tumor of the testis. Br J Urol 45:213, 1973

81. Arean VM, Kreager JA: Paratesticular rhabdomyosarcoma. Am J Clin Pathol 43:418, 1965

82. Fortune A, Bolton BR: Rhabdomyosarcoma of the paratesticular tissues. J Urol 126:563, 1981

83. Gaiger AM, Soule EH, Newton WA: Pathology of rhabdomyosarcoma. Experience of the Intergroup Rhabdomyosarcoma Study, 1972–1978. Natl Cancer Inst Monogr 56:19, 1981

84. Bale PM, Parsons RE, Stevens MM: Diagnosis of juvenile rhabdomyosarcoma. Hum Pathol 14:596, 1984

85. Altman AJ, Schwartz AD: The soft tissue sarcomas. p. 423. In Malignant Diseases of Infancy, Childhood and Adolescence, 2nd ed. W.B. Saunders. Philadelphia, 1983

86. Fleischmann J, Perinetti EP, Catalona, WJ: Embryonal rhabdomyosarcoma of the genitourinary organs. J Urol 126:389, 1981

87. Raney RB Jr, Hays DM, Lawrence W Jr et al: Paratesticular rhabdomyosarcoma in childhood. Cancer 42:729, 1978

88. Rosas-Uribe A, Luna MA, Guinn GA: Paratesticular rhabdomyosarcoma. A clinicopathologic study of seven cases. Am J Surg 120:787, 1970

89. Gonzalez-Crussi F, Black-Schaeffer S: Rhabdomyosarcoma of infancy and childhood. Problems of morphologic classification. Am J Surg Pathol 3:151, 1979

90. Miettinen M, Lehto V-P, Bradley RA, Virtanen, I: Alveolar rhabdomyosarcoma. Demonstration of the muscle type of intermediate filament protein, desmin, as a diagnostic aid. Am J Pathol 108:246, 1982

91. Raney RB Jr, Donaldson MH, Sutow WW, et al: Special considerations related to primary site in rhabdomyosarcoma: experience of the Intergroup Rhabdomyosarcoma Study, 1972–1976. Natl Cancer Inst Monogr 56:69, 1981

92. Tefft M, Hays D, Raney RB et al: Radiation to regiona nodes for rhabdomyosarcoma of the genitourinary tract in children: is it necessary? A report from the Intergroup Rhabdomyosarcoma Study #1 (IRS-1). Cancer 43:3065, 1980

93. Jereb B, Cham W, Lattin, P et al: Local control of embryonal rhabdomyosarcoma in children by radiation therapy when combined with concomitant chemotherapy. Int J Radiat Oncol 1:217, 1976

94. Heyn RM, Holland R, Newton WA Jr et al: The role of combined chemotherapy in the treatment of rhabdomyosarcoma in children. Cancer 34:2128, 1974

95. Wilbur JR: Combination chemotherapy of embryonal rhabdomyosarcoma. Cancer Chemother Rep 58:281, 1974

7

Ultrastructure of Testicular Tumors

Lawrence M. Roth and John J. Gillespie

The routine application of electron microscopy to the diagnosis of human neoplasms in the surgical pathology laboratory has increased remarkably in the past 5–10 years.[1, 2] In general, fine structural study will objectively confirm a light microscopic impression or considerably narrow a histologic differential diagnosis.[2] Within the testicular germ cell tumor group, it is essential, for therapeutic and prognostic reasons, to differentiate clearly the seminoma group of neoplasms from the embryonal variants.[3] Additionally, certain other neoplasms, particularly large cell lymphoma or metastatic carcinomas, may simulate a primary germ cell tumor in both clinical presentation and pathologic appearance. Electron microscopic study, in most instances, will aid in resolving such diagnostic problems. Studies of neoplasms of the specialized gonadal stroma of the testis have mainly concerned Leydig cell and Sertoli cell tumors.

GERM CELL TUMORS

SEMINOMAS

Description of the fine structural features of the three types of seminoma reveals that classic and the so-called "anaplastic" seminomas are comparable except for minor quantitative differences.[4-6] The seminoma cell is large and polygonal with a low nuclear/cytoplasmic ratio. (Fig. 7-1) The basal lamina, if present, is not conspicuous. Cell surface modifications such as surface microvilli are generally absent. Membrane contact specializations are simple and infrequent, consisting of small thickenings of apposed membranes. The cytoplasm is distinguished by containing pools of particulate glycogen. The usual organelles are represented with occasional parallel stacks of ribosome-bearing endoplasmic reticulum. Annulate lamellae are sometimes present (Fig. 7-2) The Golgi complex may be well developed. Lysosomes are inconsistently present. Nuclear profiles are moderately indented with dispersed chromatin. Nucleoli display a consistent configuration of a skeinlike nucleolonema associated with a pars amorpha. There are no consistent ultrastructural differences between the so-called anaplastic seminoma and the classic form (Fig. 7-3).

Spermatocytic seminomas show more differentiation at the ultrastructural level than is evident in "anaplastic" and classic testicular seminoma.[7, 8] They are considered to be composed of cells differentiating toward spermatocytes, although they have not reached that stage of differentiation.[9] Among the more distinctive differences are more uniformly rounded nuclei than found in the other forms of seminoma and occasional filamentous structures resembling chromosomes in the leptotene stage of meiotic division. Glycogen is inconspicuous. Characteristically, intercellular cytoplasmic bridges similar to those occurring between normal primary spermatocytes and spermatids are occasionally seen in spermatocytic seminoma cells.[7, 8] A larger number of organelles are present than in classic seminoma.[9]

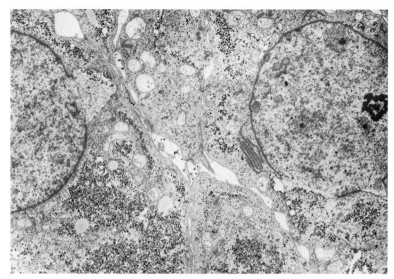

Fig. 7-1. Classic seminoma. Large cells with round nuclei and abundant cytoplasm containing glycogen and annulate lamellae are noted. × 6,400.

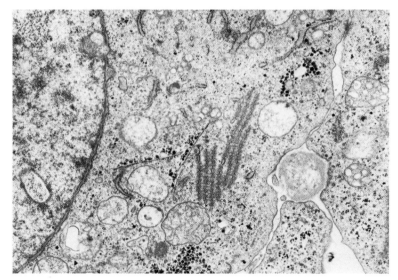

Fig. 7-2. Classic seminoma. Annulate lamellae are noted. Intercellular cell surface specializations are uncommon. A primitive junction is present at the top right of the field. × 13,000.

SOLID EMBRYONAL CARCINOMA

The ultrastructure of solid embryonal carcinomas has been studied considerably less than that of seminoma.[3, 6, 10] The cells of this neoplasm are large and rounded and also have a low nuclear/cytoplasmic ratio. In sharp contrast to seminoma, the basal lamina is conspicuous, delimiting groups of cells. Acinar formations of varying degrees of complexity are present, characterized by apically oriented junctional complexes associated with project-

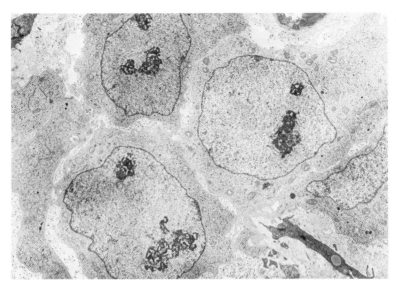

Fig. 7-3. "Anaplastic" seminoma. Skeinlike nucleoli are apparent. The overall appearance is similar to classic seminoma. × 3,800.

ing microvilli. (Fig. 7-4) Mature desmosomes are frequent and are laterally oriented. The cytoplasmic organelles show a greater degree of development than those observed in seminoma; the ribosome-bearing endoplasmic reticulum and Golgi complexes may be highly developed. Secretory products, however, are generally not observed in solid embryonal carcinoma. Particulate glycogen may be observed, though with less consistency and in less quantity than observed in seminoma. Nuclear structure and configuration are often comparable to that of seminoma.

YOLK SAC CARCINOMA (ENDODERMAL SINUS TUMOR)

There are few reported ultrastructural studies of yolk sac carcinoma of the testis; however, a testicular mixed germ cell tumor with elements of yolk sac carcinoma, immature teratoma, and seminoma has been studied and studies of four other yolk sac tumors suggest that the ultrastructural appearance of the tumor, although somewhat variable, is independent of its site of occurrence. (Roth LM, Gillespie JJ: Unpublished observations, 1979.)

The most characteristic feature of the tumor is the presence of flocculent granular material of variable density within distended cisternae of granular endoplasmic reticulum, as well as the presence of similar material extracellularly[11, 12] (Figs. 7-5, 7-6). This material appears to be condensed intracellularly to form electron-dense bodies without limiting membranes and these structures corresponding to the hyaline globules observed by light microscopy may be present intracellularly or extracellularly. These bodies are divided into two types by their electron density and inner structure: one is highly electron-dense, consisting of homogeneous or finely granular material (Fig. 7-7), and the other is moderately electron-dense and composed of finely filamentous structures, similar to basal lamina material.[13] The former corresponds to the alpha-fetoprotein (AFP)-positive hyaline globules produced by tumor cells recapitulating the visceral yolk sac; whereas the latter corresponds to the AFP-negative globules of cells of the parietal type.[13] Another significant feature is the presence of abundant glycogen particles. The tumor nuclei are markedly irregular in shape, although uniform in size. In many nuclei there is a prominent threadlike nucleo-

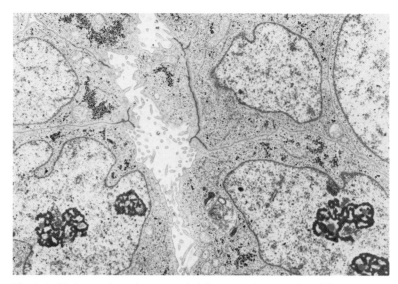

Fig. 7-4. Embryonal carcinoma. Acini lined by slender microvilli are associated with apically oriented tripartite junctional complexes. Nucleoli show multiple skeinlike filaments. Some cells contain aggregates of glycogen. × 5,100.

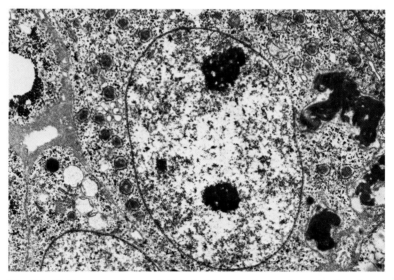

Fig. 7-5. Yolk sac carcinoma. Dilated cisternae of granular endoplasmic reticulum contain granular floccular material and aggregates of similar material are present extracellularly. × 8,100.

lonema similar to that described in seminoma cells. Where a group of tumor cells surrounds a lumen, numerous microvilli are present. Elsewhere, cells are either closely applied with frequent desmosomal attachments or are separated by extracellular electron-dense material.

INTRATUBULAR GERM CELL TUMOR

The undifferentiated intratubular germ cells, described in several studies, closely resemble early stages of germ cell differentiation.[14-17] In one case, in addition to show-

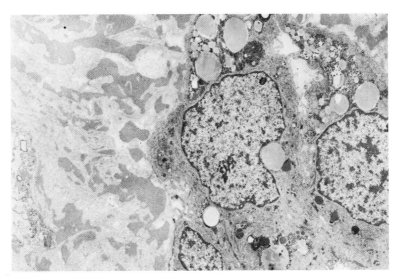

Fig. 7-6. Yolk sac carcinoma. Tumor cells have a microvillous border in the right lower portion of the field. They contain glycogen and some lipid droplets. The extracellular space contains amorphous granular material as well as reduplicated basal lamina. × 3,800.

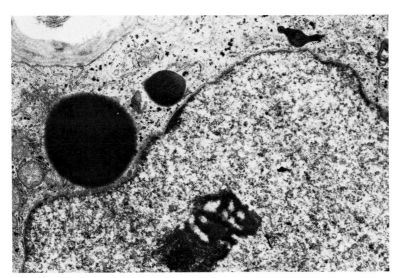

Fig. 7-7. Yolk sac carcinoma. Several dense bodies are present intracellularly composed of electron dense material without a limiting membrane. These correspond to the hyaline globules seen by light microscopy. × 13,000.

ing metastasis of the embryonal carci noma into the tunica albuginea, foci of intratubular undifferentiated germ cell tumor, as well as intratubular seminoma and embryonal carcinoma, were seen.[15] These cells of intratubular seminoma and embryonal carcinoma resemble the corresponding cells of invasive tumors, differing only in location.

The process of development of invasive classic seminoma from intratubular germ cell tumors has been described.[18] In the earliest stage of invasion, neoplastic cells covered by basal

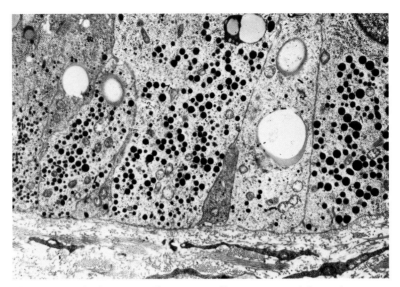

Fig. 7-8. Carcinoid tumor. The tumor cells are separated from the stroma by a basal lamina. The basilar portion of the cells contains numerous round electron dense neurosecretory granules, as well as some lipofuchsin pigment. × 5,100.

lamina protrude into evaginations of the tubule or directly invade the tubular basal lamina. At the site of tumor cell migration, the basal lamina is thickened and multilayered. Tumor cells devoid of basal lamina are seen; however, transmigration of tumor cells through the basal lamina is not observed.

MONODERMAL DEVELOPMENT OF TERATOMA

CARCINOID

Four carcinoid tumors considered primary in the testis, unassociated with a teratoma, have been described.[19-22] Three contained polymorphous neurosecretory granules characteristic of midgut carcinoids, and one contained round granules of foregut–hindgut type (Fig. 7-8). Due to the presence of cutaneous metastases considered characteristic of foregut carcinoids, the latter origin was favored.[22] These tumors are considered most likely to represent monodermal development of a teratoma.[21] A metastatic carcinoid could have a similar ultrastructural appearance. The fine structure of a neoplasm interpreted as an atypical thyroid adenoma arising in struma testis has been described.[23]

TUMORS OF SPECIALIZED GONADAL STROMA

SERTOLI CELL TUMOR

The ultrastructure of well-differentiated Sertoli cell tumors of the testis resembles that of normal Sertoli cells.[24] The most characteristic features include basal lamina around solid tubules and the presence of smooth endoplasmic reticulum, lipid droplets, cytoplasmic granules, pinocytotic vesicles, and frequent desmosomes of the macula adherens type.[25] Charcot-Böttcher filaments and annulate lamellae, although features of normal Sertoli cells, have only occasionally been described in testicular Sertoli cell tumors. A less well

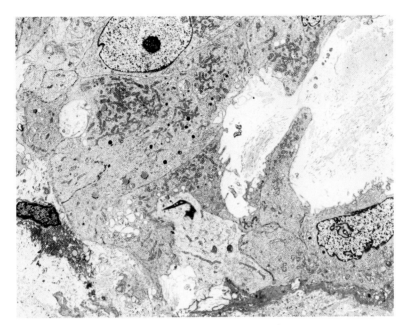

Fig. 7-9. Large-cell calcifying Sertoli cell tumor. Tubular structures are present surrounded by a basal lamina. Note the pseudolumen containing collagen and reduplicated basal lamina to the right (courtesy of G. Richard Dickersin, M.D., Boston, MA). × 1,800.

differentiated Sertoli cell tumor had a discontinuous basal lamina and lacked desmosomes, although tight junctions were present.[26]

The fine structure of a large-cell calcifying Sertoli cell tumor of the testis has been described.[27] It showed features compatible with a Sertoli cell tumor, including solid tubular structures surrounded by a basal lamina and tubular structures containing pseudolumens, that is, basal lamina also lining the pseudolumens (Fig. 7-9). Smooth endoplasmic reticulum, lipid, and lipofuscin were also present (Fig. 7-10). Another case had similar features but, in addition, showed lumina lined by microvilli with cilia and ribosome–lamella complexes.[28]

LEYDIG CELL TUMOR

The ultrastructure of testicular Leydig cell tumors resembles that of normal Leydig cells.[29-34] Similarities include abundant smooth endoplasmic reticulum, lipid droplets, and microbodies. Tubular mitochondrial cristae which, along with abundant smooth endoplasmic reticulum, are one of the major features of steroid hormone secreting cells, are present in some but not all Leydig cell tumors (Fig. 7-11). Crystalloids of Reinke, which are characteristic of Leydig cells on light or electron microscopy, have been described in several reported cases of Leydig cell tumors[29, 32, 34] (Fig. 7-12). Membranous whorls are present in some Leydig cell tumors,[29, 30] although they are extremely uncommon in the testes of normal men.

Areas of intercellular matrix containing collagenous fibrils and fusiform cells have been described by two authors, although the appearance differed somewhat.[33, 34] Carr[34] believed the stromal matrix was produced by the tumor cells, whereas Sohval et al.[33] suggested that host connective tissue was altered by a hormonal effect originating from the tumor cells.

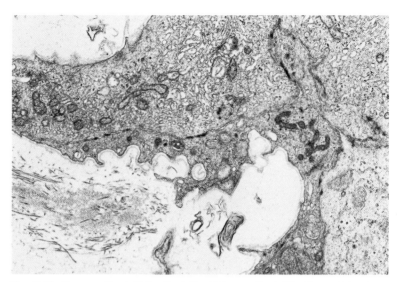

Fig. 7-10. Large-cell calcifying Sertoli cell tumor. Sertoli' cells contain abundant smooth endoplasmic reticulum and are joined by primitive junctions. The groups of tumor cells are separated from the stroma by a basal lamina (courtesy of G. Richard Dickersin, M.D., Boston, MA). × 8,300.

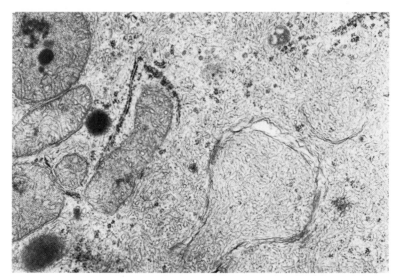

Fig. 7-11. Leydig cell tumor. Prominent smooth endoplasmic reticulum and mitochondria with tubular cristae are characteristic of steroid hormone secreting cells. × 13,000.

Of two reported cases interpreted as malignant Leydig cell tumors,[35, 36] neither contained crystalloids of Reinke. One, considered clinically malignant on the basis of persistently elevated urinary steroid levels after bilateral orchiectomy, showed the presence of multiple and irregular nuclei, multiple nucleoli, and nucleolar margination in the neoplastic Leydig cells morphologically, suggesting an active, probably malignant, lesion.[35] The other metastasized to the peritoneum and caused the patient's death 3 years after diagnosis.[36]

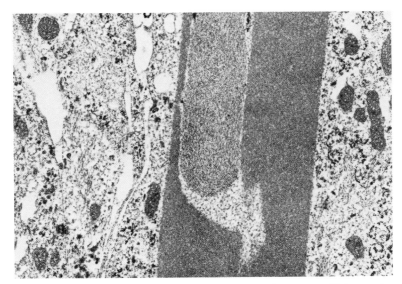

Fig. 7-12. Leydig cell tumor. A crystalloid of Reinke is present which contains precrystalline elementary material. Paraffin extraction × 13,000.

GONADAL STROMAL TUMOR, UNCLASSIFIED

Evans and Glick[37] have reported an unusual gonadal stromal tumor, the cells of which most closely resemble peritubular contractile cells.

MISCELLANEOUS TUMORS

HEMANGIOENDOTHELIOMA

An intratesticular benign hemangioendothelioma in a 26-year-old man has been reported.[38] Well-defined vascular lumens were infrequently seen by light microscopy, thus the case presented a diagnostic challenge. Ultrastructural study was helpful in defining the vascular nature of the tumor, which was considered to be derived from nonspecialized gonadal mesenchyme.

MALIGNANT LYMPHOMA, LARGE-CELL TYPE

As mentioned earlier, a reticuloendothelial neoplasm, particularly large-cell lymphoma, may present as a testicular mass.[39-41] The his-

tologic study of the neoplasm may closely simulate that of anaplastic seminoma or solid embryonal carcinoma. The diagnostic ultrastructural features of large-cell ("histiocytic") lymphoma have been described and appear to be comparable in all sites.[42-44] The tumor cells have been shown to represent large transformed lymphocytes rather than to be of monocyte–macrophage origin.[45] Cell contact sites, membrane modifications, and basal lamina are consistently absent. The cytoplasm contains a monotonous and dense array of polyribosomes (Fig. 7-13); other organelles are inconspicuous. Glycogen is invariably absent. The chromatin is dispersed, and one to two large dense nucleoli are present.

LEUKEMIA

Clinically apparent leukemic involvement of the testis is most commonly seen in children with acute lymphoblastic leukemia and may be unilateral or bilateral. It may be the first site of relapse after bone marrow remission, and the diagnosis can be established by testicular biopsy. On ultrastructural study, the nuclei are hyperlobated with prominent heterochro-

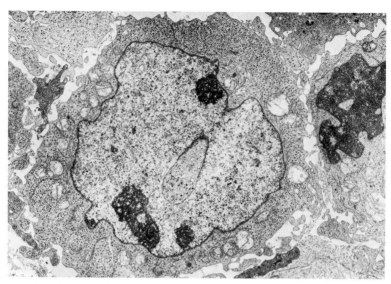

Fig. 7-13. Large-cell lymphoma. Tumor cells contain abundant free polyribosomes. Nuclei are large and irregular with prominent nucleoli. Cell junctions are absent. × 5,100.

matin and nucleoli (Fig. 7-14). Cytoplasm is scant and contains free ribosomes, mitochondria, and occasional lipid droplets. Only rarely does leukemic infiltration of the testis present as a testicular mass for which orchiectomy is performed. In granulocytic sarcoma, the immature granulocytic cells contain a prominent Golgi complex and variable numbers of primary granules (Fig. 7-15).

METASTATIC CARCINOMA

Metastatic carcinoma involving the testes can clinically simulate a primary testicular neoplasm. We have seen two cases of metastatic oat cell carcinoma involving the testis in which the primary lung tumor was not recognized initially and orchiectomy was performed.[4] Demonstration of neurosecretory granules within the cytoplasm of the tumor cells confirmed the diagnosis (Fig. 7-16). A case of transitional cell carcinoma of the urinary bladder metastatic to the testis has been reported.[46] In some areas, complex intercellular interdigitation, frequent desmosomes, and tonofilament–desmosome complexes were observed.

SUMMARY

In summary, diagnostic electron microscopy can often clearly differentiate seminoma from the nonseminomatous germ cell group. The ultrastructure of yolk sac tumors appears to be characteristic. A large-cell lymphoma or metastatic small-cell carcinoma simulating a germ-cell neoplasm can clearly be distinguished at the fine structural level. The ultrastructural diagnostic features of germ cell tumors are summarized in Table 7-1.

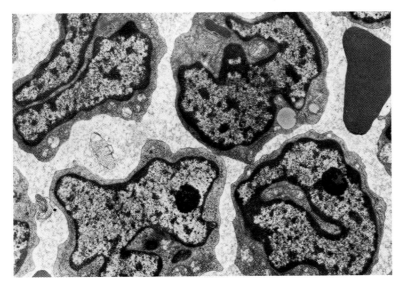

Fig. 7-14. Acute lymphoblastic leukemia. Nuclei have markedly irregular contours with prominent heterochromatin and small nucleoli. Nuclear cytoplasmic ratios are high. Cytoplasm consists mainly of free polyribosomes with an occasional lipid droplet. × 3,800.

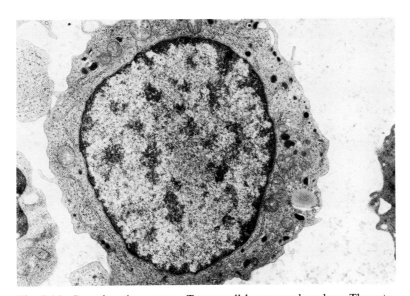

Fig. 7-15. Granulocytic sarcoma. Tumor cell has an oval nucleus. The cytoplasm contains many variably sized but generally large dense primary granules, some strands of granular endoplasmic reticulum, free ribosomes, and a lipid droplet. × 5,100.

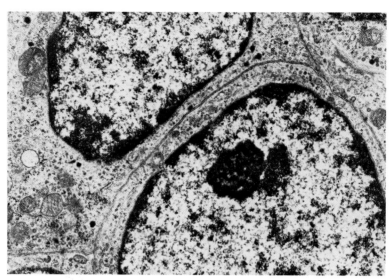

Fig. 7-16. Metastatic oat cell carcinoma. Tumor cells have high nuclear cytoplasmic ratios. A few membrane-bound dense core neurosecretory granules are present in the periphery of the cytoplasm. × 6,400.

Table 7-1. Ultrastructural Diagnosis of Germ Cell Tumors

	Seminoma	Solid Embryonal Carcinoma	Yolk Sac Carcinoma	Large Cell Lymphoma
Basal lamina	±; poorly developed	++; Conspicuous	++; Conspicuous	−
Microvilli	±; Infrequent; poorly formed	++; Frequent; well-formed	++; Frequent; well-formed	−
Cell contacts	+; Infrequent; small desmosomes	++; Frequent complex tripartite junctions; mature desmosomes	++; Frequent complex tripartite junctions; mature desmosomes	−
Acinar formation	−	+	+	−
Organelles	Heterogeneous; moderately developed	Heterogeneous; highly developed	Heterogeneous; highly developed	Homogeneous; polyribosomes
Glycogen	++	±	+	−
Secretion granules	±; small lysosome	−	++; "Hyaline bodies"	−

REFERENCES

1. Bonikos DS, Bensch KG, Kempson RL: The contribution of electron microscopy to the differential diagnosis of tumors. Beitr Pathol Bd 158:417, 1976
2. Mackay B, Osborne BM: The contribution of electron microscopy to the diagnosis of tumors. Pathobiol Annu 8:359, 1978
3. Roth LM, Gillespie JJ: Pathology and ultra-structure of germinal tumors of the testis. p. 1. In Einhorn LH (ed): Testicular Tumors. Management and Treatment. National Cancer Institute Monograph. Masson, New York, 1980
4. Holstein AF, Körner F: Light and electron microscopical analysis of cell types in human seminoma. Virchows Arch (A) Pathol Anat 363:97, 1974
5. Janssen M, Johnston WH: Anaplastic semi-

noma of the testis. Ultrastructural analysis of three cases. Cancer 41:538, 1978

6. Romanenko AM, Persidskii IUV: Ultrastructural characteristics of seminoma and embryonal cancer of the testis. Arkh Pathol 43:40, 1981

7. Rosai J, Khodadoust K, Silber I: Spermatocytic seminoma. II. Ultrastructural study. Cancer 24:103, 1969

8. Walter P: Séminome spermatocytaire. Etude de huit observations et revue de la littérature. Virchows Arch (A) Pathol Anat 386:175, 1980

9. Talerman A, Fu YS, Okagaki T: Spermatocytic seminoma. Ultrastructural and microspectrophotometric observations. Lab Invest 51:343, 1984

10. Pierce GB Jr: Ultrastructure of human testicular tumors. Cancer 19:1963, 1966

11. Nogales-Fernandez F, Silverberg SG, Bloustein PA, et al: Yolk sac carcinoma (endodermal sinus tumor). Ultrastructure and histogenesis of gonadal and extragonadal tumors in comparison with normal human yolk sac. Cancer 39:1462, 1977

12. Gonzalez-Crussi F, Roth LM: The human yolk sac and yolk sac carcinoma. An ultrastructural study. Hum Pathol 7:675, 1976

13. Nakanishi I, Kawahara E, Kajikawa K et al: Hyaline globules in yolk sac tumor. Histochemical, immunohistochemical and electron microscopic studies. Acta Pathol Jpn 32:733, 1982

14. Nielsen H, Nielsen M, Skakkabaek NE: The fine structure of a possible carcinoma in-situ in the seminiferous tubules in the testis of four infertile men. Acta Pathol Microbiol Scand (A) 82:235, 1974

15. Akhtar M, Sidiki Y: Undifferentiated intratubular germ cell tumor of the testis. Light and electron microscopic study of a unique case. Cancer 43:2332, 1979

16. Albrechtsen R, Nielsen MH, Skakkebaek NE, Wewer U: Carcinoma *in situ* of the testis. Some ultrastructural characteristics of germ cells. Acta Pathol Microbiol Immunol Scand (A) 90:301, 1982

17. Gondos B, Berthelsen JG, Skakkebaek NE: Intratubular germ cell neoplasia (carcinoma *in situ*): a preinvasive lesion of the testis. Ann Clin Lab Sci 13:185, 1983

18. Schulze C, Holstein AF: On the histology of human seminoma: development of the solid tumor from intratubular seminoma cells. Cancer 39:1090, 1977

19. Weitzner S, Robison JR: Primary carcinoid of testis. J Urol 116:821, 1976

20. Wurster K, Brodner O, Rossner JA, Grube D: A carcinoid occurring in the testis. Virchows Arch (A) Pathol Anat 370:185, 1976

21. Talerman A, Gratama S, Miranda S, Okagaki T: Primary carcinoid tumor of the testis: case report, ultrastructure and review of the literature. Cancer 42:2696, 1978

22. Sullivan JL, Packer JT, Bryant M: Primary malignant carcinoid of the testis. Arch Pathol 105:515, 1981

23. Waxman M, Vuletin JC, Pertschuk LP et al: Pleomorphic atypical thyroid adenoma arising in struma testis: light microscopic, ultrastructural and immunofluorescent studies. Mt Sinai J Med (NY) 49:13, 1982

24. Able ME, Lee JC: Ultrastructure of a Sertolicell adenoma of the testis. Cancer 23:481, 1969

25. Goellner JR, Meyers RP: Sertoli cell tumor: case report with ultrastructural findings. Mayo Clin Proc 50:459, 1975

26. Wiederhold MD, Gonzalez-Crussi F, Ou DW, Yokoyama MM: Ultrastructure of an undifferentiated Sertoli cell tumor of the testicle. Urol Int 37:297, 1982

27. Proppe KH, Dickersin GR: Large-cell calcifying Sertoli cell tumor of the testis: light microscopic and ultrastructural study. Hum Pathol 13:1109, 1982

28. Perez-Atayde AR, Nunez AE, Carroll WL et al: Large-cell calcifying Sertoli cell tumor of the testis. An ultrastructural, immunocytochemical, and biochemical study. Cancer 51:2287, 1983

29. Beals TF, Pierce GB Jr, Schroeder CF: The ultrastructure of human testicular tumors. I. Interstitial cell tumors. J Urol 93:64, 1965

30. Kay S, Fu YS, Koontz WW, Chen ATL: Interstitial-cell tumor of the testis: tissue culture and ultrastructural studies. Am J Clin Pathol 63:366, 1975

31. Sohval AR, Churg J, Suzuki Y et al: Electron microscopy of a feminizing Leydig cell tumor of the testis. Hum Pathol 6:621, 1977

32. Murakami M, Gohara S, Yoshida T, Shigematsu S: Elektronenmikroskopische Beobachtung bei einem Leydigzelltumor eines Erwachsenen. Endokrinologie 52:335, 1968

33. Sohval AR, Churg J, Gabrilove JL et al: Ultrastructure of feminizing testicular Leydig cell tumors. Ultrastruct Pathol 3:335, 1982

34. Carr I: The ultrastructure of an interstitial-cell neoplasm of testis that produced large amounts of ground-substance. J Pathol 107:223, 1972

35. Sworn MJ, Buchanan R: Malignant interstitial cell tumor of the testis. Hum Pathol 12:72, 1981

36. Feldman PS, Kovacs K, Horvath E, Adelson GL: Malignant Leydig cell tumor: clinical, histologic and electron microscopic features. Cancer 49:714, 1982

37. Evans HL, Glick AD: Unusual gonadal stromal tumor of the testis. Case report with ultrastructural observations. Arch Pathol Lab Med 101:317, 1977

38. Hargreaves HK, Scully RE, Richie JP: Benign hemangioendothelioma of the testis: case report with electron microscopic documentation and review of the literature. Am J Clin Pathol 77:637, 1982

39. Givler RL: Testicular involvement in leukemia and lymphoma. Cancer 23:1290, 1969

40. Silvert MA, Gray CP: Reticulum cell sarcoma of testes. Urology 8:395, 1976

41. Woolley PV III, Osborne CK, Levi JA et al: Extranodal presentation of non-Hodgkin's lymphomas in the testis. Cancer 38:1026, 1976

42. Gillespie JJ: The ultrastructural diagnosis of diffuse large-cell ("histiocytic") lymphoma. Fine structural study of 30 cases. Am J Surg Pathol 2:9, 1978

43. Glick AD, Leech JH, Waldron JA et al: Malignant lymphomas of follicular center cell origin in man. II. Ultrastructural and cytochemical studies. J Natl Cancer Inst 54:23, 1975

44. Levine GD, Dorfman RF: Nodular lymphoma: an ultrastructural study of its relationship to germinal centers and a correlation of light and electron microscopic findings. Cancer 35:148, 1975

45. Lukes RJ, Collins RD: A functional classification of malignant lymphomas. p 213 In Rebuck, JW, Berard CW, Abell MR (eds): The Reticuloendothelial System. International Academy of Pathology Monograph. Williams & Wilkins, Baltimore, 1975

46. Binkley WF, Seo IS: Metastatic transitional cell carcinoma of the testis. A case report. Cancer 54:575, 1984

8

Immunohistochemistry of Testicular Germ Cell Tumors

R. Scott Klappenbach and Robert J. Kurman

In the past two decades, considerable progress has been achieved in the diagnosis and treatment of testicular germ cell tumors (GCT). Serial measurement of circulating tumor products, especially alpha-fetoprotein (AFP) and human chorionic gonadotropin (HCG) by radioimmunoassay in conjunction with multiagent chemotherapy has revolutionized the management of patients with testicular cancer.[1-3] Application of immunocytochemical techniques has furthered our understanding of the histogenesis and biological behavior of these neoplasms as well as aided in their diagnosis. Although a variety of substances have been localized within testicular GCT by immunocytochemistry, HCG and AFP are the only markers in routine clinical use and, hence, these will be emphasized in this chapter. The principal objectives of this chapter are (1) to outline the methodology of the immunoperoxidase technique; (2) to review the literature with respect to the immunocytochemical characteristics of testicular germ cell tumors; and (3) to relate the contribution of immunocytochemistry to the understanding of tumor histogenesis and to patient management.

IMMUNOSTAINING METHODS

For a more detailed discussion on the methods used in immunocytochemistry, the reader may refer to two reviews.[4, 5] The peroxidase antiperoxidase and biotin avidin methods are the most frequently employed methods in diagnostic pathology because they are the most sensitive. In addition, these techniques can be performed on formalin-fixed, paraffin-embedded tissue, thereby eliminating the need for fresh or frozen tissue, and permitting retrospective studies.

Briefly, the peroxidase antiperoxidase (PAP) method depends on the addition of a primary rabbit antihuman antibody, followed by the addition of excess swine antirabbit immunoglobulin which links the primary antibody to the rabbit PAP immune complex (consisting of rabbit antibody to horseradish peroxidase and horseradish peroxidase antigen). The sites where the PAP complex is bound to the tissue are visualized by developing the sections with diaminobenzidine and hydrogen peroxide. The appropriate dilutions of the primary antibody are determined using a checkerboard titration method that permits selection of the optimal dilution, that is, the most intense specific staining and the least nonspecific background staining.

The biotin avidin technique was developed by Hsu et al.[6] and is the more sensitive of the two techniques. The method utilizes a rabbit antihuman primary antibody, followed by a biotinylated antirabbit secondary antibody, and a preformed avidin–biotin complex (consisting of avidin DH and a biotinylated horseradish complex). The remainder of the procedure is identical to the PAP technique. The sensitivity of this method is due to the high affinity of avidin, an egg white glycoprotein, for biotin, which is a vitamin B analogue. The binding of avidin to biotin is one million times greater than that of an antibody to an antigen.[6] This permits use of the primary antibody at higher dilutions, which results in lower background staining. With certain primary antisera, such as AFP, a greater number of positive cells are identified with the biotin avidin technique than with the PAP method. Occasionally, we have found that a tumor that is negative with the PAP method is positive with the biotin avidin method. In view of the enhanced sensitivity, the biotin avidin technique is generally the method of choice in our laboratory.

IMMUNOHISTOCHEMICAL CHARACTERISTICS OF TESTICULAR GERM CELL TUMORS

SEMINOMA

Although most studies have demonstrated that seminoma is not associated with the synthesis of HCG, detectable levels in the sera or urine have been reported in 6 to 20 percent of patients with "pure" seminomas.[7-10] When examined carefully, the source of the HCG is the multinucleated or syncytiotrophoblastic giant cell (STGC). The reported frequency of this finding varies[9, 11-14] from 2 to 14 percent. The STGCs seen in seminomas are typically found adjacent to hemorrhagic areas. They contain abundant cytoplasm and large, clear cytoplasmic vacuoles.[9, 15] Several investigators have localized immunoreactive HCG within the cytoplasm of STGC[9, 16-17] but not within the cytoplasmic vacuoles[9] (Fig. 8-1).

The immunocytochemical localization of HCG in STGC of seminoma provides a reliable means for distinguishing these cells from the stromal giant cells seen in 20 percent of seminomas.[9] Two reports of HCG localization within mononucleate seminoma cells suggest that STGC may not be the exclusive source of HCG production in these tumors.[18, 19] Al-

though this may explain some cases in which serum HCG is elevated in the absence of demonstrable STGCs, in the majority of these instances inadequate tissue sampling is the explanation for this apparent discordance. The presence of elevated serum HCG associated with HCG positive STGC in what is otherwise a pure seminoma does not appear to alter the prognosis from that of a typical seminoma of comparable stage.[19]

"Pure" seminoma is not usually associated with elevated serum AFP levels nor has AFP been demonstrated within these neoplasms using immunocytochemical techniques.[8, 9, 12, 17, 20-22] The finding of an elevated serum AFP level in a patient with a poorly differentiated tumor with features suggesting seminoma should alert the pathologist to the possibility that the tumor is an embryonal carcinoma, yolk sac tumor with a solid pattern, or a mixed germ cell tumor that has been inadequately sampled.[23] The presence of yolk sac or embryonal carcinoma elements in a tumor consisting predominantly of seminoma is a poor prognostic feature that significantly alters patient management.[24] Preoperative serum tumor marker levels should therefore be measured even if there is high index of suspicion that seminoma is present.

Several other markers have been demonstrated in seminomas but are not clinically useful at present. Pregnancy specific beta-1 glycoprotein (SP-1) is normally produced by the placenta and is localized in syncytiotrophoblastic elements in germ cell tumors.[25] It parallels the distribution of HCG in most but not all cases.[26, 27]

Serum placental alkaline phosphatase (Regan isoenzyme) (PLAP) elevation has been associated with a variety of malignant neoplasms[25-30] and has been reported in 40–60 percent of patients with seminoma.[8, 31] Wahren et al. first demonstrated PLAP in cytologic preparations of seminoma by immunofluorescence.[32] Since then, Uchida et al., using immunoperoxidase techniques, localized PLAP in 90 percent of seminomas primarily along the cytoplasmic membranes of tumor

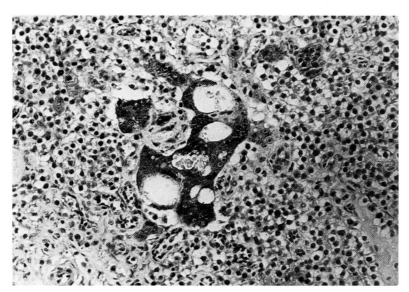

Fig. 8-1. Seminoma with STGC. Note localization of HCG within STGC. Immunoperoxidase–HCG with hematoxylin counterstain × 400.

cells.[33] In this series, there were no morphologic differences between tumors that were positive for PLAP localization and those that were negative.[33] The high frequency of PLAP localization in seminoma corresponds to enzyme histochemical studies in which 100 percent of seminomas contained detectable alkaline phosphatase although the isoenzyme was not specified.[34] Recent evidence suggests that serial measurement of serum PLAP may be useful in the management of patients with seminoma, especially when combined with measurement of HCG.[31]

Elevation of serum lactate dehydrogenase isoenzyme 1 (LD-1) has been reported in patients with testicular neoplasms by several investigators.[35-37] Murakami reported immunocytochemical localization of LD-1 in 100 percent of seminomas studied.[38] The enzyme was localized both within the cytoplasm as well as on the cell membrane. Both nonseminomatous germ cell tumors as well as a variety of nongonadal neoplasms also contain LD-1, thus limiting its usefulness as a specific testicular tumor marker.

The iron-binding protein, ferritin, has been localized immunocytochemically in more than 90 percent of seminomas and nonseminomatous germ cell tumors alike.[39] Elevated serum ferritin levels in patients with germ cell tumors have been reported, but since ferritin levels may be elevated in response to a variety of conditions, the value of this protein as a tumor marker remains to be determined.[40]

EMBRYONAL CARCINOMA

The association of elevated serum levels of alpha-fetoprotein (AFP) and testicular germ cell neoplasms was first recognized in 1967 by Abelev and co-workers.[41] Studies of the relationship of AFP production and the specific morphologic pattern of germ cell tumors indicated that the production of AFP corresponded to the presence of yolk sac elements in the tumors.[42] Since 75 percent of patients with nonseminomatous germ cell tumors have elevated serum AFP and yolk sac elements were identified in only 40 percent of cases,[43] it was evident that there was an additional source of AFP production. An immunohistochemical study of testicular germ cell tumors by Kurman et al. localized AFP within the

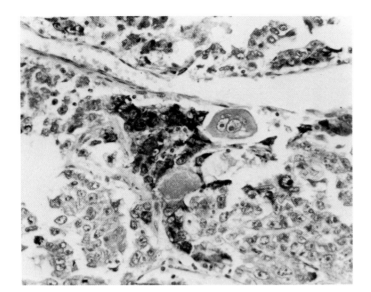

Fig. 8-2. AFP localization in embryonal carcinoma. Note negative staining of STGC. Immunoperoxidase–AFP with hematoxylin counterstain × 400.

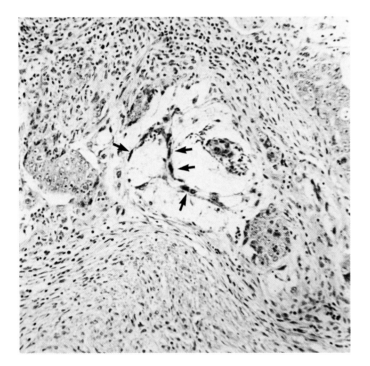

Fig. 8-3. AFP localization within spindle cells of YST elements (arrows) adjacent to nonstaining EC cells. Immunoperoxidase–AFP with hematoxylin counterstain × 100.

cytoplasm of embryonal carcinoma (EC) cells[44] (Fig. 8-2). The localization of AFP in EC is most often focal, involving individual cells or clusters of cells with frequent positive staining of cells lining glandlike clefts.[21, 44] The localization of AFP within EC cells is most often seen when EC is accompanied by yolk sac elements in mixed embryonal and yolk sac tumors.[45, 46] Alpha-fetoprotein is often concentrated in areas where EC cells assume a spindle shape forming microcystic spaces that merge with areas having a typical yolk sac appearance[21, 47] (Fig. 8-3). The localization of AFP in EC cells therefore represents

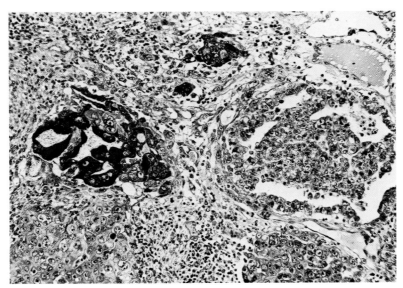

Fig. 8-4. HCG localization within STGC found in embryonal carcinoma. Immunoperoxidase–HCG with hematoxylin counterstain × 100.

biochemical differentiation towards yolk sac differentiation which precedes morphologic differentiation, thus highlighting the role of immunocytochemistry in elucidating the histogenesis of germ cell tumors. The frequency of demonstrable AFP in pure embryonal carcinoma reported in the literature varies from 0 in a series of pediatric patients[48] to 56 percent in adults.[47] Nonetheless, serial AFP measurement remains a reliable indicator of tumor recurrence. Although false-positive levels have not been reported, recurrence of tumor that has lost the capacity to produce AFP may be associated with AFP levels in the normal range.

In 71 percent of patients with EC, the serum level of HCG is elevated and correlates with the presence of STGC within the neoplasm[44] (Fig. 8-4). We have recently observed HCG in mononucleate cells in addition to STGC in a retroperitoneal EC, indicating that biochemical differentiation toward trophoblast (HCG production) may also precede morphologic differentiation. As in seminoma, the distribution of HCG in STGC parallels that of SP-1 in many, but not all cases.[27]

Alpha-1 antitrypsin (A1AT) is normally present in fetal liver and embryonic yolk sac[49] and has been reported to be elevated in the serum of patients with testicular germ cell tumors especially those with yolk sac elements (see below).[50, 51] A1AT has also been localized in EC cells in cases in which embryonal and yolk sac elements coexist.[47, 51]

A variety of other antigens have been localized within the cytoplasm of EC cells including ferritin,[47, 52] LDH isoenzyme 1,[38] and carcinoembryonic antigen (CEA).[47] Future immunocytochemical studies of these markers may provide insight into the role of EC in the histogenesis of other germ cell elements. Studies correlating serum levels of these antigens with response to treatment may also define a role for these markers in the management of patients with these tumors.

YOLK SAC TUMOR

The yolk sac tumor (endodermal sinus tumor) (YST) is the most common testicular germ cell tumor in children under 3 years of age.[24, 53] In adults, yolk sac elements are usually combined with embryonal carcinoma or teratocarcinoma.[17, 24] The reported frequency of yolk sac elements in testicular GCT ranges[17, 43, 54] from 25 to 44 percent.

The association of serum AFP and yolk sac elements in gonadal germ cell tumors was recognized[42, 55] in 1974 and was followed by immunocytochemical localization of AFP using immunofluorescence[56] and later by immunoperoxidase studies.[17, 47, 57-61] The demonstration that the human fetal yolk sac also synthesizes AFP[62] confirmed the yolk sac origin of the neoplasm as originally proposed by Teilum.[63] Besides AFP, A1AT, albumin, prealbumin, ferritin, transferrin, IgG, and hemoglobin F have been localized in the yolk sac by immunohistochemical methods.[64, 65] The frequency of demonstrable AFP in YST is more than[17, 47, 48, 61] 90 percent.

The localization of AFP in YST occurs in cells of all five morphologic patterns.[66, 67] Cytoplasmic staining of epithelial cells lining microcystic spaces is the most consistent finding although neither the distribution nor the intensity of staining is always uniform within a single tumor.[9] In addition to diffuse, granular cytoplasmic localization, intracellular and extracellular hyaline droplets may occasionally stain for AFP.[9, 47, 50]

Not all hyaline droplets are positive for AFP,[51] and other proteins synthesized by the human yolk sac, notably A1AT, have also been localized in these droplets.[65] There are no morphologic differences between cells or droplets that stain for AFP and those that do not.[9] An unusual variant of yolk sac tumor, which has only been reported in pure form in rodents, is the so-called parietal yolk sac tumor characterized by the production of abundant hyaline matrix substance rich in collagen.[68] Neither the parietal fetal yolk sac nor the parietal yolk sac tumor synthesizes AFP.[69] One case has been reported of a patient presenting with a classic YST and elevated serum AFP level who experienced a recurrent tumor with parietal yolk sac morphology and normal levels of serum AFP.[69]

Another variant of yolk sac tumor in which

AFP has been localized is the hepatoid yolk sac carcinoma, a yolk sac neoplasm with features that resemble hepatocellular carcinoma.[70] Localization of AFP in this tumor as well as the observation that AFP is synthesized by the fetal liver and gut in addition to the yolk sac[62] suggest that the synthesis of AFP may reflect endodermal differentiation rather than yolk sac differentiation specifically.[71]

In addition to AFP localization, A1AT is also found frequently within yolk sac elements of testicular GCT.[47, 50, 57, 65] The distribution of A1AT localization is similar to that of AFP including its presence in hyaline droplets.[47, 50, 51] Since A1AT is a normal constituent of adult serum and its level is subject to fluctuation in a variety of clinical settings, its value as a reliable serum marker for YST appears limited.

Yolk sac tumor does not stain for antigens typically associated with trophoblastic differentiation: HCG, SP-1, and human placental lactogen (HPL).[47, 67]

Teratoma

Patients with testicular teratoma may have slightly elevated serum levels of AFP in the absence of detectable yolk sac or EC elements.[72] Alpha-fetoprotein has been localized by immunocytochemistry in 20 percent of pure teratomas and 47 percent of teratomatous components of mixed germ cell tumors.[20] It is generally localized in cells lining mucinous glandular structures.[21] These findings correlate with the reported 41 to 60 percent frequency of elevated serum AFP in patients with teratoma.[41, 72-74] Since levels of serum AFP are lower in patients with teratoma than in patients with EC or YST, high serum levels of AFP should alert the pathologist to search carefully for YST or EC tumor as their presence would significantly alter the prognosis and such patients may be managed differently. Other proteins that have been localized within

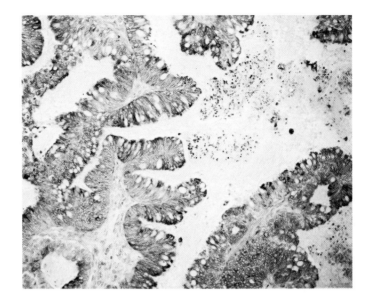

Fig. 8-5. CEA localization within intestinal type epithelium of mixed germ cell tumor. Immunoperoxidase–CEA with hematoxylin counterstain × 100.

epithelial cells of teratomas include A1AT, ferritin, carcinoembryonic antigen, and intestinal alkaline phosphatase.[16, 22, 33, 47, 51, 75] The latter two antigens are usually localized in areas of intestinal differentiation[16] (Fig. 8-5). Pregnancy-specific beta-1 glycoprotein, typically associated with trophoblastic elements, has been localized occasionally within columnar epithelial cells.[47]

CHORIOCARCINOMA

Pure choriocarcinoma of the testis is an extremely rare entity; more often choriocarcinoma is a component of a mixed germ cell tumor.[53]

Immunocytochemical localization of HCG is almost invariably present within the syncytiotrophoblast,[9] whereas cytotrophoblast has been reported to localize HCG less frequently.[47] Other placental proteins such as SP-1 and HPL have also been localized within syncytiotrophoblast.[1, 47] In certain instances, the distinction between cytotrophoblast of choriocarcinoma and mononucleate EC cells, can be accomplished by immunolo-

calization of AFP, since AFP has not been demonstrated in cytotrophoblast.[59]

MIXED GERM CELL TUMORS

Approximately 60 percent of testicular germ cell tumors contain more than one histologic type.[17] These mixed germ cell tumors most often contain EC, YST, and teratoma with mature and immature components.[17] The presence of serum markers in these patients is dependent upon the nature of the tumor components: AFP in tumors containing EC or YST and HCG in tumors composed of choriocarcinoma or containing STGC alone.

CORRELATION OF TISSUE LOCALIZATION AND SERUM MEASUREMENT OF TUMOR MARKERS IN NONSEMINOMATOUS GERM CELL TUMORS

Several studies have compared the frequency of immunocytochemical localization of AFP or HCG and elevated serum levels of these markers.[9, 17, 18, 45] Jacobsen et al.

found that 85 percent of patients with immunocytochemical localization of AFP and 61 percent of those with immunocytochemical localization of HCG had elevated serum levels of these markers.[18] The frequency[9, 18, 45] of localizing AFP and/or HCG in patients with elevated serum levels is greater than 70 percent. Kurman and McIntire found that HCG was consistently localized in tissue sections when serum levels were as low as 5 ng/ml, whereas localization of AFP was seen only when serum levels were greater than 800 ng/ml using an indirect immunoperoxidase technique.[71] With the use of the PAP and biotin avidin techniques, lower levels of AFP can be detected but the precise sensitivity of the AFP assay has not yet been determined.

Inadequate sampling must always be considered when elevations of AFP and HCG are observed in the absence of tissue localization. It is therefore recommended that two to three blocks of tissue for each centimeter of maximum tumor diameter be submitted for routine histologic and immunocytochemical testing.[71] In cases where sampling error appears remote, the presence of residual tumor or metastatic disease must be suspected.

CONCLUSION

This chapter has summarized the current information regarding the immunocytochemical features of testicular germ cell neoplasms. Although still in a relative state of infancy, these techniques have already provided a considerable fund of knowledge about the histogenesis of these tumors and the relationships between morphology and function. Indeed, with continued investigation of the antigenic characteristics of neoplastic germ cells, a revised classification of these tumors, combining both their morphologic and biochemical qualities, may prove necessary in the future. The identification of additional tumor specific antigens through immunohistochemical studies would be of great benefit in the treatment of patients with these tumors.

REFERENCES

1. Javadpour N, McIntire KR, Waldmann TA, et al: The role of the radioimmunoassay of serum alpha-fetoprotein and human chorionic gonadotropin in the intensive chemotherapy and surgery of metastatic testicular tumors. J Urol 119:759, 1978
2. Lange P, Fraley E: Serum alpha-fetoprotein and human chorionic gonadotropin in the treatment of patients with testicular tumors. Urol Clin North Am 4:393, 1977
3. Perlin E, Engeler J, Edson M et al: The value of serial measurement of both human chorionic gonadotropin and alpha-fetoprotein for monitoring germinal cell tumors. Cancer 37:215, 1976
4. Kurman RJ, Casey C: Immunoperoxidase techniques in surgical pathology: Principles and practice. p. 60. In Rose NR, Friedman H (eds): Manual of Clinical Immunology, 2nd ed. American Society for Microbiology, Washington D.C., 1980
5. Taylor C: Immunoperoxidase techniques. Practical and theoretical aspects. Arch Pathol Lab Med 102:113, 1978
6. Hsu S, Raine L, Fanger H: Use of avidin-biotin-peroxidase complex (abc) in immunoperoxidase techniques: a comparison between abc and unlabeled antibody (pap) procedures. J Histochem Cytochem 29:577, 1981
7. Hobson BM: The excretion of chorionic gonadotrophin by men with testicular tumours. Acta Endocrinol 49:337, 1965
8. Javadpour N: Multiple biochemical tumor markers in seminoma. A double blind study. Cancer 52:887, 1983
9. Kurman RJ, Scardino PT: Alpha-fetoprotein and human chorionic gonadotropin in ovarian and testicular germ cell tumors. p. 277. In DeLellis RA (ed): Diagnostic Immunocytochemistry. Masson, New York, 1981
10. Kurohara SS, George FW, Dykhuisen RF, Leary KL: Testicular tumors. Analysis of 196 cases treated at the U.S. Naval Hospital in San Diego. Cancer 20:1089, 1967
11. Hedinger C, von Hochstetter AR, Egloff B: Seminoma with syncytiotrophoblastic giant cells. A special form of seminoma. Virchows Arch Pathol [A] 383:59, 1979
12. Javadpour N, McIntire KR, Waldmann TA: Human chorionic gonadotropin (hCG) and al-

pha-fetoprotein (AFP) in sera and tumor cells of patients with testicular seminoma. A prospective study. Cancer 42:2768, 1978

13. Thackray AC, Crane WAJ: Seminoma. p. 164. In Pugh RCB (ed): Pathology of the Testis. Blackwell Scientific Publications, Oxford, 1976

14. Wurster K: Klassifizierung testikularer Keimzellgeschwulste. Neue Gesichtspunkte auf Grund morphogenetischer Studien. Normale und pathologische Anatomie. Heft 31. Georg Thieme, Stuttgart, 1976

15. Dixon FJ, Moore RA: Tumors of the male sex organs. In Atlas of Tumor Pathology, section 8, fascicles 31b, 32. Armed Forces Institute of Pathology, Washington, D.C., 1952

16. Heyderman E: Multiple tissue markers in human malignant testicular tumors. Scand J Immunol 8: Suppl. 8, 119, 1978

17. Mostofi FK, Sesterhenn IA, Davis CJ: Evaluation of World Health Organization international classification of testicular tumors and correlation with tumor markers (HCG, HPL, and AFP) in 1000 testicular tumors (abstr). Lab Invest 50:41A, 1984

18. Jacobsen GK: Alpha-fetoprotein (AFP) and human chorionic gonadotropin (HCG) in testicular germ cell tumors. A comparison of histologic and serologic occurrence of tumour markers. Acta Path Microbiol Immunol Scand [Sect A] 91:183, 1983

19. Nochomovitz LE, Lange PH, Fraley EE, Rosai J: Testicular seminoma associated with human chorionic gonadotropin (HCG) production: a study of 16 cases, with special reference to anaplastic seminoma (abstr). Lab Invest 42:140, 1980

20. Jacobsen GK, Jacobsen M: Alpha-fetoprotein (AFP) and human chorionic gonadotropin (HCG) in testicular germ cell tumors. Acta Path Microbiol Immunol Scand [Sect A] 91:165, 1983

21. Wagener C, Menzel B, Breuer L et al: Immunohistochemical localization of alpha-fetoprotein (AFP) in germ cell tumors: evidence for AFP production by tissues other than endodermal sinus tumor. Oncology 38:236, 1981

22. Wahren B: Multiple fetal antigens in germ cell tumors. Scand J Immunol 8, Suppl. 8:131, 1978

23. Prat J, Bhan AK, Dickersin GR, Robboy SJ, Scully RE: Hypothesis: when is a seminoma not a seminoma? (Letter to the Editor) J Clin Pathol 34:1308, 1981

24. Nochomovitz LE, Rosai J: Current concepts on the histogenesis, pathology and immunochemistry of germ cell tumors of the testis. Pathol Annu 13:327, 1978

25. Bohn H: Isolation and characterization of pregnancy specific beta-1 glycoprotein. Blut 24:292, 1972

26. Javadpour N: Radioimmunoassay and immunoperoxidase of pregnancy specific beta-1 glycoprotein in sera and tumor cells of patients with certain testicular germ cell tumors. J Urol 123:514, 1980

27. Javadpour N, Utz M, Soares T: Immunocytochemical discordance in localization of pregnancy specific beta-1 glycoprotein, alpha-fetoprotein and human chorionic gonadotropin in testicular cancers. J Urol 124:615, 1980

28. Belliveau RE, Yamamoto LA, Wassell AR, Wiernik PH: Regan isoenzyme in patients with hematopoietic tumors. Am J Clin Pathol 62:329, 1974

29. Nathanson L, Fishman WH: New observations on the Regan isoenzyme of alkaline phosphatase in cancer patients. Cancer 27:1388, 1971

30. Stolbach LL: Clinical application of alkaline phosphatase isoenzyme analysis. Ann NY Acad Sci 166:760, 1969

31. Lange PH, Millan JL, Stigbrand T et al: Placental alkaline phosphatase as a tumor marker for seminoma. Cancer Res 42:3244, 1982

32. Wahren B, Holmgren PA, Stigbrand T: Placental alkaline phosphatase, alpha-fetoprotein and carcinoembryonic antigen in testicular tumors. Tissue typing by means of cytologic smears. Int J Cancer 24:749, 1979

33. Uchida T, Shimoda T, Miyata H et al: Immunoperoxidase study of alkaline phosphatase in testicular tumor. Cancer 48:1455, 1981

34. Beckstead JH: Alkaline phosphatase histochemistry in human germ cell neoplasms. Am J Surg Pathol 7:341, 1983

35. Bosl GJ, Lange PH, Nochomovitz LE et al: Tumor markers in advanced non-seminomatous testicular cancer. Cancer 47:572, 1981

36. Liu F, Fritsche HA, Trujillo JM, Samuels ML: Serum lactate dehydrogenase isoenzyme 1 in patients with advanced testicular cancer. Am J Clin Pathol 78:178, 1982

37. Wampler GL, Hazra T: Use of LDH isoenzyme 1 as a serum marker for seminoma. Proc Am Assoc Cancer Res 18:339, 1977

38. Murakami SS, Said JW: Immunohistochemical

localization of lactate dehydrogenase isoenzyme 1 in germ cell tumors of the testis. Am J Clin Pathol 81:293, 1984

39. Jacobsen GK, Jacobsen M: Ferritin (FER) in testicular germ cell tumors. An immunohistochemical study. Acta Pathol Microbiol Immunol Scand [Sect A] 91:177, 1983

40. Grail A, Bates G, Ward AM et al: Serum ferritin as a third marker in germ cell tumors. Eur J Cancer Clin Oncol 18:261, 1982

41. Abelev GI, Assecritova IV, Kraevsy NA et al: Embryonal serum alpha-globulin in cancer patients: diagnostic value. Int J Cancer 2:551, 1967

42. Norgaard-Pedersen B, Albrechtsen R, Teilum G: Serum alpha-fetoprotein as a marker for endodermal sinus tumour (yolk sac tumour) or a vitelline component of teratocarcinoma. Acta Pathol Microbiol Scand [Sect A] 83:573, 1975

43. Talerman A: Endodermal sinus (yolk sac) tumor elements in testicular germ-cell tumors in adults. Cancer 46:1213, 1980

44. Kurman RJ, Scardino PT, McIntire KR et al: Cellular localization of alpha-fetoprotein and human chorionic gonadotropin in germ cell tumors of the testis using an indirect immunoperoxidase technique. A new approach to classification utilizing tumor markers. Cancer 40:2136, 1977

45. Fowler JE, Sesterhenn I, Stutzman RE, Mostofi FK: Localization of alpha-fetoprotein and human chorionic gonadotropin to specific histologic types of non-seminomatous testicular cancer. Urology 22:649, 1983

46. Wittekind C, Wichmann T, von Kleist S: Immunohistological localization of AFP and HCG in uniformly classified testis tumors. Anticancer Res 3:327, 1983

47. Jacobsen GK, Jacobsen M, Clausen PP: Distribution of tumor-associated antigens in the various histologic components of germ cell tumors of the testis. Am J Surg Pathol 5:257, 1981

48. Wold LE, Kramer S, Farrow GM: Testicular yolk sac and embryonal carcinomas in pediatric patients: comparative immunohistochemical and clinicopathologic study. Am J Clin Pathol 81:427, 1984

49. Gitlin D, Perricelli A: Synthesis of serum albumin, pre-albumin, alpha-feto-protein, alpha-1-antitrypsin and transferrin by the human yolk sac. Nature 228:995, 1970

50. Palmer PE, Safaii H, Wolfe HJ: Alpha-1-antitrypsin and alpha-fetoprotein. Protein markers in endodermal sinus (yolk sac) tumors. Am J Clin Pathol 65:575, 1976

51. Cardoso de Almeida PC, Scully RE: Diffuse embryoma of the testis. A distinctive form of mixed germ cell tumor. Am J Surg Pathol 7:633, 1983

52. Wahren B, Alpert E, Esposti P: Multiple antigens as marker substances in germinal tumors of the testis. J Natl Cancer Inst 58:489, 1977

53. Mostofi FK, Price EB: Tumors of the male genital system. In Atlas of Tumor Pathology, 2nd series, fascicle 8. Armed Forces Institute of Pathology, Washington D.C., 1973

54. Talerman A: The incidence of yolk sac tumor (endodermal sinus tumor) elements in germ cell tumors of the testis in adults. Cancer 36:211, 1975

55. Talerman A, Haije WG: Alpha-fetoprotein and germ cell tumors: a possible role of yolk sac tumor in production of alpha-fetoprotein. Cancer 34:1722, 1974

56. Teilum G, Albrechtsen R, Norgaard-Pedersen B: Immunofluorescent localization of alpha-fetoprotein synthesis in endodermal sinus tumor (yolk sac tumor). Acta Pathol Microbiol Scand [Sect A] 82:586, 1974

57. Beilby JOW, Horne CHW, Milne GD, Parkinson C: Alpha-fetoprotein, alpha-1-antitrypsin and transferrin in gonadal yolk-sac tumours. J Clin Pathol 32:455, 1979

58. Kurman RJ, Norris HJ: Embryonal carcinoma of the ovary. A clinicopathologic entity distinct from endodermal sinue tumor resembling embryonal carcinoma of the adult testis. Cancer 38:2420, 1976

59. Kurman RJ, Scardino PT, McIntire KR et al: Cellular localization of AFP and HCG in germ cell tumors of the testis and ovary. Scand J Immunol 8 (Suppl. 8): 127, 1978

60. Palmer PE, Wolfe HJ: Immunocytochemical localization of oncodevelopmental proteins in human germ cell and hepatic tumors. J Histochem Cytochem 26:523, 1978

61. Rimbaut C, Caillaud JM, Caillou B et al: Alpha-1-fetoprotein (AFP) and germ cell tumors: biological and histological correlation. Scand J Immunol 8 (Suppl. 8):201, 1978

62. Gitlin D, Perricelli A, Gitlin GM: Synthesis of alpha-fetoprotein by liver, yolk sac and gas-

trointestinal tract of the human conceptus. Cancer Res 32:979, 1972

63. Teilum G: Endodermal sinus tumor of the ovary and testis. Comparative morphogenesis of the so-called mesonephroma ovarii (Schiller) and extra-embryonic (yolk-sac-allantoic) structures of the rat's placenta Cancer 12:1092, 1959

64. Jacobsen GK, Jacobsen M, Henriksen OB: An immunohistochemical study of a series of plasma proteins in the early human conceptus. Oncodeve Biol Med 2:399, 1981

65. Endo Y, Urano Y, Tsuchida Y et al: Protein synthesis in yolk sac tumor: histochemical studies of human and rat yolk sac tumor. Scand J Immunol 8 (Suppl. 8):171, 1978

66. Teilum G: Classification of endodermal sinus tumour (mesoblastoma vitellinum) and so-called "embryonal carcinoma" of the ovary. Acta Pathol Microbiol Scand 64:407, 1965

67. Kurman RJ, Norris HJ: Endodermal sinus tumor of the ovary. A clinical and pathologic analysis of 71 cases. Cancer 38:2404, 1976

68. Pierce GB, Midgley AR, Sri Ram J, Feldman JD: Parietal yolk sac carcinoma: clue to the histogenesis of Reichert's membrane of the mouse embryo. Am J Pathol 41:549, 1962

69. Damjanov I, Amenta PS, Zarghami F: Transformation of an AFP-positive yolk sac carcinoma into an AFP-negative neoplasm. Evidence for in vivo cloning of the human perietal yolk sac carcinoma. Cancer 53:1902, 1984

70. Prat J, Bhan AK, Dickersin GR et al: Hepatoid yolk sac tumor of the ovary (endodermal sinus tumor with hepatoid differentiation). A light microscopic, ultrastructural and immunohistochemical study of seven cases. Cancer 50:2355, 1982

71. Kurman RJ: Immunocytochemistry of testicular cancer. p. 92. In Donohue JP (ed): Testis Tumors. Williams and Wilkins, Baltimore, 1983

72. Grigor KM, Detre, SI, Kohn J, Neville AM: Serum alpha-1-fetoprotein levels in 153 male patients with germ cell tumors. Br J Cancer 35:52, 1977

73. Kohn J, Orr AH, McElwain TJ et al: Serum alpha-fetoprotein in patients with testicular tumors. Lancet 2:433, 1976

74. Shepheard BGF: Alpha-fetoprotein and teratomas of the testis. Proc R Soc Med 67:307, 1974

75. Jacobsen GK, Jacobsen M: Possible liver cell differentiation in testicular germ cell tumours. Histopathology 7:537, 1983

9

Intermediate Filaments in Testicular Germ Cell Tumors

Markku Miettinen, Ismo Virtanen, and Aleksander Talerman

Virtually all nucleated cells of eukaryotes contain a cytoplasmic fibrillary network, the cytoskeleton, composed of the following fibrillar structures: microfilaments (6 nm), intermediate filaments (10 nm), and microtubuli (25 nm). While most cells have similar microfilaments and microtubuli, different cell types contain biochemically and immunologically distinct intermediate filaments (IF) differing in the protein composition of their subunits.[1-5] The expression of IF proteins is genetically controlled and reflects the origin and the state of differentiation of the cells. Thus, epithelial cells express keratins/cytokeratins; mesenchymal nonmuscular cells, vimentin; muscle cells, desmin; neural cells, neurofilaments; and astrocytes and some ependymal cells, glial fibrillary acidic protein (GFAP).[2-5] The constant and highly predictable expression of IF proteins concurs with the histologic classification of cells and tissues. The expression of IF is preserved also in malignant cells, and this makes IF proteins suitable cell-type-specific markers for cell biology and surgical pathology.[2-7] As a general rule, different types of carcinomas contain keratins/cytokeratins; sarcomas of nonmuscular origin, lymphomas, and melanomas, vimentin; leiomyosarcomas and rhabdomyosarcomas, desmin; and neural and glial tumors, neurofilaments and GFAP, respectively.[5-8]

Cytokeratins are a complex group of related polypeptides. To date, 19 biochemically and immunologically different cytokeratin polypeptides are known to occur in various keratinizing and nonkeratinizing epithelia.[9-10] In addition, antibodies recognizing different keratins/cytokeratins show various reactivities with different epithelial cells. Epidermal keratin antibodies, the first antikeratin antibodies used in research, react strongly with the epidermis and other stratified epithelia, and may react with some simple epithelial cells, but generally do not react with epithelia of certain internal organs, such as hepatocytes, renal tubular cells, or acinar cells of the pancreas.[11,12] In contrast, antibodies raised against liver cytokeratins[13] or antibodies to renal tubular cell cytokeratins[14] react with these epithelial cells. Monoclonal cytokeratin antibodies with different specificities have recently been produced and used to characterize normal tissues and tumors.[8,15-17] Such antibodies may either present a broad-spectrum reacting with a number of different cytokeratin polypeptides, or they may have a narrow reactivity with only a single polypeptide.[15] A set of different cytokeratin antibodies enables us to distinguish between various epithelial tumors and acts as an aid to diagnosis. For example, squamous and nonsquamous cell carcinomas, cholangiocarcinomas and hepatocellular carcinomas, and thyroid papillary and follicular carcinomas can be differentiated with the aid of different cytokeratin antibodies.[15, 18, 19]

In this chapter, we present the results of our studies concerning the distribution of intermediate filaments in testicular germ cell tumors.

METHODOLOGY

In the immunohistochemical analysis of intermediate filaments, both polyclonal and monoclonal antibodies are useful when they are adequately characterized and tested with known cells and tissues to exclude cross reactions between different types of intermediate filaments. Monoclonal antibodies may show less background staining than polyclonal antibodies, but they are more vulnerable to nonoptimal fixation as they react only with a single antigenic site (epitope). While the use of frozen sections is most desirable, formalin-fixed and paraffin-embedded material may also be suitable but often requires special pretreatment of the sections. Mild proteolytic digestion is useful in such material, probably by exposing the masked antigens.[20, 21] Pepsin, trypsin, and pronase[22] have all been successfully used, but we have mostly used pepsin (0.4 percent in 0.01 N HCl for 30 minutes to 2 hours at 37°C). As an alternative for immunohistochemical analysis, intermediate filaments of tumors can also be analyzed biochemically by polyacrylamide gel electrophoresis. In homogeneous tumors this works well, while in heterogeneous tumors it poses problems and necessitates microdissection of the various components.[10]

The antibodies to intermediate filaments used in this study have been described elsewhere [rabbit antibodies to epidermal keratin,[6] vimentin,[6] desmin,[23] and mouse monoclonal antibodies to cytokeratin (PKK 1 and PKK 2), vimentin, neurofilaments, and GFAP].[8]

The epidermal keratin antibodies recognize numerous high-molecular-weight keratin polypeptides, whereas the cytokeratin antibodies recognize low-molecular-weight keratin polypeptides.

NORMAL TESTIS

The normal testes studied (n=7) were from orchiectomies performed in patients with prostatic cancer or from autopsies in cases of accidental death. The Sertoli cells in the seminiferous tubules, like the connective tissue elements, are vimentin-positive (Fig. 9-1A), as described by Franke.[24] Only some of the germ cells in the seminiferous epithelium are vimentin-positive, while in cytologic specimens the spermatozoa show a narrow rim of vimentin-positivity in their equatorial segment region.[25] Antibodies to desmin disclose positivity in the cell layer encircling the seminiferous tubules, corresponding to the myoid cell layer, while other components are negative. Antibodies to epidermal keratin react only with the epithelium of the rete testis (Fig. 9-1B), while all other components of the seminiferous tubules are negative. However, the cytokeratin antibodies, while reacting with the rete testis epithelium, also react with intratubular epithelial cells in structures present between the rete testis and the seminiferous tubules which probably represent the tubuli recti (Fig. 9-1C). It may be of interest that occasional cells scattered in the lumina of some seminiferous tubules also stain positively with monoclonal cytokeratin antibodies (Fig. 9-1D). The identity of these cytokeratin-positive cells remains a question, but they may represent a special type of Sertoli cell.

TESTICULAR TUMORS

Classic Seminomas

Forty-one classic seminomas, five of which were obtained at frozen section, were studied. In both frozen and paraffin sections all cases show vimentin-positive tumor cells (Fig. 9-

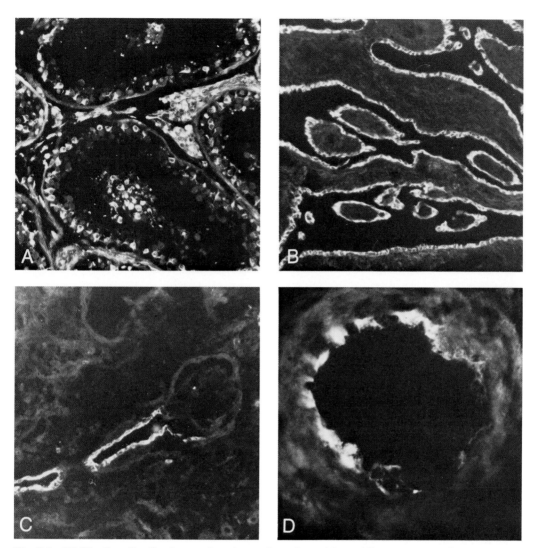

Fig. 9-1. (A) The Sertoli cells of normal testis are vimentin-positive, while most germ cells are negative. Note also the vimentin positivity of the Leydig cells (center right). (B) The rete testis epithelium is labeled with cytokeratin antibodies as are (C) the tubuli recti structures between the rete testis and seminiferous tubules. (D) Single cells within some seminiferous tubules show cytokeratin positivity. Immunofluorescent stain.

2A,B), although usually only a small number of the tumor cells are positive, suggesting a poorly developed intermediate filament system in these tumors. The connective tissue septa, blood vessels, and infiltrating lymphoid cells are also vimentin-positive. Epidermal keratin antibodies do not react with the tumor cells, but monoclonal cytokeratin antibodies show isolated or small groups of positive cells in nearly half of the cases (17/41) (Fig. 9-2C,D). Many of the cytokeratin-positive tumor cells are larger than other tumor cells, and some of them represent multinucleated giant cells (Fig. 9-2D).

The nature of the single cytokeratin-positive epithelial cells found in nearly half of the semi-

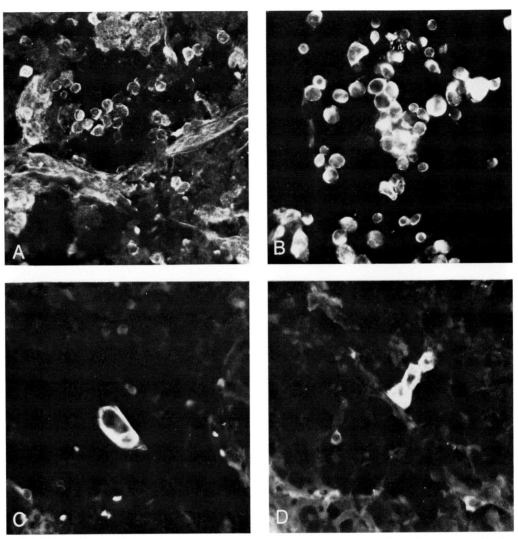

Fig. 9-2. In classic seminoma, (A) some tumor cells, the vascular septa and lymphatic cells, are labeled with antibodies to vimentin. (B) In cytologic imprint preparations, the cytoplasmic vimentin positivity is more clearly seen in seminoma. (C) Single cytokeratin-positive large cells or (D) small groups/multinucleated cytokeratin-positive cells are seen in many seminomas. Immunofluorescent stain.

nomas is intriguing. These cells may represent an early differentiation into embryonal carcinoma or choriocarcinoma, both of which express cytokeratin. It is well recognized that syncytiotrophoblastic giant cells occur in seminomas,[26, 27] and such cells may be positive for chorionic gonadotropin when stained by immunofluorescent or immunoperoxidase techniques.[28] The cytokeratin-positivity of such cells is further evidence of their trophoblastic nature. The occurrence of cytokeratin-positive cells in seminomas also suggests that seminomas may occasionally differentiate further in both embryonal and extraembryonal directions. Some further evidence also suggests that choriocarcinoma-like differentiation may occur in some seminomas. Occasional patients with pure seminomas have developed

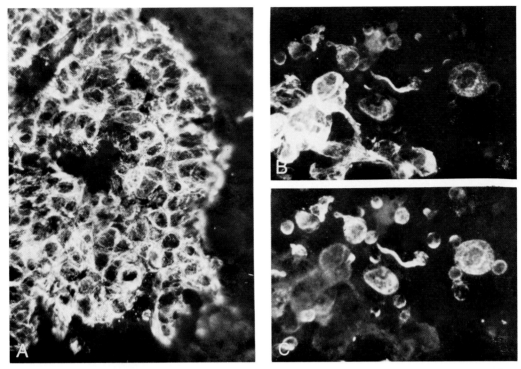

Fig. 9-3. (A) Solid areas of embryonal carcinoma show cytokeratin positivity. (B) In imprint preparations of an embryonal carcinoma, cytokeratin-positive tumor cells are found, and (C) a portion of these cells also contain vimentin. Immunofluorescent stain.

choriocarcinomatous metastases[29] and, furthermore, patients with seminoma containing syncytiotrophoblastic giant cells invariably have elevated serum titers of chorionic gonadotropin.[27, 30]

SPERMATOCYTIC SEMINOMAS

In common with classic seminoma, the seven spermatocytic seminomas studied show vimentin-positive tumor cells. Cytokeratin-positivity was found only in one of the seven cases, compared with 40 percent of the classic seminomas. The rarity of cytokeratin-positive cells in spermatocytic seminoma suggests that further differentiation of the cells is rare and indicates that the large cells in spermatocytic seminoma are different from the large syncytiotrophoblast-like cells observed in some classic seminomas.

EMBRYONAL CARCINOMAS

Eighteen embryonal carcinomas (5 pure and 13 combined with other neoplastic germ cell elements mainly immature teratoma) were studied. The embryonal carcinoma cells differ from those of a classic seminoma by showing cytokeratin positivity in most tumor cells. This is observed in solid, undifferentiated (Fig. 9-3A), as well as in papillary, areas of embryonal carcinoma. When epidermal keratin antibodies are used they reveal only a small number of positive cells (this was observed in 10 of 15 cases), and solid undifferentiated areas of the tumor are generally totally negative. By their selective cytokeratin positivity, embryonal carcinoma cells resemble the early embryonal cells that only express cytokeratin, and do not acquire vimentin positivity until the time when the primary mesenchymal elements are formed.[31]

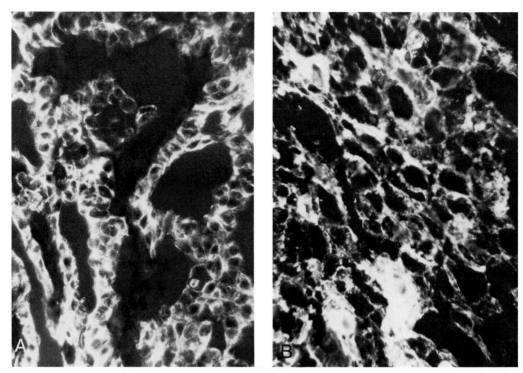

Fig. 9-4. The tumor cells in the (A) glandular as well as (B) solid and microcystic areas of endodermal sinus tumor show cytokeratin positivity. Immunofluorescent stain.

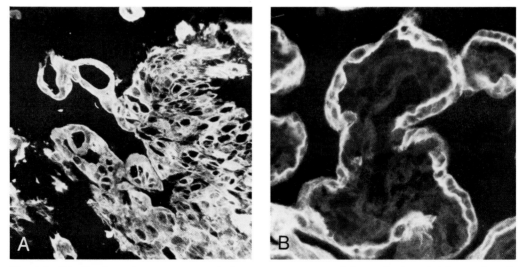

Fig. 9-5. (A) Choriocarcinomatous areas in immature teratoma of the testis show bright cytokeratin positivity, similar to that of (B) trophoblastic cells lining the chorionic villi in normal placenta. Immunofluorescent stain.

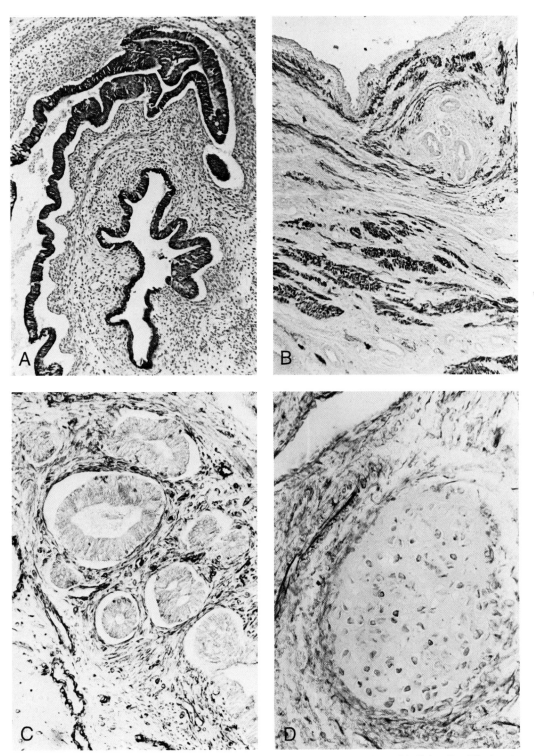

Fig. 9-6. (A) Immature teratoma of the testis displays cytokeratin in the epithelial cells, (B) desmin only in the bundles and fascicles of smooth muscle cells, and (C) vimentin in the stromal fibroblasts and vascular endothelial cells but not in the epithelia. (D) Vimentin is also seen in the cartilage cells. Immunofluorescent stain.

187

In 9 of 18 cases, vimentin-positive tumor cells were also found in embryonal carcinomas, and some cells appear to express cytokeratin and vimentin reactivity when stained for both substances simultaneously (Fig. 9-3B,C). Such expression, being rare in normal tissues,[3-5] has been revealed in parietal endodermal cells of early embryos.[32] It is possible that the tumor cells expressing cytokeratin and vimentin in embryonal carcinomas represent parietal endoderm-like differentiation.

The cytokeratin positivity in undifferentiated embryonal carcinomas and the vimentin positivity in seminomas can be used as a differential diagnostic feature, as also suggested by Battifora et al.[33] However, the frequent presence of occasional cytokeratin-positive cells in seminomas must be taken into account and the findings treated with a certain degree of caution.

ENDODERMAL SINUS TUMORS

The 10 endodermal sinus tumors studied showed cytokeratin positivity in most tumor cells, while they were negative when examined with epidermal keratin antibodies (Fig. 9-4A,B). Vimentin is observed in the septal fibroblasts, endothelial cells, and macrophages.

CHORIOCARCINOMAS

The trophoblastic tumor cells present in the choriocarcinomatous component of the three malignant teratomas examined showed cytokeratin positivity, but were only weakly epidermal keratin-positive (Fig. 9-5A). In their cytokeratin positivity, choriocarcinoma cells were similar to the trophoblastic cells present in the normal placenta (Fig. 9-5B). The choriocarcinoma cells were negative for vimentin.

TESTICULAR TERATOMAS

Nineteen testicular teratomas with varying patterns composed of admixture of mature and immature components were studied. The

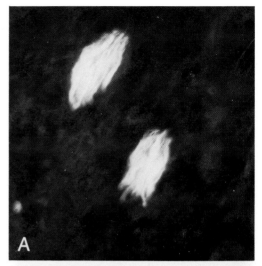

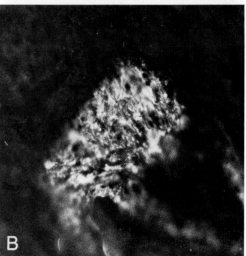

Fig. 9-7. (A) The neural tissue within immature teratoma shows neurofilament positivity, and (B) the glial areas show positivity with antibodies to GFAP. Immunofluorescent stain.

intermediate filament expression in these tumors is similar to the findings observed in corresponding normal tissues, as well as in ovarian teratomas.[34] Thus, epithelial elements show cytokeratin, stromal fibroblasts, cartilage and vascular endothelial cells, vimentin, and smooth muscle elements, desmin (Fig. 9-6). Furthermore, antibodies to neurofilaments reveal positivity in neural tissue, and antibodies to GFAP show a positive reaction in glial-

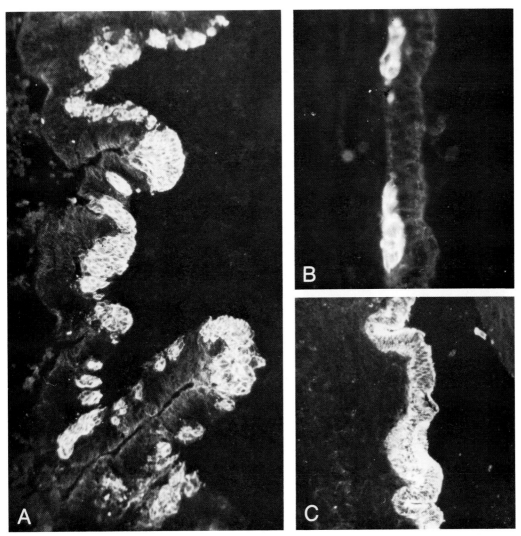

Fig. 9-8. (A&B) Many stratified columnar epithelia in immature teratomas show epidermal keratin-like immunoreactivity restricted to the basal cells while (C) widely reacting cytokeratin antibodies label the whole thickness of the epithelium. Immunofluorescent stain.

like areas, which were found in three cases (Fig. 9-7).

The epithelial components show an interesting diversity in their reactivity to different types of keratin and cytokeratin antibodies. Squamous-epithelium-lined cyst-like structures are labeled equally with epidermal keratin and cytokeratin antibodies. Many columnar epithelia show epidermal keratin positivity only in their basal cells (Fig. 9-8A,B), while cytokeratin antibodies stain the whole thickness of such epithelia (Fig. 9-8C). A similar situation is seen in some normal epithelia, for example, in prostatic epithelium where only basal cells are labeled with epidermal keratin antibodies, while the widely reactive cytokeratin antibodies can react with all epithelial cells (Virtanen et al., in preparation).

CONCLUSION

The varying patterns of cellular differentiation in testicular germ cell tumors are also reflected in their expression of intermediate filaments, making the IF proteins valuable differentiation markers for these tumors. Antibodies to IF also reveal an interesting polymorphism in many tumors, not easily apparent on conventional histologic methods. In selected cases, differential diagnosis between tumors resembling each other when examined light microscopically can be possible: for example, seminomas can be differentiated from embryonal carcinomas by the constant cytokeratin positivity present in the cells of the latter. Our findings, by demonstrating the presence of cytokeratin-positive cells in some classic seminomas, lend further support to the view that classic seminomas in some cases may be capable of differentiation to embryonal carcinoma and further.

REFERENCES

1. Weber K, Osborn M: Cytoskeleton: definition, structure and gene regulation. Pathol Res Pract 175:128, 1982
2. Anderton BH: Intermediate filaments: a family of homologous structures. J Muscle Res Cell Motil 2:141, 1981
3. Franke WW, Schmid E, Schiller DL et al: Differentiation-related patterns of expression of proteins of intermediate filaments in tissues and cultured cells. Cold Spring Harbor Symp Quant Biol 46:431, 1982
4. Lazarides E: Intermediate filaments: a chemically heterogeneous developmentally regulated class of proteins. Annu Rev Biochem 51:219, 1982
5. Osborn M, Weber K: Biology of disease. Tumor diagnosis by intermediate filament typing: a novel tool for surgical pathology. Lab Invest 48:372, 1983
6. Virtanen I, Lehto V-P, Lehtonen E et al: Expression of intermediate filaments in cultured cells. J Cell Sci 50:45, 1981
7. Ramaekers FCS, Puts JJG, Moesker O et al: Antibodies to intermediate filament proteins in the immunohistochemical identification of human tumors: an overview. Histochem J 15:691, 1983
8. Virtanen I, Miettinen M, Lehto V-P et al: Diagnostic application of monoclonal antibodies to intermediate filaments. Ann NY Acad Sci, in press
9. Franke WW, Schiller DL, Moll R et al: Diversity of cytokeratins: differentiation specific expression of cytokeratin polypeptides in epithelial cells and tissues. J Mol Biol 153:933, 1981
10. Moll R, Franke WW, Schiller DL et al: The catalog of human cytokeratins: patterns of expression in normal epithelia, tumors and cultured cells. Cell 31:11, 1982
11. Franke WW, Appelhans B, Schmid E et al: Identification and characterization of epithelial cells in mammalian tissues by immunofluorescence microscopy using antibodies to prekeratin. Differentiation 15:7, 1979
12. Sun T-T, Shih C, Green H: Keratin cytoskeletons in epithelial cells of internal organs. Proc Natl Acad Sci USA 76:2813, 1979
13. Franke WW, Denk H, Kalt R, Schmid E: Biochemical and immunological identification of cytokeratin proteins present in hepatocytes of mammalian liver tissues. Exp Cell Res 131:299, 1981
14. Holthofer H, Miettinen A, Paasivuo R et al: Cellular origin and differentiation of renal carcinomas: a fluorescence microscopic study with kidney-specific antibodies, and lectins. Lab Invest 49:317, 1983
15. Ramaekers F, Huysmans A, Moesker O et al: Monoclonal antibody to keratin filaments, specific for glandular epithelia and their tumors. Use in surgical pathology. Lab Invest 49:353, 1983
16. Debus E, Weber K, Osborn M: Monoclonal cytokeratin antibodies that distinguish simple from stratified squamous epithelia: characterization on human tissues. EMBO J 1:1641, 1982
17. Van Muijen GNP, Ruiter DJ, Ponec M, et al: Monoclonal antibodies with different specificities against cytokeratins. An immunohistological study of normal tissues and tumors. Am J Pathol 114:9, 1984
18. Krepler R, Denk H, Artlieb U et al: Antibodies to intermediate filament proteins as molecular markers in clinical tumor pathology. Differen-

tiation of carcinomas by their reaction with different cytokeratin antibodies. Pathol Res Pract 175:212, 1982

19. Miettinen M, Franssila K, Lehto V-P, Paasivuo R: Expression of intermediate filaments in thyroid gland and thyroid tumors. Lab Invest 50:262, 1984

20. Brozman M: Immunohistochemical analysis of formaldehyde- and trypsin- or pepsin-treated material. Acta Histochem 63:25, 1978

21. Miettinen M, Lehto V-P, Badley RA, Virtanen I: Alveolar rhabdomyosarcoma—demonstration of desmin, the muscle-type of intermediate filament, as a diagnostic aid. Am J Pathol 108:246, 1982

22. Kaku T, Ekem K, Lindayem C et al: Comparison of formalin- and acetone-fixation for immunohistochemical detection of carcinoembryonic antigen (CEA) and keratin. Am J Clin Pathol 80:806, 1983

23. Badley RA, Woods A, Carruthers L, Rees DA: Cytoskeleton changes in fibroblast adhesion and detachment. J Cell Sci 43:379, 1980

24. Franke WW, Grund C, Schmid E: Intermediate-sized filaments present in Sertoli cells are of vimentin-type. Eur J Cell Biol 19:269, 1979

25. Virtanen I, Badley RA, Paasivuo R, Lehto V-P: Distinct cytoskeletal domains revealed in sperm cells. J Cell Biol 99:1083, 1984

26. Mostofi FK, Price EB: Tumors of the Male Genital System. Armed Forces Institute of Pathology, Washington D.C., 1973

27. Talerman A: Germ cell tumors of the testis. In Fenoglio CM, Wolff M (eds): Progress in Surgical Pathology, vol 1. Masson, New York, 1980

28. Rosai J: Ackerman's Surgical Pathology, vol 2. CV Mosby, St. Louis, 1981

29. Crook JC: Morphogenesis of testicular tumours. J Clin Pathol 21:71, 1968

30. Hobson BM: The excretion of chorionic gonadotrophin by men with testicular tumours. Acta Endocrinol 49:337, 1965

31. Franke WW, Grund C, Kuhn C et al: Formation of cytoskeletal elements during mouse embryogenesis. III. Primary mesenchymal cells and the first appearance of vimentin filaments. Differentiation 23:43, 1983

32. Lehtonen E, Lehto V-P, Paasivuo R, Virtanen I: Parietal and visceral endoderm differ in their expression of intermediate filaments. EMBO J 2:1023, 1983

33. Battifora H, Sheibani K, Tubbs RR et al: Antikeratin antibodies in tumor diagnosis. Distinction between seminoma and embryonal carcinoma. Cancer 54:843, 1984

34. Miettinen M, Lehto V-P, Virtanen I: Expression of intermediate filaments in ovarian epithelial, sex cord-stromal and germinal tumors. Int J Gynecol Pathol 2:64, 1983

10

Spontaneous and Experimental Testicular Tumors in Animals

Ivan Damjanov

Testicular tumors of animal origin have been studied in great detail, particularly since they represent excellent replicas of the equivalent human tumors and could thus provide valuable information directly relevant to the understanding of the histogenesis and overall biology of human testicular tumors. Several extensive reviews[1-7] pertaining to this topic have already been published, and the reader is referred to these articles for a more exhaustive overview of the older literature and details that might not be covered in this brief summary of the present day knowledge on spontaneous and experimentally induced testicular tumors in animals.

CLASSIFICATION OF ANIMAL TUMORS

Testicular tumors found in various animals can be histologically classified into the same categories as the human neoplasms. Three major groups are recognized: germ cell tumors, tumors of specialized gonadal stroma, and tumors of the nonspecific stroma and supporting structures, including the mesothelium of the testicular tunica.

Germ Cell Tumors

Spontaneous germ cell tumors are, with notable exceptions, rare in common laboratory or domestic animals. These exceptions include

seminomas of dogs, teratomas in stallions,[3] and spontaneous congenital teratomas in strain 129 mice.[2] Spontaneous teratomas have been occasionally recorded in cockerels, rabbits, rats, and many other animals, but they represent isolated occurrences and have been recorded more as curiosities than as tumors that could provide experimental material or data relevant for the understanding of the overall pathogenesis of germ cell neoplasia.

Seminoma

Seminomas occur most commonly in dogs, forming approximately one-third of all testicular tumors in this species,[4] and only occasionally in other species.[8] The tumors appear as solitary nodules or as multinodular and even separate masses within scrotal or cryptorchid testes of older dogs. On gross examination canine seminomas resemble human tumors and appear as clay-colored, yellowish-white, or pinkish gray, lobulated moderately soft masses, which bulge from the cut surface.[3, 4] Histologically and ultrastructurally, the tumors also resemble human seminomas and are composed of clear cells filled with abundant cytoplasmic glycogen.[9] Tumor cells are large with a centrally located nucleus surrounded by clear cytoplasm that contains abundant glycogen (Fig. 10-1). Cells are arranged in broad sheaths delineated by scant intervening stroma or form broad lobules without distinct boundaries. The stroma often contains lym-

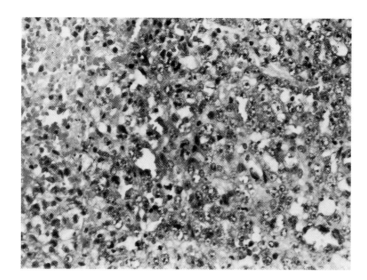

Fig. 10-1. Canine seminoma.

phocytes, plasma cells, and foamy histiocytes. Lymphocytes are most prominent around blood vessels. The tumor occasionally contains multinucleated giant cells.[4] The nature of these cells has not been determined, although some of them may be multinucleated histiocytes or reactive sustentacular cells seen inside the tubules in the testes of many experimental animals following chemical or mechanical injury (Fig. 10-2). On the other hand, some of these giant cells may represent equivalents of human syncytiotrophoblastic cells seen in some seminomas.[10] Finally, it is possible that the large cells of canine seminomas represent the equivalent of large cells in human spermatocytic seminomas,[11] a possibility that deserves additional studies, especially in view of the observation made by Scully[12, 13] about the similarity of some canine tumors to human spermatocytic seminomas.

In addition to frankly invasive tumors, canine testes may also contain foci of preinvasive, intratubular seminoma.[4] Intratubular seminoma is often multifocal and consists of large, polygonal slightly basophilic cells with vesicular nuclei and prominent nucleoli (Fig. 10-3). It is not clear whether the multifocal nature of intratubular seminoma indicates the mode of growth of these tumor cells or whether these foci represent widespread de

novo neoplastic transformation of germ cells. On the other hand, the preinvasive nature of these intratubular atypical germ cells is reflected not only in the nuclear atypia and their enlarged size but also in the frequently obvious transition from the intratubular to frankly invasive mode of growth. Disruption of tubular basement membranes and penetration of tumor cells through the wall of seminiferous tubules are frequently observed.

In contrast to human seminomas, which may be combined with other neoplastic germ cell elements, the seminomas of dogs are not combined with teratomas or embryonal carcinomas. On the other hand, in almost one-third of the cases, canine seminomas are combined with Sertoli cell or interstitial cell tumors.[4]

Although canine seminomas may attain considerable size, invasion of extratesticular tissue, usually the lymphatics and the veins of the pampiniform plexus, is only rarely seen. In a series of 125 canine seminomas collected by Nielsen and Lein,[4] only five tumors showed infiltration beyond testicular boundaries, and only seven tumors had metastasized.

Although spontaneous seminomas represent a rather common testicular tumor in dogs, there are no experimental methods to produce these tumors at will in either dogs or other laboratory animals. There are also

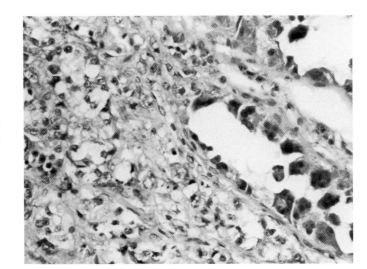

Fig. 10-2. Invasive tumor and intratubular giant cells in a canine seminoma.

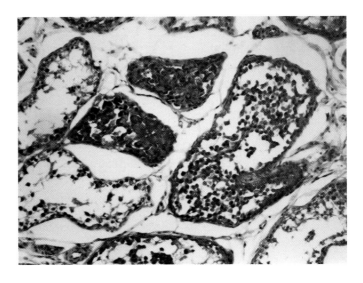

Fig. 10-3. Intratubular seminoma in a canine testis.

no seminoma-derived cell lines of either animal or human origin that could be used to characterize further these tumors and study in vitro their biological properties.

Teratoma

Spontaneous teratomas are extremely rare tumors in most animal species with the exception of humans, strain 129 mice, horses, and poultry.[2] In contrast to human testicular teratomas, which are predominately malignant, spontaneous teratomas in other species are usually benign. Nevertheless, malignant testicular teratomas occur spontaneously in strain 129 mice, and the data obtained on these retransplantable tumors, along with the cell lines derived from them, represent the foundations of our present knowledge about the biology and histogenesis of teratomas in general.[14-16]

The tendency of strain 129 mice to form spontaneous testicular teratomas was reported for the first time in 1954, when Stevens and Little[17] noted that 1 percent of all males in this strain had testicular tumors. By introducing several mutant genes into the genome of strain 129 mice, Stevens and his associates[2] have raised the incidence of spontaneous testicular tumors to 10 percent. Using techniques of selective inbreeding, Stevens[18] developed a new subline of the original 129 strain (called 129/Sv-ter) characterized by an exceptionally high (30 percent) incidence of spontaneous testicular teratomas. Thus, it was proven beyond any doubt that the predisposition to testicular teratoma formation is inherited and that it is determined by several genetic factors, although some genes may be more influential than the others. The very high rate of tumor formation in the 129/Sv-ter subline points to a single gene mutation resulting in a heritable trait and suggests that spontaneous tumors occurring at random could also be explained by some previously unidentified changes involving the genome of primordial germ cells.

In contrast to human teratomas of the testis, which are most often found in postpubertal individuals, spontaneous mouse tumors are present at birth, and their development can be traced to the fetal gonad. Studying fetal gonads of strain 129 mice, Stevens found that the first recognizable teratomas appear on day 15 of pregnancy.[19] This prompted him to hypothesize that the initiation of tumorigenesis must have occurred 2 to 3 days earlier.

To prove this hypothesis, Stevens transplanted the genital ridges of 11 to 15-day male fetuses of strain 129 mice into the testis of adult syngeneic recipients and showed that the early genital ridges indeed contain germ cells which can be stimulated to form teratomas.[20] Transplantation of 15-day-old gonads or older fetal testes did not result in the formation of teratomas. This not only proved that the congenital teratomas originate from relatively immature germ cells but also showed that teratocarcinogenesis can be initiated only during a given "critical" period of gonadogenesis.

Transplantation of fetal genital ridges to the testes of adult syngeneic testes proved to be a most efficient method for the production of teratomas, since 75 to 80 percent of all grafts formed tumors. It was also shown that testicular teratomas may be produced not only from the gonads of strain 129 mice but also from some other mouse strains, most notably strain A/He which normally shows no tendency for spontaneous teratoma formation. In the strain 129, grafting of fetal gonads could thus have had an *enhancing* effect on the spontaneous tumorigenesis; whereas in strain A/He, which does not develop teratomas spontaneously, one could definitively state that the grafting has actually *induced* tumor formation de novo, since teratomas would never have occurred in the testes of this mouse strain spontaneously. However, there are other mouse strains, such as CH3, in which it is not possible to induce teratomas by any type of manipulation of the fetal gonads, which suggests again that a certain genetic predisposition or "permissiveness" has to be present for the experimental procedure to initiate tumor formation.

In addition to the genetic factors regulating the tumor formation in fetal genital ridges of strain 129 mice, Stevens[2] has shown that the environmental factors also play an important role in the initiation of tumorigenesis. By transplanting fetal genital ridges to extratesticular sites, Stevens[2] showed that only the testicular sites exert the proper tumorigenic influence on the graft. Genital ridges transplanted to abdominal organs did not form more teratomas than one would expect in the intact nonmanipulated gonad of this mouse strain. Stevens[21] concluded that the scrotal site promotes teratocarcinogenesis by virtue of the lower temperature in this anatomical site, a notion supported by the fact that more tumors were produced from genital ridges transplanted to scrotal than the experimentally cryptorchid testes.

The histogenesis of murine testicular teratomas has been studied in fetal gonads transplanted to the adult testis.[22] Although the nature of the initial stimulus leading to the initiation of tumorigenesis remains incompletely understood, it has been convincingly shown that the tumors originate from intratu-

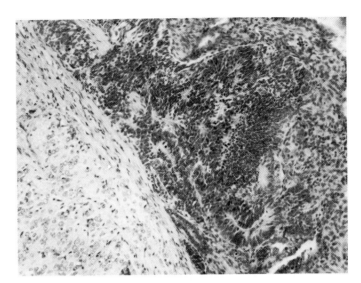

Fig. 10-4. Benign teratoma of a mouse composed of mature and immature neural tissue.

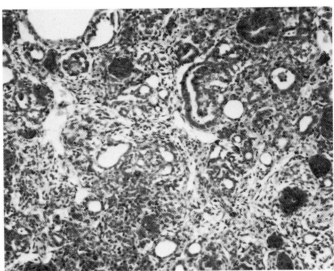

Fig. 10-5. Teratocarcinoma of a mouse.

bular germ cells. These cells give rise to undifferentiated embryonal-like cells which, in turn, either retain this undifferentiated phenotype or differentiate into various somatic and extraembryonal tissues. Tumors composed of somatic fully differentiated tissues have a limited growth span and behave like benign teratomas (Fig. 10-4). On the other hand, tumors that retain the embryonal-like cells, the undifferentiated descendants of the activated germ cells, continue to grow and finally kill the host (Fig. 10-5). These malignant teratomas, or teratocarcinomas, behave like malignant tumors, and their malignancy resides in the self-renewing pool of stem cells.

Stem cells of murine teratocarcinomas are undifferentiated embryonic cells showing a striking resemblance to the undifferentiated embryonic cells of the early mouse embryo. Stem cells of murine teratocarcinomas share with the normal embryonal cells not only a common phenotype, but also many cell membrane surface characteristics, and, most importantly, a uniquely broad developmental po-

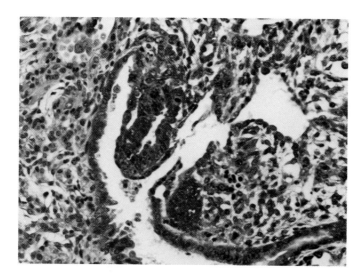

Fig. 10-6. Embryoid body from a mouse teratocarcinoma resembling a mouse egg-cylinder, that is, 6-day implanted embryo.

tential. Similarly to the early embryonic cells, the stem cells of teratocarcinoma can give rise to various somatic tissues and extraembryonic membranes corresponding to the parietal and visceral yolk sac. If injected into the blastocyst, the malignancy of these cells may be regulated and they may be induced to differentiate into essentially all somatic tissues.[15] This again shows that these tumor stem cells are indeed closely related to normal embryonic cells.

The embryonic nature of embryonal carcinoma cells has made them a popular model for the study of phenomena relevant to the understanding of normal embryogenesis and differentiation (see the recent monograph edited by Silvers, et al.[25] which illustrates various aspects of teratocarcinoma research). On the other hand, it also became soon apparent that embryonal carcinoma cells can not only be generated from activated germ cells in fetal genital ridges but also can be derived directly from early murine embryonic cells by either transplanting the early embryos into extrauterine sites[26] or by culturing embryos under conditions which would allow selective proliferation of undifferentiated cells.[27] Embryonal carcinoma cells derived from manipulated mouse embryos are biologically indistinguishable from testicular or ovarian embryonal carcinoma cells. This indicates that teratocarci-

nomas originating from various anatomical sites apparently share a common developmental pathway, which invariably includes morphogenetic events closely resembling early embryogenesis. Furthermore, the stem cells of these tumors retain a capacity to recapitulate and/or mimic some of the morphogenetic events of early embryogenesis, the most striking of which is the formation of so-called embryoid bodies in solid tumors (Fig. 10-6). Similar complex structures resembling early embryos can be produced by growing embryonal carcinoma cells in an ascites form or in vitro under conditions that prevent the cells from attaching themselves to the surface of the culture dishes[28] (Fig. 10-7).

From the perspective of comparative pathology, mouse teratomas and teratocarcinomas are fairly good, although not perfect, replicas of their human counterparts. Morphologically, the similarity is most striking at the light-microscopic level. Embryonal carcinoma cells, the primitive stem cells of both human and murine teratocarcinoma, are morphologically almost indistinguishable. The somatic tissues found in human and murine teratomas are essentially similar as all simple tissues in all stages of differentiation may be found. In contrast to human tumors, which often contain highly organized structures such as teeth or thyroid, histologically complex

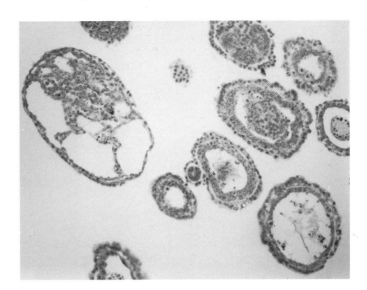

Fig. 10-7. Embryoid bodies obtained in culture from mouse embryonal carcinoma cells.

structures are not found in murine teratomas. Other differences are also seen, such as embryoid bodies which are quite common in mouse tumors but are uncommon in human teratoid tumors.

There are major differences in the cell surface antigenic properties of human and mouse embryonal carcinoma cells.[29] However, probably the most important difference between human and murine teratocarcinomas is that the malignancy of murine tumors resides in most instances in the embryonal carcinoma cells. Other malignant stem cells such as yolk sac carcinoma, choriocarcinoma, or various somatic-tissue-derived carcinomas and sarcomas are rare and have been recorded only as secondary phenomena upon retransplantation of malignant teratocarcinomas.[16] Mouse tumors frequently contain immature neural tissue, but this component is invariably benign in contrast with immature neural tissue of human teratomas, which may have considerable malignant potential.

Embryonal Carcinoma

In humans, embryonal carcinoma cells either form monomorphic neoplasms or are admixed with other components of typical germ cell tumors. In the complex nonseminomatous germ cell tumors, human embryonal carcinomas are usually capable of differentiating into various somatic and extraembryonic tissues and thus correspond to the developmentally pluripotent mouse embryonal carcinoma cells. The embryonal carcinoma cells forming monomorphic tumors are developmentally "nullipotent" cells because they have either never acquired or have somehow lost their capacity for differentiation.

In mice, "nullipotent" embryonal carcinomas do not occur spontaneously in the testis, ovary, or extragonadal sites. Several embryonal carcinoma cell lines have been isolated[25] from spontaneous or embryo-derived teratocarcinomas, and claims have been made that these cells do not differentiate, and thus represent nullipotent embryonal carcinoma cells. However, it has been shown that many of these "nullipotent" embryonal carcinoma cells differentiate spontaneously at a slow rate[30] and that their differentiation can be hastened with inducers of differentiation such as retinoic acid.[31] Since embryonal carcinoma cells grow faster than other components of the tumor and since the differentiation into somatic tissues may be minimal, many solid tumors produced from cultured murine teratocarcinoma stem cells injected into the living animals will

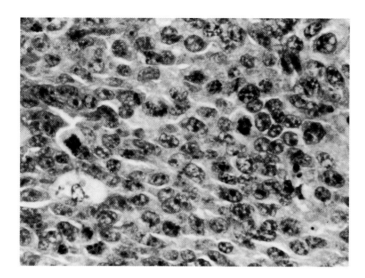

Fig. 10-8. Embryonal carcinoma. Section of a solid tumor produced by intramuscular injection of clonal embryonal carcinoma cells.

predominantly have the appearance of embryonal carcinoma (Fig. 10-8).

Yolk Sac Carcinoma

Yolk sac carcinoma (endodermal sinus tumor), as originally described by Teilum,[32] does not occur in experimental animals. However, yolk sac carcinomas have been described in mice,[33] rats,[34] and hamsters,[35] and their equivalence to human yolk sac carcinomas has been fully documented. The morphologic differences between human and laboratory animal tumors could, in this case, be explained by invoking the differences in the morphogenesis of yolk sac formation. Since the human yolk sac differs from the murine and hamster yolk sac, and since the yolk sac carcinomas reduplicate features expressed during normal formation of these vitelline membranes, it is understandable that the human tumors will differ from tumors found in laboratory animals.

Yolk sac tumors most commonly occur upon transplantation of teratocarcinomas. Experimentally, it is also possible to induce these tumors from transplanted embryos, especially when working with rat embryos,[34] or from placentas by leaving the placentas attached to the uterus following surgical removal of the fetus.[36] Tumors obtained in this manner

have a fairly typical appearance. In most instances the tumor cells correspond to the parietal yolk sac epithelium. These highly differentiated cells secrete basement membrane material corresponding to the so-called Reichert's membrane[33] and extracellular matrix: laminin, collagen type IV, or other structural proteins characterizing epithelial basement membranes.[37] Typically, tumor cells form small groups or strands surrounded by copious basement-membrane-like material (Fig. 10-9). Ultrastructurally, these cells contain prominent profiles of rough endoplasmic reticulum filled with the basement membrane material (Fig. 10-10).

While yolk sac carcinomas found in mice are almost invariably composed only of parietal yolk sac cells, those found in rats additionally contain visceral yolk sac cells. These cells, corresponding to the visceral yolk sac epithelium of the mouse embryo, are known to secrete alpha-fetoprotein[34] (Fig. 10-11). Yolk sac carcinomas of the rat also form complex structures which bear some resemblance to the Schiller-Duval bodies of human yolk sac carcinomas.[36] All this suggests that the rat parietovisceral yolk sac carcinoma represents a better replica of human tumor than the pure parietal yolk sac carcinoma of the mouse. Nevertheless, it appears that in some human yolk sac carcinomas the parietal yolk sac compo-

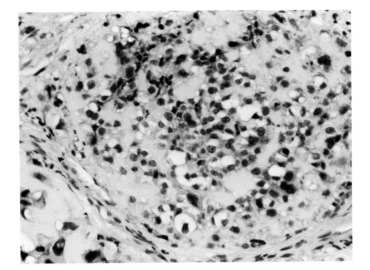

Fig. 10-9. Rat yolk sac carcinoma.

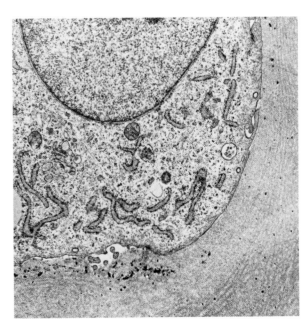

Fig. 10-10. Ultrastructural appearance of rat yolk sac carcinoma.

nent may selectively proliferate, and these tumors may then resemble the pure parietal yolk sac carcinoma of rodents.[38]

Choriocarcinoma

Tumors displaying the typical biphasic cellular composition of human choriocarcinomas and/or tumors secreting large amounts of cho-

rionic gonadotropin have not been described in laboratory animals. In this respect it should be noted that mouse and rat trophoblastic cells do not secrete chorionic gonadotropin[36] and that the antibody to human chorionic gonadotropin does not react with placental cells of the rodents. Trophoblastic giant cells are also not a common feature of murine teratocarcinomas, but the exact data on the occurrence of trophoblastic cells in mouse teratocarcino-

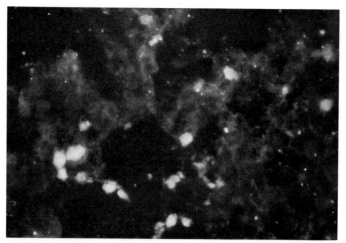

Fig. 10-11. Section of rat yolk sac carcinoma stained with fluorescein-isothiocyanate-labeled antibodies to alpha-fetoprotein, showing focally immunoreactive cells.

mas are not available since special histochemical techniques to identify these cells have so far not been applied systematically. The tumor labeled by Nicolas et al.[39] as trophoblastoma probably represents the only well-characterized mouse equivalent of human choriocarcinoma. Trophoblastic giant cells are present in the rat yolk sac carcinomas produced by fetectomy from midgestational placentas left behind in the uterus.[36]

Tumors of Specialized Gonadal Stroma

Sertoli cell tumors and interstitial (Leydig) cell tumors form a small fraction of human testicular tumors. On the other hand, these tumors of specialized gonadal stroma account for at least two-thirds of all canine testicular tumors[4] and are not infrequently, at least in dogs, combined with seminomas. Exact statistics on the occurrence of these tumors are, however, hard to compile because many male domestic animals are spayed and tumors noted clinically are not always examined histologically by veterinarians. Additionally, in those testes examined histologically, it is not always possible to distinguish small tumors from hy-

perplastic nodules representing either precursor lesions or a nonspecific reaction related to hormonal changes of senility. Systemic studies such as the Danish study of bulls[40] disclosed that, at least in that species, testicular tumors do occur, but only rarely.

Sertoli Cell Tumors

Sertoli cell tumors have been recorded in many domestic and zoo animals,[3] but they most often occur in old dogs. In this species Sertoli cell tumors occasionally induce feminization manifested by the loss of libido, homosexuality, enlargement of the nipples, and symmetrical loss of hair.[4] Histologically, the tumors occur in two forms: tubular and diffuse (Fig. 10-12). Both patterns can be seen in the same tumors. Also, quite frequently the atrophic seminiferous tubules in the vicinity of the main tumor mass contain foci of Sertoli cell hyperplasia. The tumor cells are usually elongated and, frequently, at least in the tubular variety, form cords with their longer axes perpendicular to the basement membrane and arranged tightly in rows or ribbons. Mitoses are rare, and the nuclear features rarely show marked atypia. Many cells have lipid-rich

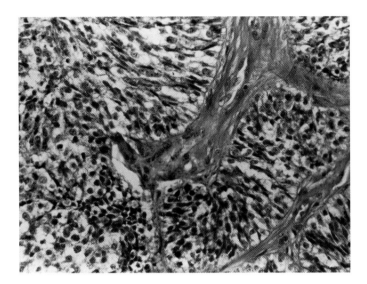

Fig. 10-12. Sertoli cell tumor of a dog.

foamy and vacuolated cytoplasm, and the cell borders are not distinct. Metastases are rare. Continuous cell lines have been established in vitro from at least one canine Sertoli cell tumor.[3] There are no acceptable methods for producing Sertoli cell tumors experimentally.

Interstitial Cell Tumors

Since these tumors occur quite frequently in dogs, rats, mice, and many other animals the pathology of interstitial cell tumors has been reviewed extensively.[1-7] Histologically, interstitial cell tumors cannot be differentiated from hyperplastic nodules, which are quite common in testes of many old animals because they exhibit similar histologic features. The distinction between these two lesions is arbitrary and usually based on size. Cotchin[3] designates canine testicular nodules larger than 1 cm as tumors, and anything smaller than that as hyperplasia. In rats and mice, one could apply the same criteria but use smaller dimensions to draw the arbitrary line between neoplasia and hyperplasia. The presence of metastatic foci sometimes encountered in old mice and rats serves as a definite sign of neoplasia.[1] Interstitial cell tumors of dogs are invariably benign and do not metastasize.

Histologically, three patterns of growth are typically recognized in the canine tumors:[4] solid–diffuse, cystic–vascular (angiomatoid), and pseudoadenomatous (Fig. 10-13). The tumor cells are polygonal or elongated and have centrally located round, vesicular, or even elongated nuclei. The texture of the cytoplasm varies. In some tumors the cells are granular and have eosinophilic cytoplasm. In others, the cells contain more lipid and are vacuolated or rich in lipofuscin.

Interstitial cell tumors can be induced in rats or mice using several experimental methods such as administration of carcinogenic hydrocarbons, hormones, subtotal castration, mechanical trauma, transplantation of testes to the spleen of castrated animals, irradiation, injection of caustic metals into the testis, or a combination of several of these approaches.[5] It has been shown that some mouse strains are more susceptible to hormonal induction of interstitial cell tumors than others.[6] Experimentally induced tumors, as well as some spontaneous interstitial cell tumors, have been used to obtain cell lines which can be propagated in vitro ad infinitum.

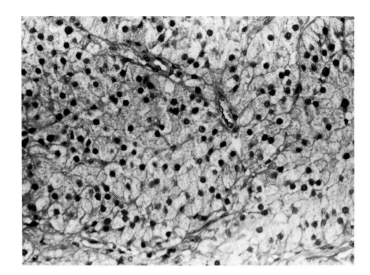

Fig. 10-13. Interstitial tumor from a 2-year-old rat.

Mixed Sertoli Cell–interstitial Cell Tumors

Some tumors of canines show features of both Sertoli cells and interstitial cells and cannot be properly classified.[4] Although rare, these tumors are of considerable interest because they indicate a common histogenesis and a possible common ancestral cell of origin for both Sertoli cells and interstitial cells.

TUMORS OF NONSPECIFIC STROMA AND SUPPORTING STRUCTURES

Benign and malignant tumors originating from the connective tissue cells of the testis do not differ from similar tumors spontaneously arising or experimentally induced in other anatomical sites. These include various benign neoplasms such as fibromas, hemangiomas, adenomatoid tumors (benign localized mesothelioma), or malignant soft tissue sarcomas such as fibrosarcomas, angiosarcomas, leiomyosarcomas, etc.[5, 6] Even rhabdomyosarcomas have been experimentally induced in the testis,[42] which suggests that these tumors probably arise from undifferentiated mesenchymal, developmentally pluripotent cells of

the supporting structures of the testis or the testicular stroma.

ACKNOWLEDGMENTS

Some of the material photographed for this article was contributed by Dr. W.-C. Hall. Ms. Jacklyn Powell typed the manuscript.

The author's original work was supported by NIH grants CA 23097 and CA 38405.

REFERENCES

1. Lacassagne A: Revue critique des tumeurs expérimentales des cellules de Leydig, plus particulièrement chex le rat. Bull Cancer 58:235, 1971
2. Stevens LC: The biology of teratomas. Adv Morphogen 6:1, 1967
3. Cotchin E: Spontaneous and experimentally-induced testicular tumours in animals. p. 371. In Pugh RCB (ed): Pathology of the Testis. Blackwell, Oxford, 1976
4. Nielsen SW, Lein DH: VI. Tumours of the testis. Bull WHO 50:71, 1974
5. Mostofi FK, Bresler VM: Tumours of the testis. p. 135. In Turusov VS (ed): Pathology of Tumours in Laboratory Animals, vol. 1. Tumours

of the Rat, part 2. International Agency for Research on Cancer, Lyon, 1976

6. Mostofi FK, Bresler VM: Tumours of the testis. p. 325. In Turusov VS (ed) Pathology of Tumours in Laboratory Animals, vol. 2. Tumours of the Mouse. International Agency for Research on Cancer, Lyon, 1979

7. Damjanov I, Solter D: Experimental teratoma. Curr Topics Pathol 59:69, 1974

8. Trigo FJ, Miller RA, Torbeck RL: Metastatic equine seminoma: report of two cases. Vet Pathol 21:259, 1984

9. von Bomhard D, Pospisch A: The ultrastructure of testicular tumors in the dog. I. Germinal cells and seminomas. J Comp Pathol 88:49, 1978

10. Zaloudek CJ, Tavassoli FA, Norris HJ: Dysgerminoma with syncytiotrophoblastic giant cells. Am J Surg Pathol 5:361, 1981

11. Talerman A, Fu YS, Okagaki T: Spermatocytic seminoma: ultrastructural and microspectrophotometric observations. Lab Invest 51:343, 1984

12. Scully RE: Spermatocytic seminoma of the testis. Cancer 14:788, 1961

13. Scully RE, Coffin DL: Canine testicular tumors, with special references to their histogenesis, comparative morphology, and endocrinology. Cancer 5:788, 1961

14. Solter D, Damjanov I: Teratocarcinoma and the expression of oncodevelopmental genes. Methods Cancer Res 18:277, 1979

15. Mintz B, Fleischman RA: Teratocarcinoma and other neoplasms as developmental defects in gene expression. Adv Cancer Res 34:211, 1981

16. Martin GR: Teratocarcinomas and mammalian embryogenesis. Science 209:768, 1980

17. Stevens LC, Little CC: Spontaneous testicular teratomas in an inbred strain of mice. Proc Natl Acad Sci USA 40:1080, 1954

18. Stevens LC: A new inbred subline of mice (129/ter SV) with a high incidence of spontaneous congenital testicular teratomas. J Natl Cancer Inst 50:235, 1973

19. Stevens LC: Testicular teratomas in fetal mice. J Natl Cancer Inst 28:247, 1962

20. Stevens LC: Experimental production of teratomas in mice of strains 129, A/He, and their F_1 hybrids. J Natl Cancer Inst 44:929, 1970

21. Stevens LC: Environmental influences on ex-

perimental teratocarcinogenesis in testes of mice. J Exp Zool 174:407, 1970

22. Pierce GB Jr, Stevens LC, Nakane PK: Ultrastructural analysis of the early development of teratocarcinoma. J Natl Cancer Inst 39:755, 1967

23. Damjanov I, Andrews PW: Ultrastructural differentiation of a clonal human embryonal carcinoma cell line in vitro. Cancer Res 43:2190, 1983

24. Pierce GB, Abell MR: Embryonal carcinoma of the testis. Pathol Annu 5:27, 1970

25. Silver LM, Martin GR, Strickland S (eds): Teratocarcinoma Stem Cells. Cold Spring Harbor Laboratory, Cold Spring Harbor, NY, 1983

26. Damjanov I, Bagasra O, Solter D: Genetic and epigenetic factors regulate the evolving malignancy of embryo-derived teratomas. p. 501. In Silver LM, Martin GR, Strickland S (eds) Teratocarcinoma Stem Cells. Cold Spring Harbor Laboratory, Cold Spring Harbor, NY, 1983

27. Evans MJ, Kaufman MH: Pluripotent cells grown directly from normal mouse embryos. Cancer Surveys 2:185, 1983

28. Martin GR, Wiley LM, Damjanov I: The development of cystic embryoid bodies in vitro from clonal teratocarcinoma stem cells. Dev Biol 61:230, 1977

29. Andrews PW, Goodfellow PN, Damjanov I: Human teratocarcinoma cells in culture. Cancer Surveys 2:41, 1983

30. Sherman MI, Miller RA: F9 embryonal carcinoma cells can differentiate into endoderm-like cells. Dev Biol 63:27, 1978

31. Strickland S, Smith KK, Marotti KR: Hormonal induction of differentiation in teratocarcinoma stem cells: generation of parietal endoderm by retinoic acid and dibutyryl cAMP. Cell 21:347, 1980

32. Teilum G: Endodermal sinus tumor of the ovary and testis: comparative morphogenesis of the so-called mesonephroma ovarii and of extraembryonic (yolk sac, allantoic) structures of rat's placenta. Cancer 12:1092, 1959

33. Pierce GB Jr, Midgley AR Jr, Ram JS, Feldman JD: Parietal yolk sac carcinoma: clue to the histogenesis of Reichert's membrane of the mouse embryo. Am J Pathol 41:549, 1962

34. Damjanov I: Yolk sac carcinoma (endodermal sinus tumor). Am J Pathol 98:569, 1980

35. Sobis H, Vadeputte M: Yolk sac derived terato-

mas and carcinomas in hamsters. Eur J Cancer 13:1175, 1977

36. Sobis H, van Hove L, Vandeputte M: Trophoblastic and mesenchymal structures in rat yolk sac carcinoma. Int J Cancer 29:181, 1982

37. Martinez-Hernandez A, Miller EJ, Damjanov I, Gay S: Laminin-secreting yolk sac carcinoma of the rat. Lab Invest 47:247, 1982

38. Damjanov I, Amenta PS, Zarghami F: Transformation of an AFP-positive yolk sac carcinoma into an AFP-negative neoplasm: evidence for in vivo cloning of the parietal yolk sac carcinoma. Cancer 53:1902, 1984

39. Nicolas JF, Avner P, Gaillard J et al: Cell lines derived from teratocarcinomas. Cancer Res 36:4224, 1976

40. Blom E, Christensen NO: Sertoli cell tumour combined with lack of epididymis in a bull. Acta Pathol Microbiol Scand [A] 90:283, 1982

41. Weaver AD: Survey with follow-up of 67 dogs with testicular Sertoli cell tumours. Vet Rec 113:105, 1983

42. Damjanov I, Sunderman FW Jr, Mitchell JM, Allpass PR: Induction of testicular sarcomas in Fischer rats by intratesticular injection of nickel subsulfide. Cancer Res 38:268, 1978

11

Clinical Management of Patients with Testicular Tumors

Nicholas J. Vogelzang

Germ cell tumors of the testes present unique and challenging problems to the pathologist, surgeon, and oncologist. This chapter will define areas of clinical management about which there is general agreement, but it will also highlight areas of controversy in the clinical management of these patients.

Germ cell tumors of the testis are the most common malignancy[1] in men between the ages of 15 and 34. Malignant ovarian germ cell tumors occur with a much lower frequency, in approximately 1:10 testicular tumors but are much more common than extragonadal tumors arising in the mediastinum, retroperitoneum, and pineal gland (Table 11-1).

While the cause of testicular germ cell tumors is unknown, any hypothesis concerning their origin must take into account these unique host factors. In the first place, the majority of patients with this disease are young, postpubertal males. Second, these patients have an increased frequency of minor congenital anomalies such as cryptorchidism, inguinal hernia, and supranumerary nipples; bone abnormalities such as spina bifida occulta; and urologic tract anomalies such as duplicated urinary collecting systems[2-4] (Table 11-2). These patients are also unique in that they appear to experience an excess of preexisting psychological abnormalities compared to patients with acute leukemia.[5] Patients with germ cell tumors are commonly of northern European ancestry; Denmark has the highest incidence[6] of testicular cancer in the world,

with a rate of 8–9:100,000 men. A genetic predisposition to germ cell tumor is also suggested by the reports of testicular cancer occurring in individuals of certain HLA haplotype and by reports of testicular cancer in multiple family members over several generations.[3] There does not appear to be an association between exposure to diethylstilbestrol (DES) in utero and the subsequent development of germ cell cancer, although careful case–control studies have not yet been performed.[4, 7] Patients with Klinefelter's syndrome and hypogonadism appear to have an increased frequency of mediastinal germ cell tumors,[8] but they apparently do not have an increased risk of testicular cancer.

CLINICAL PRESENTATION

Patients with testicular cancer have a mean age of 32 years.[9] In a series of 335 patients, 87 percent of men with the disease had a testicular symptom (i.e., pain, swelling, or a mass). Other symptoms such as gynecomastia (5 percent) or metastatic symptoms, which include cough or an abdominal mass, (10.5 percent) were usually present in men with nonseminomatous cancer. There are several important aspects to underscore in the clinical presentation of patients with testicular cancer. First, patients with seminomas may have different signs from patients with other germ cell tumors. For example, recent studies report that

Table 11-1. Incidence, Site, and Histologic Type of Germ Cell Tumors

Histologic type	% of Total	Site of Origin				
		Testis	Ovary	Retroperitoneum	Mediastinum	Pineal
Seminoma	50	869	77	14	14	3
Embryonal	25	449	33	5	10	1
Teratoma	19	284	65	6	20	1
Choriocarcinoma	6	107	3	1	3	0
Total	100	1709	178	26	47	5

An analysis of 1973 cases of germ cell cancer seen within a population base of 20 million over a 5-year period (case rate = 395/year). Areas analyzed: Connecticut, Iowa, New Mexico, Utah, Hawaii, Puerto Rico, Detroit, Atlanta, New Orleans, Seattle and San Francisco.

Abstracted from Young JL, Perry CL, Asire AJ, et al: Cancer incidence and mortality in the United States 1973–77. Surveillance, epidemiology and end results program (SEER). National Cancer Institute Monograph No. 57, 1982.

most seminomas are larger than other germ cell tumors,[9, 10] which are generally less than 5 cm. In one study, 11 of 15 patients with tumors larger than 5 cm which did not metastasize were found to have seminomas.[10] It is not clear if patients with seminoma have different symptoms than those with other germ cell tumors. Many textbooks of physical diagnosis emphasize the painless nature of testicular cancer, yet in the series of 335 patients 45 percent did complain of pain.[9] A large study comparing symptoms of patients with different types of germ cell tumors is needed. Second, patients with seminomas have a median age of 36 years, while those with other types of germ cell tumors have a median age of 26–28 years. Third, seminomas are more likely to involve the entire testis and to present

as smooth, symmetrical masses whereas other tumors have a propensity to be focal and nodular within the substance of the testis. Fourth, delay in diagnosis of testicular cancer is associated with a worsening prognosis.[9, 11] In the same study mentioned above, stage I and II disease patients had a median delay from symptom onset to diagnosis of 2.5–3.3 months, while patients with stage III disease (metastatic) had a median delay from symptoms to diagnosis of 4.5 months.[9] Finally, the primary testicular lesions may be extremely small or detectable only by testicular ultrasound, and yet widespread metastatic disease may be present. An example of this is found in the following case report.

A 27-year-old man presented to his local physician with abdominal pain and a neck

Table 11-2. Congenital Anomalies of the Genitourinary Tract in 138 Patients with Germ Cell Tumors

Abnormality	No. with Finding/ No. of Patients	Expected Incidence in a "Normal" Population
Renal agenesis	2/138	1/600–1/1000
Renal tract duplication	6/138	2/100
Extrarenal pelvis	3/138	?
Ureterocele	1/138	1/500–1/4000
Medullary sponge kidney	1/138	1/5000–1/20,000
Total (%)	14/138 (10.1)	5/100 (5)

All patients were seen at the University of Minnesota and underwent intravenous pyelography during pretreatment evaluations.

mass. Computed tomographic scan disclosed a mass involving the pancreas and retroperitoneum. A biopsy specimen of the neck mass disclosed an undifferentiated carcinoma, and he was referred to the University of Chicago with the diagnosis of pancreatic adenocarcinoma. Review of the pathologic specimen disclosed a tumor consistent with embryonal carcinoma. Serum human chorionic gonadotropin (HCG) level was 610 mIU/ml, and the alpha-fetoprotein (AFP) level was less than 5 ng/ml. A testicular ultrasound examination disclosed a small, clinically undetectable mass in the right testis. The testis was explored and both seminoma and teratoma were found. Chemotherapy for testis cancer was begun, a complete remission was achieved, and the patient is alive and free of disease 2 years after the diagnosis. Based on ultrasound this patient's diagnosis was changed from a pancreatic tumor or primary retroperitoneal germ cell tumor to a primary testicular cancer.

Thus, any young man who presents with a primary retroperitoneal tumor, a metastatic cancer of uncertain origin, or a widespread malignancy should have serum drawn for measurement of AFP and HCG as well as having testicular ultrasound performed to rule out any primary testicular lesion.

INITIAL CLINICAL AND LABORATORY EXAMINATION

The patient with a clinically suspicious testicular mass should have a complete physical examination and a chest radiograph followed by measurement of serum AFP, HCG, and lactate dehydrogenase (LDH). A standard inguinal orchiectomy should be performed next. Pathologic evaluation of the specimen will determine the further work-up as shown in Figure 11-1, which, although complex, summarizes the clinical decision-making by the urologists, oncologists, and radiotherapists. A transscrotal biopsy or an inguinal biopsy approach and reinsertion of the testes risks contamination or seeding of the inguinal and scrotal areas with tumor cells; such an approach must be avoided.

MANAGEMENT OF SEMINOMA

Orchiectomy followed by radiotherapy has cured more than 95 percent of cases diagnosed as stage I seminoma[12] and 84 to 100 percent of those diagnosed as stage IIA (small-volume retroperitoneal metastases) seminoma.[13] Lymphangiograms only need be done in patients with seminoma defined as clinical stage I by all other criteria. For patients who have palpable abdominal masses or metastatic disease, computed tomography of the retroperitoneum is sufficient evaluation, and lymphangiogram need not be performed. There is considerable debate as to the management of patients with bulky abdominal seminomas, that is, masses >10 cm in diameter. Although radiotherapy alone can cure such patients, a substantial relapse rate of 35 to 60 percent exists.[12, 13] Cisplatin-based therapy is highly effective in curing stage III seminoma.[14] We suggest that stage IIC seminomas (i.e., bulky, >10 cm abdominal seminomas) be treated initially with chemotherapy as this approach allows best tolerance of the chemotherapy and further surgery or radiotherapy as needed.

Classic seminomas are associated with elevated serum HCG and AFP levels in 5 to 10 percent of patients. In the Danish series of 381 seminomas, preoperative serum HCG levels were increased in 28 (7.3 percent)[15] as follows: 17/307 patients with stage I, 7/67 with stage II, and 2/7 with stage III disease. The elevated preoperative serum levels correlated with stage of disease. Because an elevated serum AFP level is diagnostic of a nonseminomatous germ cell tumor, the tumor should be treated as such, in spite of the histologic appearance of "seminoma"[16, 17]; in fact, autopsy or further pathologic evaluation has disclosed "nonseminomatous foci" in many cases. In the Danish series nine patients with "seminoma" were found to be AFP-positive. Of those patients, two had died of disease at

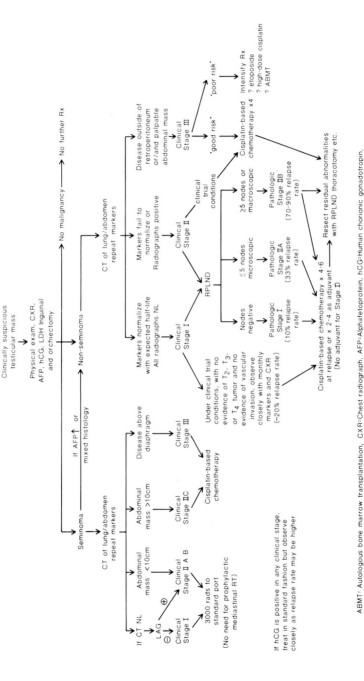

Fig. 11-1. Steps in the pathologic evaluation of a clinically suspicious testicular mass.

ABMT= Autologous bone marrow transplantation, CXR=Chest radiograph, AFP=Alphafetoprotein, hCG=Human chorionic gonadotropin, LDH=Lactate dehydrogenase, Rx=Treatment, ↑=elevated, NL=Normal, Markers=AFP/hCG//LDH, CT=Computed tomography, LAG=Lymphangiogram, RT=Radiotherapy, RPLND=Retroperitoneal lymph node dissection the time of publication, two had had recurrences of the disease, and five were free of disease. Thus, these data support the finding that seminoma patients with significantly elevated serum AFP levels in the blood should be treated as having nonseminomatous tumors. Recently, Lange et al. have demonstrated that placental alkaline phosphatase is a marker for pure seminoma.[18]

In conclusion, seminomas rarely require treatment with chemotherapy, but when it is necessary, cisplatin-based therapy is highly effective. Patients who have marker-positive seminomas apparently have a worse prognosis than those with marker-negative disease. Alpha-fetoprotein-positive seminomas may portend a much worse prognosis. However, patients with HCG-positive seminomas may not have worse prognosis than those who have similar-stage disease. For the present, the management of HCG-positive seminoma patients should be similar to those without a marker, although there must be careful follow-up with recording and analysis of the data whenever possible. The value of placental alkaline phosphatase as a marker in patients with seminoma has not yet been determined.

MANAGEMENT OF STAGE I AND II NONSEMINOMATOUS GERM CELL TUMOR

Careful attention must be paid to distinguishing clinical stage from pathologic stage of disease. In seminomas this is not a consideration as virtually no patients are pathologically (i.e., surgically) staged. In nonseminomas all radiographic procedures, blood tests, or physical examinations are considered to be part of the clinical stage. With the advent of tumor markers, computed tomography, and magnetic resonance imaging,[19] such clinical staging tests are extremely accurate. Yet, despite such advances, clinical staging will fail to detect retroperitoneal disease in approximately 15 percent of patients with clinical stage I disease.

Pathologic examination of the retroperitoneal lymph nodes continues to be warranted for patients with clinical stage I cancer. The retroperitoneal lymph node dissection is valuable for the following indications:

1. Surgical removal of five or fewer microscopically involved lymph nodes (pathologic stage IIA) is curative in 60 to 70 percent of patients.[20]

2. Failure to detect retroperitoneal lymph node involvement by nonseminomatous germ cell tumor confers an excellent prognosis. Only 8 to 10 percent of patients with pathologic stage I disease will relapse. These relapses will virtually all be within the lung parenchyma and are detectable at an early stage by routine monthly chest radiographs. Some cases will be detected only because of a rise in serum AFP or HCG levels. This 8 to 10 percent incidence of relapse probably reflects the true incidence of primary hematogenous dissemination from a primary testicular germ cell cancer.

3. Complete surgical removal via a retroperitoneal lymph node dissection of five or fewer microscopically involved nodes or removal of macroscopic disease less than 5 cm (pathologic stage IIB) is associated with a less than 5 percent chance of recurrence in the retroperitoneum.[21] This surgical "sterilization" of an anatomically hidden area is reassuring to the oncologist who may later need to treat the patient for metastatic pulmonary disease. Few aspects of the clinical care of testicular cancer patients are more distressing than attempting to palliate patients who have bulky abdominal masses that recurred after a technically inadequate retroperitoneal lymph node dissection.

4. The patient who undergoes a retroperitoneal lymph node dissection has a precisely defined prognosis. The relapse rate and time to relapse are a function of the extent of the retroperitoneal tumor (Table 11-3). The need or lack thereof for adjuvant chemotherapy following surgical dissection can be clearly defined.

Table 11-3. Relapse Rate (No. Relapsed/Total No. of Patients) of Stage II Disease Treated with Retroperitoneal Lymph Node Dissection with or without Adjuvant Radiotherapy

Stage II Substage	Relapse Rate	Percentage	Median Time to Relapse (Days)
N_1	5/13	38	190
N_2	6/11	55	76
N_3	23/25	92	26
N_4	4/4	100	34
Total	38/53	72	36

N_1, Microscopic metastases in less than five lymph nodes.
N_2, Macroscopically enlarged lymph nodes less than 2 cm or more than five nodes microscopically involved.
N_3, Any resected nodal disease > 2 cm.
N_4, Residual microscopic disease.
Summarized from Vogelzang NJ, Fraley EE, Lange PH, et al: Stage II nonseminomatous testicular cancer: a 10-year experience. J Clin Oncol 1:171, 1983.

The major drawback to the retroperitoneal lymph node dissection is the 40 to 80 percent postoperative incidence of impaired ejaculatory function, usually retrograde ejaculation. Although this common complication has been reduced by improved surgical techniques to avoid damage to the hypogastric sympathetic plexus, located at the aortic bifurcation,[22] for some patients retrograde ejaculation is still an extremely distressing symptom. Additionally, the lymph node dissection is a major operation with all the attendant surgical risks. Suitable patients with clinical stage I nonseminomatous germ cell tumors may enter clinical trials of observation alone following orchiectomy.[23-25] Because of these two concerns, meticulous follow-up with markers and radiographic studies is needed to detect early relapse in such patients.

Follow-up requires diligence and care on the part of both the patient and the physician. Not only should careful attention be paid to the psychological background of patients selected for such an approach,[5] but also patients with spermatic cord invasion and other evidence of extensive local tumor invasion should be excluded from such trials because of the high rate of metastases in this group.[10] As summarized by Raghavan et al.,[24] patients selected for this "observation only" approach should fulfill the following entry criteria: (1) they should be diagnosed as having clinical stage I disease according to intensive noninvasive staging; (2) they must have a T stage of less than 2; that is, patients with spermatic cord invasion, tunica albuginea invasion, or scrotal wall invasion are not suitable for such "observation alone" approach; (3) the patient must have normal circulating levels of AFP and/or HCG, or the levels must be decreasing at the expected half-life decay rate;[26] (4) there must be no transscrotal procedure that could contaminate the inguinal lymph nodes; (5) the patient must be cooperative and reliable and must attend follow-up visits meticulously; and (6) there must be no evidence of vascular invasion in the primary pathologic specimen. It would be unwise to place patients with pure choriocarcinoma in such a clinical study.

An area of continuing controversy in the treatment of patients with stage IIB nonseminomatous disease is outlined in Figure 11-1. This recommends that patients with stage IIB disease undergo adjuvant chemotherapy. There is evidence that surgery alone will cure 60 to 70 percent of patients with stage IIA disease, but less than 20 percent of patients with stage IIB disease.[20] Thus, we recommend adjuvant chemotherapy for any patient who has stage IIB disease. There are, however, some patients for whom the prospects of chemotherapy and its attendant toxicities of nausea, vomiting, alopecia, and loss of bodily image are so forbidding as to preclude its immediate acceptance. For these patients, there may be a role for close observation, with the hope that they will be among the less than 50 percent of patients in whom the disease is cured with retroperitoneal lymph node dissection alone. The current results of the Testis Cancer Intergroup Study suggest that of the patients given immediate postoperative adjuvant chemotherapy, there has been 1 relapse among 86 treated patients and no deaths from recurrent testicular cancer. In the patients randomized to receive no adjuvant chemotherapy, there have been 40 relapses in 82 treated patients and 4 deaths from testicular cancer. Based on these preliminary data and other prior data, the recommendation for adjuvant chemotherapy in stage IIB disease can be made quite strongly.

MANAGEMENT OF STAGE III SEMINOMA AND NONSEMINOMATOUS GERM CELL TUMOR

As outlined in Figure 11-1 and Table 11-3, the following groups of patients will receive chemotherapy: those who either present with metastatic disease or relapse after receiving prior therapy for low stage disease or who require adjuvant chemotherapy. All groups together compose 20 to 40 percent, and sometimes up to 50 percent of germ cell testicular cancer patients.

Chemotherapy is the mainstay of management for stage III disease. The history of chemotherapy of testicular cancer is unique and bears repeating. In 1960, Li et al.,[27] at Memorial Sloan-Kettering Cancer Center reported that 23 patients with metastatic testicular tu-

mors were treated with "triple therapy" which consisted of an antimetabolite (either methotrexate, the glutamine antagonist 6-diazo-5 oxo-L-norleucine [DON], or 6-mercaptopurine), actinomycin-D, and an alkylating agent (either nitrogen mustard or chlorambucil).[27] Of the 23 treated patients, 12 patients had objective shrinkage of tumor, and 4 remain alive and well more than 20 years after initiation of chemotherapy.[28] That paper was remarkable in several aspects: first, it established that metastatic germ cell testicular cancer could regress following chemotherapy; second, it was the first report of successful combination chemotherapy for any "solid tumor" malignancy; third, it indicated that patients could be cured with chemotherapy; and fourth, the paper reported that both seminomas and nonseminomatous germ cell tumors regressed following chemotherapy. These general findings of Li et al.[27, 28] have been repeatedly confirmed since that initial report. Multiple drugs have been tested and found to cause regression of metastatic testicular cancer.[29]

The most important advance in the 1960s and early 1970s was reported by Melvin Samuels at M.D. Anderson Hospital.[30] He reported that the combination of vinblastine and bleomycin induced responses in 36 of 51 patients (71 percent), with 17 of the patients (33 percent) experiencing complete disappearance of disease. In 1974, Higby et al., at the Roswell Park Memorial Institute, reported the effectiveness of cis-diamminedichloroplatinum II (cisplatin). Eleven patients with testis cancer were treated, nine of whom responded.[31] Then in 1977, Einhorn and Donohue from Indiana University, using the combination of vinblastine, bleomycin, and cisplatin, successfully induced regressions in 100 percent of patients with metastatic germ cell cancer.[32] Of the first 47 patients treated, 70 percent remained alive and disease-free 5 or more years after the initiation of therapy. In a randomized study the addition of doxorubicin to the vinblastine, bleomycin, and cisplatin (VBP) regimen did not improve the results, and a reduction in the vinblastine dosage from 0.2 mg/kg to 0.15

mg/kg on day 1 and 2 was associated with a dramatic decrease in toxicity, and no decrease in efficacy, of the drug combination.[33] Multiple institutions around the United States and the world have found the "Einhorn regimen" to be an effective, tolerable, and safe regimen able to cure between 60 and 90 percent of patients. It is a tribute to the pioneering effort of all investigators that cisplatin-based chemotherapy for metastatic germ cell cancer is now both standard and curative.

Table 11-4 describes six series using the VBP regimen in which long-term patient follow-up is available. Note that the average patient with metastatic germ cell cancer treated with the VBP regimen will have approximately a 75 percent chance of achieving a complete remission of disease and that in some institutions up to 90 percent of patients attain a complete remission. The average patient treated with VBP for metastatic testicular cancer is now surviving more than 4 years without evidence of recurrent disease.

During the development of VBP, other drug regimens were found equally able to eradicate metastatic testicular cancer. These alternative regimens have been popularized by Drs. Newlands and Bagshawe at the Charing Cross Hospital in London[40] and by Golbey and associates[41-44] at Memorial Sloan-Kettering Cancer Center (MSKCC). In the current MSKCC regimen, called VAB-6, VAB stands for vinblastine, actinomycin-D, and bleomycin, which were the active drugs used in the initial trials. Recent results using the VAB-6 regimen are indistinguishable from those using the VBP regimen. The feature common and essential to the two regimens is that high dosages of cisplatin be used in the treatment of these patients. In a recent elegant study performed by the Southwestern Oncology Group, randomized patients with metastatic germ cell cancer received either a low (13–15 mg/m²) or a high (20 mg/m²) dosage of cisplatin daily for 5 days, combined with vinblastine and bleomycin.[45] There was unequivocal evidence that complete remission and survival rates were improved in the patients receiving the high-dosage cisplatin regimen. There is every indication that cisplatin in a dosage of 100–120 mg/m² every 3–4 weeks is the cornerstone of therapy of metastatic testicular germ cell cancer.

In spite of the 70 to 85 percent cure rate of metastatic testicular cancer with cisplatin-based chemotherapy, a minority of patients continued to relapse and die. However, in the past 4–5 years etoposide (VP-16-213) has

Table 11-4. Combination Chemotherapy with Vinblastine, Bleomycin and Cisplatin: Results of Treatment

Study Center	No. of Patients	Percentage Achieving Complete Remission (Chemotherapy ± Surgery)	Percentage Alive	Median Follow-Up (Years)	Reference
Indiana and Southeastern Cancer Study Group	181	74	77	4+	32–34
Minnesota	28	82	86	4+	35
Harvard	39	90	87	3+	36
Netherlands	40	N.A.	65	3+	37
Royal Marsden	41	N.A.	50[a]	2+	38
Southwestern Oncology Group	143	59	46[b]	2+	39

[a] Many patients had undergone prior radiotherapy which compromised the ability to give full-dosage chemotherapy.
[b] Patients only received low-dosage (13 mg/m² intravenously on days 1–5) cisplatin.
N.A., Not available.

been found to be effective as second-line treatment.[46-48] This drug, a derivative of the mitotic inhibitor podophyllin, has minimal organ toxicity and is synergistic with cisplatin. Up to one half of the patients whose disease relapses on VBP or VAB-6 will be rendered free of disease with etoposide-/cisplatin-containing regimens.

The management of patients receiving such chemotherapy is complex and should be the exclusive domain of medical oncologists familiar with the treatment. Following the baseline assessment of tumor markers and metastatic disease sites, the patients can be stratified into good- and poor-risk groups. Exact assignment of a patient to a "good-" or "poor-" risk group has been difficult in the past.[49] However, based on the recent studies by Bosl et al.,[50] patients with high serum levels of HCG or LDH or more than two sites of metastatic disease (i.e., lung, bone, and liver) have a poor prognosis, that is, a less than 50 percent chance of achieving a complete remission.[50] On the other hand, patients with a good prognosis are those who have a greater than 50 percent chance of obtaining a complete remission with chemotherapy and surgery (Table 11-5). Thus, there is an excellent rationale for intensifying the current therapy offered to poor-risk patients and reducing the toxicity of chemotherapy to the good-risk patients. Other institutions have devised similar but less exact stratification parameters for these patients. At the National Cancer Institute, Ozols et al.[51] have randomized "poor-risk" patients to receive either VBP or VBP modified by the addition of VP-16 and higher dosages of cisplatin (40 mg/m² per day for 5 days) with hypertonic saline diuresis.[51] The series is not yet ready for full analysis but current results suggest that there is a higher complete remission rate in the VP-16 and high-dosage cisplatin group. There is also a lower relapse rate in the group receiving intensive therapy. There is not yet, however, a survival advantage. The study has only been reported in abstract form and further follow-up is eagerly anticipated. Bosl et al.[50] have reported on preliminary results using their mathematical stratification model. The poor-risk patients, as reported by Israel et al.[52] continue to do poorly in spite of the addition of VP-16 and cisplatin to the standard VAB-6 regimen. The study of good-risk patients includes a randomization in which patients receive either the VAB-6 regimen which contains cyclophosphamide, actinomycin-D, bleomycin, vinblastine, and cisplatin, or etoposide and cisplatin (Bosl GJ, Vogelzang NJ: unpublished findings 1985).[53] The rationale behind the study is that chronic toxicity

Table 11-5. Probability of Achieving a Complete Remission (CR) with Chemotherapy with or without Surgical Resection of Residual Disease for Specific Values of LDH and HCG

LDH (IU/ml)	HCG (1 ng/ml)	HCG (10 ng/ml)	HCG (100 ng/ml)	HCG (500 ng/ml)
300	0.91	0.88	0.81	0.75
	0.78	0.70	0.58	0.49
500	0.87	0.82	0.73	0.66
	0.69	0.60	0.48	0.39
1000	0.79	0.72	0.60	0.51
	0.55	0.46	0.33	0.26
2000	0.67	0.58	0.46	0.37
	0.41	0.32	0.22	0.16

Upper value, one site of metastases; lower value, two or more sites.
Summarized from Bosl GJ, Geller NL, Cirrincone C et al: Multivariate analysis of prognostic variables in patients with metastatic testicular cancer. Cancer Res 43:3403, 1983.

should be associated less with the etoposide group than with the VAB-6 group. It is hoped that complete remission rates will be equivalent in the two arms but that the chronic toxicity of VAB-6 or VBP chemotherapy such as sterility, pulmonary dysfunction, neuropathy, and hyperpigmentation of the skin will be less common and less disabling in the etoposide/cisplatin group.

In virtually 100 percent of the patients who receive chemotherapy, normalization of the tumor markers AFP, LDH, and HCG is expected. Normalization of the markers and disappearance of metastatic disease signify a complete remission. However, if a complete remission is not obtained radiographically, in spite of tumor marker normalization, it is possible to resect the residual disease in a majority of patients. These postchemotherapy surgical procedures often disclose evidence of fibrosis or benign teratoma. Complete surgical extirpation of malignant teratoma is necessary to prevent relapse of the disease. The complete remission after surgery confers an excellent prognosis as does complete remission with chemotherapy alone. Patients in whom residual embryonal carcinoma is found after surgical procedure must receive an additional two cycles of chemotherapy,[36] and their prognosis is not as good as those patients in whom no evidence of residual cancer in the surgically excised specimen[26, 53] can be found. The operations required to resect all disease vary from transabdominal retroperitoneal lymph node dissection to median sternotomies with concomitant abdominal explorations.

An important consideration in patients with metastatic testicular cancer is an assessment of long-term therapy-related toxicity. These patients are young and have an additional 40–50-year life expectancy. Chronic drug toxicity such as sterility, cardiomyopathy, neuropathy, and vascular disease must be carefully assessed, and reports of such toxicity must be sought.[54, 55] It is also important to reduce the toxicities from surgery and radiotherapy as much as possible. In addition to the chronic toxicity, one must be alert to late relapses that occur in chemotherapy-treated patients.[56] Although late relapses apparently occur most commonly in patients who have not had all disease resected, there are some patients in whom chemotherapy has not been successful in eradicating disease. Thus, patients who have been given chemotherapy must be evaluated for an extended period of time.

FUTURE DIRECTIONS

The cause of germ cell testicular cancer is not known. Evidence has been presented by Atkin and Baker[57] that a specific chromosome abnormality, isochromosome 12p, is involved in testicular tumors. Cooper et al.[58] have shown that the c-ras oncogene is apparently amplified in some tissue-culture maintained human germ cell tumor lines. Finally, Jhanwar et al.[59] have localized the c-ras oncogene family to chromosomes 11 and 12, specifically the short arm of chromosome 12 (12p). If a group of high-risk patients (i.e., patients with cryptorchidism) was prospectively analyzed for this specific chromosomal marker i (12) or for amplification of the c-ras oncogenes, a clear understanding of the mechanisms of testicular carcinogenesis could result.

The recent development of monoclonal antibody technology has allowed the clinical use of radiolabeled antibodies and thus radioimmunodetection of metastatic testicular cancer.[60] These studies have been pursued in the animal systems using antibodies directed at the testicular-cancer-specific markers known as stage-specific embryonic antigens 1 and 3 (SSEA-1 and SSEA-3).[61] Radioimmunolocalization and detection of germ cell tumors can also be accomplished with antibodies directed at other antigens, such as AFP.[62] This technology may allow for precise localization of metastatic disease in patients who are otherwise not known to have active cancer.

In conclusion, the clinical management of patients with testicular tumors has undergone a dramatic revolution within the past decade. The development of sophisticated tumor imaging modalities has allowed clear definition of disease extent. The development and widespread use of the tumor markers HCG, AFP, and LDH have allowed early diagnosis of metastatic disease and early detection of relapsing disease after initial treatment for low-stage disease. Lastly, the striking development of effective chemotherapeutic agents, especially cisplatin and etoposide, has now made metastatic testicular cancer curable in all cases except in those with very far advanced disease. Further improvement in treatment can be expected in the small subgroup of patients who are not currently curable by available methods, and reduction in toxicity associated with radiotherapy, surgery, and chemotherapy can be expected in all subgroups of patients. Lastly, the application of new techniques in molecular biology may lead to the elucidation of the cause of testicular cancer.

ACKNOWLEDGMENTS

The author thanks Pamela Jones and Deborah Gifford for secretarial assistance. Grant support was provided in part by the American Cancer Society Junior Faculty Fellowship (JFCF 639) and Gould Faculty Fellowship.

REFERENCES

1. Silverberg E: Cancer in young adults (ages 15–34). CA 32:32, 1982
2. Johnson DE, Woodhead DM, Pout DR et al: Cryptorchidism and testicular tumorigenesis. Surgery 63:919, 1968
3. Tollerud DJ, Blattner WA, Fraser MC et al: Familial testicular cancer and urogenital developmental anomalies. Cancer 55:1849, 1985
4. Depue RH, Pike MC, Henderson BE: Estrogen exposure during gestation and risk of testicular cancer. J Natl Cancer Inst 71:1151, 1983
5. Gorzynski G, Lebovits, Holland J, Vugrin D: A comparative study of psychosexual adjustment in men with testicular cancer and acute leukemia. Cancer Detect Prev 4:1731, 1981
6. Schultz HP, et al: Testicular carcinoma in Denmark 1976–1980. Personal communication
7. Gill WB, Schumacher GFB, Bibbo M et al: Association of diethylstilbestrol exposure in utero with cryptorchidism, testicular hypoplasia and semen abnormalities. J Urol 122:36, 1979
8. Sogge MR, McDonald SD, Cofold PB: The malignant potential of the dysgenetic germ cell in Klinefelter's syndrome. Am J Med 66:515, 1979
9. Bosl GJ, Vogelzang NJ, Goldman A et al: Impact of delay in diagnosis on clinical stage of testicular cancer. Lancet 2:970, 1981
10. Raghavan D, Vogelzang NJ, Bosl GJ et al: Tumor classification and size in germ cell testicular cancer: influence on the occurrence of metastases. Cancer 50:1591, 1982
11. Scher H, Bosl GJ, Geller N et al: Impact of symptomatic interval on prognosis of patients with stage III testicular cancer. Urology 21:559, 1983
12. Thomas GM, Rider WD, Dembo AJ et al: Seminoma of the testis: results of treatment and patterns of failure after radiation therapy. Int J Radiat Oncol Biol Phys 8:165, 1982
13. Walther PJ, Paulson DF: Testicular seminoma revisited: time for a multimodal therapeutic approach. World J Urol 2:68, 1984
14. Stanton GF, Bosl GJ, Whitmore WF et al: VAB-6 as initial treatment of patients with advanced seminoma. J Clin Oncol 3:336, 1985
15. Norgaard-Pedersen B, Schultz H, Arends J, et al: Biochemical markers for testicular germ cell tumors in relation to histology and stage: some experiences from the Danish testicular cancer (DATECA) study from 1976–1981. Ann NY Aca Sci 417:390, 1983
16. Lange PH, Nochomovitz LE, Rosai J et al: Serum alphafetoprotein and human chorionic gondotropin in patients with seminoma. J Urol 124:472, 1980
17. Ball D, Barrett A, Peckham MJ: The management of metastatic seminoma testis. Cancer 50:2289, 1982
18. Lange PH, Millan JL, Stigbrand T et al: Placental alkaline phosphatase as a tumor marker for seminoma. Cancer Res 42:3244, 1982
19. Hricak H, Williams RD, Spring DB et al: Anatomy and pathology of the male pelvis by magnetic resonance imaging. Am J Radiol 141:1101, 1983
20. Vogelzang NJ, Fraley EE, Lange PH et al: Stage II nonseminomatous testicular cancer:

a 10 year experience. J Clin Oncol 1:171, 1983

21. Fraley EE, Lange PH: Technical nuances of extended retroperitoneal dissection for low-stage nonseminomatous testicular germ cell cancer. World J Urol 2:43, 1984

22. Narayan P, Lange PH, Fraley EE: Ejaculation and fertility after extended retroperitoneal lymph node dissection for testicular cancer. J Urol 127:685, 1982

23. Peckham MJ, Barrett A, Husband JE et al: Orchidectomy alone in testicular stage I non-seminomatous germ cell tumours. Lancet 1:678, 1982

24. Raghavan D: Expectant therapy for clinical stage A non-seminomatous germ cell cancers of the testis? A qualified "yes." World J Urol 2:59, 1984

25. Sogani PC, Whitmore WF Jr, Herr H et al: Orchiectomy alone in the treatment of clinical Stage I non-seminomatous germ cell tumors of the testis. J Clin Oncol 2:267, 1984

26. Vogelzang NJ, Lange PH, Goldman A et al: Acute changes of alpha-fetoprotein and human chorionic gonadotropin during induction chemotherapy of germ cell tumors. Cancer Res 42:4855, 1982

27. Li MC, Whitmore WF Jr, Golbey R et al: Effects of combined drug therapy on metastatic cancer of the testis. JAMA 174:145, 1960

28. Golbey RB, Reynolds TF, Vugrin D: Chemotherapy of metastatic germ cell tumors. Semin Oncol 6:82, 1979

29. Fraley EE, Lange PH, Kennedy BJ: Germ cell testicular cancer in adults. N Engl J Med 301:1370; 1420, 1979

30. Samuels ML, Holoye PY, Johnson DE: Bleomycin combination chemotherapy in the management of testicular neoplasia. Cancer 36:318, 1975

31. Higby DJ, Wallace HJ Jr, Albert DJ, Holland JF: Diaminodichloroplatinum: a phase I study showing responses in testicular and other tumors. Cancer 33:1219, 1974

32. Einhorn LH, Donohue J: Cis-diamminedichloroplatinum, vinblastine and bleomycin combination chemotherapy in disseminated testicular cancer. Ann Intern Med 87:293, 1977

33. Einhorn LH, Williams SD: Chemotherapy of disseminated testicular cancer: a random prospective study. Cancer 46:1339, 1980

34. Einhorn LH: Testicular cancer as a model for a curable neoplasm: the Richard and Hilda Rosenthal Foundation Award Lecture. Cancer Res 41:3275, 1981

35. Bosl GJ, Lange PH, Fraley EE et al: Vinblastine, bleomycin, and cisdiamminedichloroplatinum in the treatment of advanced testicular carcinoma: possible importance of longer induction and shorter maintenance schedules. Am J Med 68:492, 1980

36. Garnick MB, Canellos G, Richie JP: Treatment and surgical staging of testicular and primary extragonadal germ cell cancer. JAMA 250:1733, 1983

37. Stoter G, Vendrik CPJ, Struyvenberg A et al: Combination chemotherapy with cis-diammine-dichloroplatinum, vinblastine, and bleomycin in advanced testicular non-seminoma. Lancet 1:941, 1979

38. Peckham MJ, Barrett A, McElwain TJ et al: Non-seminoma germ cell tumours (Malignant teratoma) of the testis: results of treatment and an analysis of prognostic factors. Br J Urol 53:162, 1981

39. Samson MK, Fisher R, Stephens RL et al: Vinblastine, bleomycin and cis-diamminedichloroplatinum in disseminated testicular cancer: response to treatment and prognostic correlations. Eur J Cancer 16:1359, 1980

40. Newlands ES, Reynolds KW: Clinical management of malignant germ cell tumours. Cancer Surv 2:21, 1983

41. Wittes RE, Yagoda A, Silvay O et al: Chemotherapy of germ cell tumors of the testis 1. Induction of remission with vinblastine, actinomycin D and bleomycin. Cancer, 37:637, 1976

42. Reynolds TF, Vugrin D, Cvitkovic E et al: VAB-3 combination chemotherapy of metastatic testicular cancer. Cancer 48:888, 1981

43. Vugrin D, Whitmore WF, Golbey RB: VAB-5 combination chemotherapy in prognostically poor risk patients with germ cell tumors. Cancer 51:1072, 1983

44. Vugrin D, Herr HW, Whitmore WF et al: VAB-6 combination chemotherapy in disseminated cancer of the testis. Ann Intern Med 95:59, 1981

45. Samson MK, Rivkin SE, Jones SE et al: Dose-response and dose-survival advantage for high versus low-dose cisplatin combined with vinblastine and bleomycin in disseminated testicular cancer: a Southwest Oncology Group Study. Cancer 53:1029, 1984

46. Vogelzang NJ, Raghavan D, Kennedy BJ: VP-

16-213 (etoposide): the mandrake root of Issyk-Kul. Am J Med 72:136, 1982

47. Williams SD, Einhorn LH, Greco FA et al: VP-16-213 salvage chemotherapy for refractory germinal neoplasms. Cancer 46:2154, 1980

48. Wade JL III, Vogelzang NJ: Use of etoposide (VP-16-213) in urologic cancer. p. 209. In Garnick MB (ed) Genitourinary Cancer: Contemporary Issues in Clinical Oncology. Vol. 5. Churchill Livingstone Inc., 1985

49. Javadpour N, Ozols RF, Anderson T et al: A randomized trial of cytoreductive surgery followed by chemotherapy versus chemotherapy alone in bulky stage III testicular cancer with poor prognostic features. Cancer 50:2004, 1982

50. Bosl GJ, Geller NL, Cirrincione C et al: Multivariate analysis of prognostic variables in patients with metastatic testicular cancer. Cancer Res 43:3403, 1983

51. Ozols RF, Ihde D, Jacob J et al: Randomized trial of PVeBV versus PVeB in poor prognosis non-seminomatous testicular cancer (NSTC). Proc Am Soc Clin Oncol 3:155, 1984

52. Israel AM, Bosl GJ, Whitmore WF: Treatment of poor prognosis germ cell tumors (GCT) with alternating cycles of VP-16/cisplatin (CDDP) and cyclophosphamide, bleomycin, actinomycin D, vinblastine, CDDP (VAB-6). Proc Am Soc Clin Oncol 3:159, 1984

53. Brenner J, Vugrin D, Whitmore WF: Cytoreductive surgery for advanced nonseminomatous germ cell tumors of the testis. Urology 19:571, 1982

54. Vogelzang NJ, Bosl GJ, Johnson K, Kennedy BJ: Raynaud's phenomenon: a common toxicity after combination chemotherapy of testicular cancer. Ann Intern Med 95:288, 1981

55. Vogelzang NJ, Frenning DH, Kennedy BJ: Coronary artery disease after treatment with bleomycin and vinblastine. Cancer Treat Rep 64:1159, 1980

56. Terebelo HR, Geyer L, Brown A et al: Late relapses of testicular cancer. J Clin Oncol, 1:566, 1983

57. Atkin NB, Baker MC: i(12p): A specific chromosomal marker in seminoma and malignant teratoma of the testis? Cancer Genet Cytogenet 10:199, 1984

58. Cooper CS, Blair DG, Oskarsson MK et al: Characterization of human transforming genes from chemically transformed, teratocarcinoma and pancreatic carcinoma cell lines. Cancer Res 44:1, 1984

59. Jhanwar SC, Neel BG, Hayward WS et al: Localization of c-ras oncogene family on human germ line chromosomes. Proc Natl Acad Sci USA 80:4794, 1983

60. Ballou B, Levin G, Hakala T, Solter D: Tumor localization detected with radioactively labeled monoclonal antibody and external scintography. Science 206:846, 1979

61. Shevinsky LH, Knowles BB, Damjanov I, Solter D: Monoclonal antibody to murine embryos defines a stage specific embryonic antigen expressed in mouse embryos and human teratocarcinoma cells. Cell 30:667, 1982

62. Lange PH, Vogelzang NJ, Fraley EE et al: Radioimmunodetection in non-seminomatous germ cell tumors. Presented at the American Urological Association Annual meeting, Kansas City, MO, 1982

12

Value of Tumor Markers in Testicular Cancer

Nasser Javadpour

Testicular cancer cells may synthesize certain proteins that may be localized in these cells and measured in the sera of patients bearing the tumor. The advent of sensitive and specific radioimmunoassay and immunocytochemical techniques makes it possible to detect minute amounts of these proteins in the serum and in the histologic sections from testicular tumors, respectively. These substances can thus be used as specific and valuable tumor markers in testicular cancer.

A number of tumor markers have been found in the serum of patients with germ cell testicular cancer (Table 12-1). Among these tumor markers, serum alpha-fetoprotein (AFP) and human chorionic gonadotropin (HCG) have been most useful in clinical application.[1-10]

Sensitive and specific radioimmunoassays (RIA) and immunocytochemical techniques that have been developed for HCG and AFP are capable of detecting minute amounts of these markers in sera and cancer cells of patients with testicular cancer. When these two

glycoproteins are utilized together, they are the best serologic and cellular markers available in the diagnosis, detection of early recurrence, accurate staging, and assessment of the adequacy of therapy of testicular cancer.[4]

FREQUENCY OF HCG AND AFP IN TESTICULAR CANCER

Human chorionic gonadotropin (HCG) is a glycoprotein secreted by the normal placenta. It is normally found in the serum only during pregnancy. Human chorionic gonadotropin has a molecular weight of 38,000 daltons and is composed of two dissimilar subunits, alpha and beta. The alpha subunit is the basic subunit of the pituitary glycoprotein hormones: luteinizing, follicle-stimulating, and thyrotropin. The beta subunit, which forms two-thirds of the molecular weight, is unique to the HCG and is distinct from the subunits of luteinizing, follicle-stimulating, and thyrotropic hormones particularly in the terminal 29 amino acids. The beta subunit has been isolated, purified, and used to immunize rabbits to produce an antibody specific for HCG which does not cross react with physiological concentrations of the other glycoprotein hormones.[11] The data from our clinical and laboratory programs indicate that 70 percent of the patients with active nonseminomatous germ cell testicular tumors had elevated serum HCG levels (Table 12-2). Elevated levels fell to normal with effective therapy. When an elevated level persisted or a level rose above

---

Table 12-1. Testicular Tumor Markers

Specific Markers
  Alpha-fetoprotein (AFP)
  Human chorionic gonadotropin (HCG)
  Placental alkaline phosphatase (PLAP)
  Gamma-glutamine transpeptidase (GGT)
  Placental Proteins 5, 10, 15
  Human placental lactogen (HPL)

Nonspecific Markers
  Lactic dehydrogenase (LDH)
  Polyamines (putrescine, spermine, spermicline)
  Carcinoembryonic antigen (CEA)

Table 12-2. Frequency of Elevated Serum HCG and AFP Levels in Patients with Testicular Cancer

	AFP		HCG		AFP and/or HCG	
	No. of Patients	Percentage of Patients	No. of Patients	Percentage of Patients	No. of Patients	Percentage of Patients
Seminoma	0/160	0	14/160	9.0	14/160	9.0
Teratoma	6/16	37.5	4/16	25.0	7/16	43.7
Embryonal Carcinoma [Including EST (YST)]	102/145	70.3	87/145	60.0	127/145	87.5
Embryonal Carcinoma with teratoma [Including EST (YST)]	36/56	64.2	32/56	57.0	48/56	85.7
Choriocarcinoma	0/5	0	5/5	100.0	5/5	100.0
Endodermal Sinus (Yolk Sac) Tumor	3/4	75.0	1/4	25.0	3/4	75.0

EST, endodermal sinus tumor; YST, yolk sac tumor.

normal after initial therapy, recurrent tumor was invariably found. Approximately 9 percent (14 of 160) of patients with testicular seminoma had an elevated serum HCG level (Table 12-2).

In 1963, Abelev et al. demonstrated a specific alpha-1-globulin (AFP) in the serum of mice bearing hepatocellular carcinoma, and later in humans with this tumor.[1] Human AFP is a glycoprotein with a molecular weight of approximately 70,000 and containing 41 percent carbohydrate. It is produced in the liver, yolk sac, and gastrointestinal tract of the fetus.[12] Alpha-fetoprotein is present in human fetal serum at a concentration of 3,000 ng/ml by the 12th week after gestation. At birth, the concentration is approximately 30 ng/ml and decreases to much lower levels by 1 year of age; in normal adults it is found in concentrations of approximately 1–16 ng/ml. Alpha-fetoprotein has been clinically useful primarily in the diagnosis of hepatocellular carcinoma and malignant germ cell tumors. Javadpour et al.,[3] using a double antibody RIA for AFP, showed that 75 percent of 101 patients with testicular germ cell tumors had elevated levels of AFP. The discovery that testicular tumors so often produce AFP is a direct result of the development of a sensitive RIA: 71 percent of the elevated levels were below 3,000 ng/ml, which was the lower limit of detectability of the previously used gel precipitation assay, and had gone undetected prior to the development of this sensitive RIA. In our series, about 70 percent of the patients had an elevated level of serum AFP.[6] If an elevated serum level of AFP persisted after therapy, recurrent metastatic tumor generally was found (Table 12-2).

STAGING OF TESTICULAR CANCER

The effective use of surgery, chemotherapy, and radiation therapy for patients with testicular cancer requires accurate staging for therapy and/or interpretation of end results. The conventional staging parameters, including the lymphangiogram, inferior venacavogram, excretory urogram, and computed tomogram yield a considerable staging error.

With the use of sensitive and specific radio-immunoassays of serum AFP and HCG in 118 patients with embryonal carcinoma with or without teratoma who were undergoing clinical and surgical staging, the staging errors have decreased to 9 to 14 percent in stage I and to 5 to 10 percent in stage II cases. Various clinical observations have been made in this group of patients: (1) persistently elevated serum markers after orchiectomy for testicular cancer invariably indicate stage II or III disease, (2) persistently elevated serum markers after positive lymphadenectomy usually suggest stage III disease, and (3) persistently elevated serum markers after lymphadenectomy negative for tumor invariably indicate stage III disease. Clearly, such determinations are important guides to further therapy and must be essential features of adjuvant trials.

RIA OF URINARY HCG

By concentrating HCG in urine specimens, its production can be more sensitively monitored with a new carboxyterminal RIA than by serum measurement. Simultaneous serum and urinary HCG levels were measured in 12 patients with disseminated testicular cancer with seminoma, embryonal carcinoma, terato-carcinoma, or choriocarcinoma of the testis. While these patients initially had elevated levels of serum HCG, after intensive chemotherapy and/or surgery the levels became undetectable. On the other hand, the 24-hour urinary HCG level measured by radioimmunoassay of urine concentrations remained elevated in 10 of 12 patients. Indeed, there were four patients in whom serum HCG was undetectable but in whom elevated levels of urinary HCG were found; these four patients were proven to have persistent tumor, which contained HCG as documented by histopathologic and immunoperoxidase staining. This highly sensitive urinary HCG radioimmunoassay has improved the detection of persistent tumor burden and has been rewarding in selecting those patients with testicular can-

cer in whom further therapy is warranted.[8]

Clinically, when these markers were considered in staging testicular tumors the staging errors decreased to 5 to 14 percent, a dramatic improvement when compared to previously reported staging errors of 35 to 53 percent. It is important to consider the biological half-lives of these markers (AFP 5 to 6 days, HCG 18 to 24 hours) to avoid any confusion from the progressively decaying markers of the already excised tumor. Preorchiectomy serum markers are not always available, but this should not disturb the proposed system since the original specimen from orchiectomy usually is available and immunohistologic techniques such as immunoperoxidase can determine the presence of cellular markers when serum is not available.

From observation of serum levels in testicular cancer patients pre and postoperatively, correlations can be seen which help both to reduce the staging error to an acceptable degree and to direct the physician in recommending appropriate therapy. A persistently elevated level of serum markers after orchiectomy for testicular cancer invariably indicates stage II or III disease. A persistently elevated level of serum markers after lymphadenectomy usually indicates stage II disease. When lymphadenectomy is negative for tumor but levels of serum markers after lymphadenectomy are persistently elevated, patients invariably have stage III disease. Persistently elevated levels of serum markers after orchiectomy and/or lymphadenectomy indicate the presence of residual tumor and therefore a need for further therapy.

The important features which tumor markers contribute to prevent the understaging of testicular cancer are the following:

1. The clinical staging based on markers is superior to conventional noninvasive staging for evaluation of therapy but is not superior to pathologic staging.
2. Persistently elevated levels of serum markers after orchiectomy for testicular cancer invariably indicate stage II or III disease.

3. Persistently elevated levels of serum markers after lymphadenectomy indicate advanced-stage disease or an inadequate lymphadenectomy.

4. When lymphadenectomy is negative for tumor but postlymphadenectomy serum markers' levels are persistently elevated, patients invariably have stage III disease. However, surgery still remains the most accurate means of assessing retroperitoneal metastasis.

5. Perhaps the most important application of these markers is in the monitoring of a testicular tumor by serial measurement.[14]

An improved technique for detecting small amounts of HCG that is 20 times more sensitive than the conventional RIA for detecting the beta subunit of HCG has been reported. This technique utilizes concentrated 24-hour urinary HCG and a highly specific RIA with an antiserum (H93) specifically prepared against the carboxyl terminus of urinary HCG.[8]

SERUM AFP AND HCG IN SEMINOMA

In a prospective study at the National Cancer Institute (NCI), 160 patients with "pure seminoma" underwent serial quantitative measurement of serum HCG and AFP by specific double-blind antibody immunoassays originally developed at the NCI. These markers were localized in different cells using techniques of immunoperoxidase or immunofluorescence on serial sections of the tumors. Fourteen of 160 patients had an elevated serum HCG level (Table 12-2). When total blocking of the tumor specimens was used, 1 of 16 patients had an element of choriocarcinoma and underwent a retroperitoneal lymph node dissection and chemotherapy; subsequently, the serum HCG level decreased to normal. There were 120 patients with normal levels of AFP. However, in one patient the serum AFP level was 152 ng/ml. On total blocking of the specimen, an element of em-

bryonal carcinoma was found and this patient has also been proven to have metastatic involvement.

In this study, we have observed the following clinical findings. First, the frequency of elevated HCG levels in the serum of patients with seminoma is approximately 9 percent (14 of 160) (Table 12-2). Second, although the synctiotrophoblastic tumor cell occasionally found in pure seminoma is capable of secreting HCG, one must look for elements of choriocarcinoma or embryonal carcinoma or both; if detected, this will change the therapeutic approach. Third, the elevated serum AFP level in patients with seminoma indicates the presence of an element of endodermal sinus (yolk sac) tumor or embryonal carcinoma and this also changes the therapeutic approach. Finally, the cases of seminoma with an elevated level of HCG reported in the literature are lacking either careful histopathologic studies or localization of cellular HCG, or both. Therefore, caution must be exercised before accepting such tumors as pure seminoma.

MULTIPLE MARKERS IN SEMINOMA

The roles of γ-glutamyl transpeptidase (GGT), placental alkaline phosphatase (PLAP), and HCG have been studied in testicular seminoma. In 89 seminoma patients with normal levels of alpha-fetoprotein, total serum GGT was measured and values of approximately 30 IG/L were considered abnormal. Serum PLAP was measured by enzyme-linked immunoabsorbent assay and values above 1.85 mg/ml were considered abnormal. Serum HCG and AFP levels were measured by double antibody radioimmunoassays (normals below 1 ng/ml and below 20 ng/ml, respectively). At the time of this study, 30 patients had detectable seminoma, 10 did not have histologic confirmation, and the remaining 49 patients had no evidence of tumor. Only 6 of 30 patients (20 percent) with active tumor had elevated levels of serum HCG. Twelve

Table 12-3. False-Positive and False-Negative Findings of Placental Alkaline Phosphatase (PLAP), γ-glutamyl Transpeptidase (GGT), and Human Chorionic Gonadotropin (HCG) in 89 Patients with Seminoma

Status of 79 Patients	Patients	PLAP (%)	GGT (%)	HCG (%)	PLAP, GGT, and/or HCG (%)
Detectable tumor	30	40	33	20	80
Nondetectable tumor	49	12	4	0	14

Ten patients who had suspected tumor, but in whom it was not confirmed histologically, were excluded for this analysis.

of 30 patients with active tumor (40 percent) had elevated serum PLAP, and 10 of 30 (33 percent) of these patients had elevated serum levels of GGT. When these three serum markers were considered together, more than 80 percent of the patients with clinically active tumors had detectable serum levels of one or more of these biochemical serum markers. Since the survival of patients with stage III seminomas treated by radiation is only 28 percent, we advocate serial measurements of these serum markers along with early utilization of new chemotherapeutic regimens in these patients. However, it should be emphasized that the false-positive and false-negative results of these markers, especially false-positive results for GGT due to occasional concomitant liver disease, and the biological half-lives of these markers, should be taken into consideration (Table 12-3).

OTHER MARKERS IN SEMINOMA

A common marker that may be useful in the management of seminoma is lactic dehydrogenase. Serum LDH is a nonspecific enzyme made up of five heterogeneous isoenzymes that can be measured electrophoretically. Cancer cells have increased glycolysis leading to an increased synthesis of lactate, and this may be utilized as a nonspecific tumor marker in several cancers. In seminoma, LDH may be particularly useful because of several factors:

1. There is a lower frequency of serum HCG elevation in seminoma than in nonseminomatous tumors.

2. The measurements of LDH are more easily available and simpler compared than radioimmunoassay studies.

3. The majority of patients with bulky stage II and III seminomas seen at the National Cancer Institute had elevated serum levels of LDH which were useful in monitoring their therapy. The preliminary results suggest that an elevation of LDH may be somewhat specific in testicular cancer compared with other neoplasms.

DISCORDANCE BETWEEN MARKERS

The discordance between various testicular tumor markers is well recognized. It may be explained on the basis of the findings that different cells produce different markers. Also, during chemotherapy in a patient with elevated levels of serum HCG and AFP, one marker may return to normal while levels of the other marker remain elevated. This may occur if some of the cells producing a given marker are resistant to the therapy (Fig. 12-1).

Furthermore, we have demonstrated the cellular source of various tumor markers utilizing immunocytochemical techniques.[3, 13]

OTHER PLACENTAL PROTEINS

Over the past several years, we have studied a number of glycoproteins and placental proteins including pregnancy-specific beta-glycoprotein (SP-1), placental proteins 5, 10, and

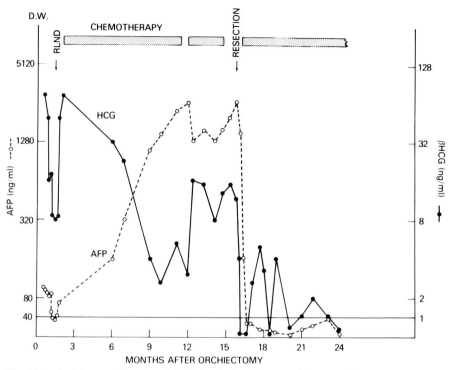

Fig. 12-1. Serial serum HCG and AFP levels in a 21-year-old man with embryonal carcinoma and an element of choriocarcinoma of the right testis. The patient underwent a retroperitoneal lymphadenectomy (RLND) and chemotherapy; the markers were still elevated. A tumor was found in the right obturator lymph nodes and resected. The markers decreased to normal levels. (Normal level of AFP in our laboratory at that time was 40 ng/ml and HCT was 1 ng/ml).

15 utilizing immunoperoxidase techniques. We have localized these markers in syncytiotrophoblastic components of the human placenta, in choriocarcinoma, and syncytiotrophoblastic giant cells found in other types of testicular cancer (Table 12-4).

STUDIES OF LACTIC DEHYDROGENASE

Lactate dehydrogenase is a glycolytic enzyme found in many human tissues and fluids. The enzyme is released into the serum due to tissue injury occurring in inflammatory conditions, degenerative processes, toxicity, or cancer.[15] Elevations of serum LDH levels have been found to reflect growth and regression of various malignant neoplasms.

Eighty patients with testicular cancer were studied with serial determinations of serum LDH, based on observation of the change in absorption of DPNH as pyruvate was converted to lactate. Normal values used were below 340 ng/ml before June 1, 1978, below 281 for June, 1978, and below 248 after July 1, 1978, due to technical improvements.

Of the 80 patients, 19 (23.8 percent) had stage I cancer (tumor confined to the testicle), another 19 patients (23.8 percent) were stage II (metastatic disease in the retroperitoneal lymph nodes only), and 42 patients (52.5 percent) were stage III (visceral or distant metastases). Because the National Institutes of

Table 12-4. Other Placental Proteins

	SP-1	Placental Protein # 5, 10, 15
Placenta	+	+
Syncytiotrophoblast	+	+
Tumor Giant Cell	+	+

SP-1, Pregnancy specific beta 1-glycoprotein.

Health specifically sought patients with bulky metastatic disease during this period for protocol purposes, patients with bulky stage III disease were more frequently represented.

Eight of the stage III patients had extragonadal tumors. Eleven patients had seminomas, while 69 patients had nonseminomatous germ cell tumors.

In this study, the frequency of elevated pretherapy levels of serum LDH in patients with germ cell testicular tumors was definitely higher in stage III patients. Only 20 percent (1:5) of stage I patients had elevated LDH levels (Table 12-3) compared to 26.3 percent (5:19) of stage II patients, and 62.5 percent (25:40) of stage III patients. However the frequency of pretherapy elevated serum HCG and AFP levels was similar when stages were compared in these patients.

In conclusion, serum LDH levels are elevated in a number of patients with bulky testicular tumors and correlate well with the course of treatment. Therefore, when elevated, they may be utilized as a guide for response to therapy. Serum LDH is not helpful in diagnosis or staging of patients with testicular tumors. However, it can be valuable in patients with seminoma with no elevation of other markers. It is a simple, inexpensive rapid hospital test that is easily available. Finally, because we have had a considerable number of patients with advanced bulky testicular tumors with poor prognostic features, we have correlated prognosis with serum LDH and it appears that an elevated serum LDH level is of value as a prognostic indicator. This perhaps reflects the bulk of tumor since large disseminated tumors have a poor prognosis. These investigations have become an important part of contemporary urologic practice.

MONITORING THE RESPONSE TO THERAPY

Serial measurements of serum HCG and AFP by RIA reflect the efficacy of surgical, radiation, and/or chemotherapeutic regimens in patients with testicular tumors. When these therapies are effective, they produce an immediate decrease in serum levels of HCG and AFP that reflects the decrease in the tumor size and could be as rapid as the catabolic rate for these markers. In our series, elevated markers were found, often months before the patients were symptomatic or recurrence was detectable by any other clinical tests. Consequently, the markers proved to be sensitive indicators of the presence of otherwise undetectable metastases.

The alpha subunit of HCG, with a short half-life of 20 minutes, is valuable in localizing a tumor that is not detectable by conventional clinical tests, including intravenous pyelogram, inferior venacavogram, and lymphangiogram, and is especially useful in the localization of metastases in the retroperitoneal area. Because tumor markers have made such important contributions, they currently constitute the basis for the management of testicular cancer (Figs. 12-2 to 12-4).

LIMITATIONS OF TUMOR MARKERS IN TESTICULAR CANCER

In spite of certain limitations in utilizing these markers, they appear to be the best available markers for any solid tumors. The current practices and recommendations to minimize certain problems and maximize the efficacy

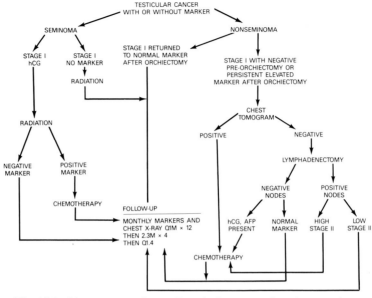

Fig. 12-2. Management of stage I testicular cancer based on markers.

of RIA measurement of serum AFP and HCG from commercial sources in testicular cancer include those discussed here.

The physician should discuss the sensitivity and specificity of a given commercial assay with the laboratory personnel. Occasional use of normal serum or serum with known levels of AFP and/or HCG as negative and positive controls is recommended.

These markers should not replace scrotal exploration and/or retroperitoneal lymphadenectomy for histopathologic diagnosis of the

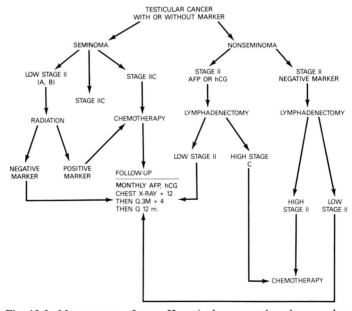

Fig. 12-3. Management of stage II testicular cancer based on markers.

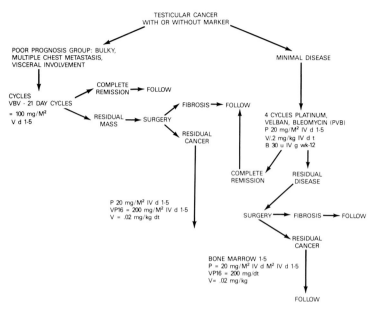

Fig. 12-4. Management of stage III testicular cancer.

primary tumor and/or for ruling out the presence of retroperitoneal metastases. However, the elevated levels of tumor markers are indicative of the presence of tumor and the necessity for further treatment. They are also helpful in monitoring the efficacy of and the need for changing therapy.

The problem of impurity of certain antisera against the subunit of the HCG or the possibility of high levels of luteinizing hormone (LH) in patients undergoing orchiectomy and/or chemotherapy causing a false-positive result should also be kept in mind. The false-positive results may be clarified by a testosterone suppression test, measurement of serum LH, and measurement of HCG by urinary concentrate utilizing a carboxy-terminal RIA that is currently available as a courtesy to all urologists through the National Cancer Institute laboratories.

In monitoring the therapy or evaluating patients with testicular tumors, one should utilize frequent physical examination, chest x-rays, and other tests as necessary, along with measurement of serum AFP and HCG. In patients receiving chemotherapy, the normalization of these serum markers does not mean

tumor-free status; on exploration of the retroperitoneum and chest, it is not unusual to find cystic fibrotic material with necrosis and tumor. Therefore, normalization of serum markers should not deter the surgeon from looking for evidence of persistent tumor. Appropriate utilization of chemotherapy, surgery, radiotherapy, and tumor markers can make a dramatic improvement in prognosis and survival of these patients.

FUTURE PERSPECTIVES

Perhaps the most important contribution of immunology has been in providing radioimmunoassay, immunocytochemical techniques, and monoclonal antibodies. Also, there is a great potential for radioimmunodetection (RID) of cancer with reliable markers. It may help to detect and localize the tumor by utilizing a specific antibody tagged with isotope that can be injected into the body and traced by scintography (Fig. 12-5). Finally, one may attach various cytotoxic or radioactive agents to the antibody against a given marker and deliver them specifically to the tumor. This

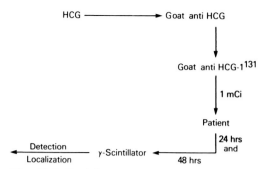

Fig. 12-5. Radioimmunodetection of HCG-producing tumor.

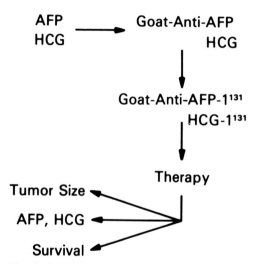

Fig. 12-6. Radioimmunotherapy of AFP- and/or HCG-producing tumor.

approach has the potential advantages of specifically killing the tumor cells and sparing the normal cells, thereby avoiding the side effects of chemotherapy and/or radiotherapy (Fig. 12-6).

REFERENCES

1. Abelev GI, Perova SD, Khramkova NI et al: Production of embryonal alpha-globulin by transplantable mouse hepatoma. Transplantation 1:174, 1963

2. Abelev GI: Alpha-protein in oncogenesis and its association with malignant tumors. Adv Cancer Res 14:295, 1971

3. Javadpour N, McIntire KR, Waldmann TA: Immunochemical determination of human chorionic gonadotropin (HCG) and alpha-fetoprotein (AFP) in sera and tumors of patients with testicular cancer. Natl Cancer Inst Monogr 49:209, 1978

4. Javadpour N, Bergman SM: Recent advances in testicular cancer. Curr Probl Surg 17:1, 1978

5. Javadpour N: Serum and cellular biologic tumor markers in patients with urologic cancer. Hum Pathol 10:557, 1979

6. Javadpour N: The role of biologic tumor markers in testicular cancer. Cancer 45:1755, 1980

7. Javadpour N: Immunocytochemical techniques in localization of tumor markers in cells and tumors: a potential for radioimmunodetection and radioimmunotherapy. Urology 11:1, 1983

8. Javadpour N, Chen HC: Improved HCG detection utilizing the beta-subunit of carboxyl-terminal radioimmunoassay of concentrated 24 hour urine in patients with testicular cancer. J Urol 126:170, 1981

9. Javadpour N, Kim EE, Deland FH: The role of radioimmunodetection in the management of testicular cancer. JAMA 246:45, 1981

10. Talerman A, Haije WG: Alphafetoprotein and germ cell tumors: a possible role of yolk sac tumor in production of alphafetoprotein. Cancer 34:1722, 1974

11. Vaitukaitis JL, Braunstein GD, Ross GF: A radioimmunoassay which specifically measures human chorionic gonadotropin in the presence of human luteinizing hormone. Am J Obstet Gynecol 113:751, 1972

12. Gitlin D, Perricelli A, Gitlin GM: Synthesis of alphafetoprotein by liver, yolk sac and gastrointestinal tract of the human conceptus. Cancer Res 32:979, 1972

13. Kurman RJ, Scardino PT, McIntire KR, et al: Cellular localization of alphafetoprotein and human chorionic gonadotropin in germ cell tumors of the testis using an indirect immunoperoxidase technique. A new approach to classification utilizing tumor markers. Cancer 40:2136, 1977

14. Perlin E, Engeler JE Jr, Edson M, et al: The value of serial measurement of both human chorionic gonadotropin and alphafetoprotein for monitoring germinal cell tumors. Cancer 37:215, 1976

15. Von Eyben FE: Biochemical markers in advanced testicular tumors. Cancer 41:648, 1978

13

Evaluation of Germ Cell Tumors Following Chemotherapy

Thomas M. Ulbright and Lawrence M. Roth

Pathologists are now confronted with the evaluation of resected metastases from patients with testicular germ cell tumors who have been treated with very effective chemotherapeutic regimens. The pathologic diagnosis of such specimens determines whether or not the patient receives additional chemotherapy, and is prognostically important as well.[1] Furthermore, the nature of treated metastases provides important insights into the mechanisms of action of chemotherapy used in the treatment of testicular germ cell tumors and the biology of "tumor maturation."

mens. With the combination of cisplatin, vinblastine, and bleomycin (PVB), complete remission rates of 70 percent are attained, and further remissions to a total of 81 percent are possible when adjuvant surgery is utilized.[6] At the Indiana University Medical Center, patients with metastatic testicular cancer of germ cell origin, excluding pure seminoma, are generally treated with four courses of PVB chemotherapy and are then evaluated for persistent disease. Pulmonary, mediastinal, and retroperitoneal masses that persist after chemotherapy are surgically excised.

CHEMOTHERAPY REGIMENS

Li and co-workers[2] reported the first effective chemotherapy for testicular cancer in 1960 using a combination of an alkylating agent (usually chlorambucil), an antimetabolite (usually amethopterin), and an antitumor antibiotic (usually actinomycin D). With this type of regimen 12 of 23 patients with metastatic testicular cancer showed tumor regression. Significant breakthroughs occurred when vinblastine[3] and bleomycin[4] demonstrated activity in the treatment of germ cell tumors. The combination of these two agents, in one study,[5] produced a 57 percent complete remission rate with 45 percent of the patients showing no evidence of disease at the time of the report. Another important step was the incorporation of cisplatin into chemotherapy regi-

SURGICAL EXCISION

Sixty-two patients who had residual pulmonary or retroperitoneal disease following chemotherapy for metastatic testicular germ cell tumors underwent surgical excision.[1] Thirteen patients (21 percent) showed only necrosis and fibrosis; 20 patients (32 percent) had mature teratoma; 5 patients (8 percent) had immature teratoma, and 22 patients (35 percent) had persistent malignant germ cell tumors other than or in addition to teratoma (i.e., embryonal carcinoma, seminoma, yolk sac tumor, and/or choriocarcinoma). Two patients had apparently unrelated pulmonary granulomas. Follow-up of at least 6 months showed that 35 of 39 patients (90 percent) who had necrosis and fibrosis, mature teratoma, or immature teratoma resected after chemotherapy were

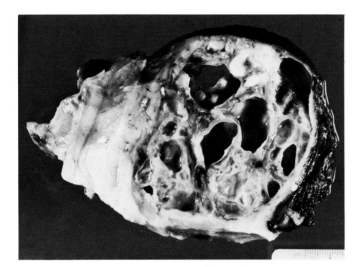

Fig. 13-1. Residual retroperitoneal teratoma excised from a patient following PVB chemotherapy is composed of multiple cysts embedded in a matrix of connective tissue. Incorporation of adjacent fat is apparent at left.

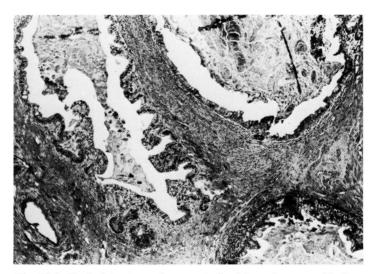

Fig. 13-2. Typical teratoma shows cysts lined by columnar epithelium which contain mucinous secretion. There is abundant smooth muscle and connective tissue in the stroma. H & E. × 27.

well. On the other hand, only 2 of 22 patients (9 percent) with residual malignant germ cell tumor remained disease-free on follow-up.

POSTTREATMENT FINDINGS

RESIDUAL TERATOMA

Residual teratoma is a common finding in postchemotherapy resections. On gross examination teratoma usually consists of well-cir-cumscribed masses of dense, gray fibrous tissue with frequent cystic foci (Fig. 13-1). The size range is considerable, varying from 1 to more than 20 cm. On microscopic examination there are numerous cysts lined by cuboidal or columnar epithelium with frequent intracytoplasmic mucin or luminal cilia (Fig. 13-2). The stroma between the cysts often consists of loose or dense fibrous tissue, although smooth muscle, cartilage, and bone occur with some frequency. In some cases

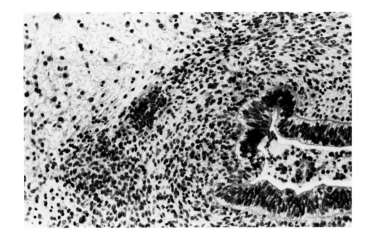

Fig. 13-3. Mucinous epithelium of this teratoma (right) is surrounded by a nonspecific, spindle-cell stroma. H & E. × 198.

there is a nonspecific stroma composed of spindle cells resembling endometrial stroma and having a periglandular distribution (Fig. 13-3). Differentiation to squamous, intestinal, and bronchial epithelial types is common. We do not require, however, the demonstration of derivatives of the three germ layers of the embryo to diagnose teratoma. Epithelium-lined glands are usually sufficient to allow a diagnosis of teratoma. The distinction between mature and immature teratoma, in our experience, rests predominantly on the assessment of the immaturity of the stroma, which demonstrates an embryonic appearance more commonly than the epithelium. However, we have been impressed by the frequency of cytologic atypia, not necessarily related to an "immature" appearance, which can occur in both the epithelial and stromal elements in resected teratomas following chemotherapy. To consider this atypia a manifestation of immaturity is not, we believe, appropriate. Most recently, therefore, we have graded teratomas based on the cytologic atypia and mitotic rate of individual teratomatous elements rather than on the amount or degree of immature tissue. With this method we found that patients who had teratomas with high-grade epithelial or stromal elements developed recurrent teratoma more frequently than patients who had teratomas with low-grade epithelial or stromal elements.[7] There was no correlation, however, between the grade of the resected teratoma

and subsequent relapse with nonteratomatous germ cell malignancies. In some cases there was a trend for atypia to become more severe in subsequent resections and, rarely, for malignant transformation of teratomatous elements to occur (see below). The situation observed in metastatic testicular teratomas, therefore, is quite different from that in ovarian teratomas, where the amount of neuroepithelium correlates closely with the clinical behavior and hence determines the grade of "immaturity" of the ovarian teratoma.[8] Immature neuroepithelial elements are rare in testicular teratomas and hence the assessment of the aggressive potential of teratomas following chemotherapy must rely on the features of other elements. One study from our institution showed no correlation between the grade of "immaturity" of a teratomatous metastasis and the subsequent course of the patient when the grade was based on an adaptation of the method of Norris et al.[8] The presence of malignant teratomatous elements was the only prognostically important feature identified (Loehrer PJ, Clark SA: Personal communication, 1983).

NECROSIS

Necrosis associated with fibrous connective tissue represents another common finding in the metastatic lesions of germ cell cancer fol-

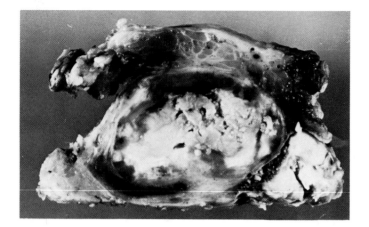

Fig. 13-4. Central tumor necrosis surrounded by a fibrous capsule and adherent fat is a common finding in the retroperitoneum following chemotherapy for metastatic germ cell tumors.

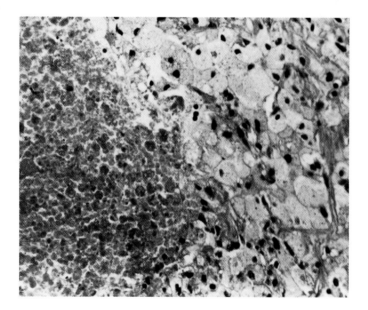

Fig. 13-5. Necrotic germ cell tumor is present at left, with "ghost-like" outlines of individual cells still visible. The necrotic zone is surrounded by prominent, foamy histiocytes. H & E. × 196.

lowing chemotherapy. We believe that many of these lesions represent lymph nodes which were previously overgrown by metastatic malignant germ cell tumors and thus became matted together. The lesions are often quite large, have a thick fibrous capsule, and contain grumous, yellow to white, necrotic material in the interior (Fig. 13-4). The microscopic features are not distinctive. The central necrotic zone appears eosinophilic and in some cases the ghost-like outlines of necrotic, malignant cells are discernible (Fig. 13-5). Fibrous connective tissue usually surrounds this central zone of necrosis and often contains an

infiltrate of foamy histiocytes, presumably cells which have phagocytosed lipid that is released from the cytoplasm of damaged germ cells. Chronic inflammatory cells and deposits of hemosiderin are also common in the area near the central zone of necrosis.

Persistent Tumor

Persistent malignant germ cell tumor may occasionally be grossly recognizable as a solid, often tan to white nodule which is frequently associated with hemorrhage. Any solid tissue

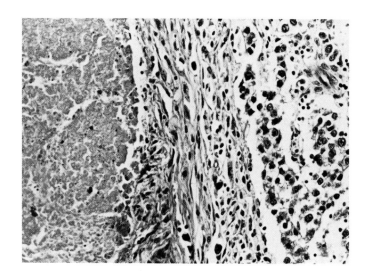

Fig. 13-6. There is both central tumor necrosis (left) and residual germ cell tumor (right) in this node resected after PVB chemotherapy. The appearance of the germ cell tumor is typical of seminoma. H & E. × 128.

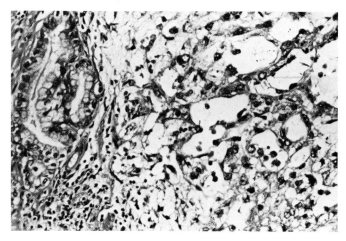

Fig. 13-7. A retroperitoneal dissection from this treated patient consists only of teratoma and a microfocus of germ cell tumor which shows the microcystic pattern of yolk sac tumor. There are several teratomatous glands in close association with the focus of yolk sac tumor. H & E. × 136.

found in resected tissue following chemotherapy for metastatic malignant germ cell tumor should be examined microscopically. The microscopic patterns encountered are similar to those found in primary testicular neoplasms (Figs. 13-6, 13-7). The argument that intact-appearing germ cells in these metastases may not be viable does not appear to be valid from a clinical standpoint. Most of the patients (91 percent) who have viable-appearing embryonal carcinoma following chemotherapy show clinical progression and are thus candidates for additional chemotherapy, whereas the great majority of patients who carry a diagnosis of teratoma or necrosis–fibrosis do not

show further progression and do not need additional chemotherapy.[1]

It is important for both the clinician and pathologist to know that persistent malignant germ cell tumor is not always accompanied by elevated serum markers of alpha-fetoprotein and/or human chorionic gonadotropin.[1] Even in patients who previously were seropositive and became seronegative following chemotherapy, the possibility of persistent malignant germ cell tumor in metastatic lesions cannot be excluded without histologic examination.[1] In the series of Einhorn and co-workers,[1] 22 patients had persistent embryonal carcinoma in pulmonary or retroperitoneal sites after receiving PVB chemotherapy, and 12 (55 percent) were seronegative at the time of operation. Furthermore, the surgeon cannot only sample the largest lymph node group and expect that the tissue biopsied represents the most aggressive component of a malignant germ cell tumor. Donohue et al.[9] showed that persistent embryonal carcinoma was distributed in a random fashion in retroperitoneal lymph nodes and frequently was small and not detectable grossly. Inspection and biopsy of lymph nodes is therefore not an acceptable substitute for a more thorough retroperitoneal dissection.

TRANSITION TO MATURE TERATOMA

Several reports in the literature document a transition of malignant germ cell tumors to mature teratoma, usually following therapeutic radiation and/or chemotherapy.[10-13] As a possible explanation for such cases, some authors have speculated that chemotherapy may induce differentiation of malignant germ cell elements to produce mature teratoma.[11, 12] Recently, Oosterhuis and co-workers[14] cogently addressed this issue. They examined groups of patients who had either been treated with chemotherapy and subsequently undergone resection of residual tumor, or who had no treatment prior to surgical resection. The primary testicular tumors were available for review in both of these groups of patients. While patients who received chemotherapy showed more metastases consisting of mature teratoma compared to the untreated patients, this finding could be related to the derivation of the metastases from primary tumors with a greater incidence of mature teratoma. In both the treated and untreated groups, however, the incidence of mature teratoma in the metastases was less than the incidence of mature teratoma in the primary testicular tumors. This finding suggests that chemotherapy does not induce differentiation of a noncommitted, totipotential cell (generally regarded as the embryonal carcinoma cell).[15] One

would expect, in that case, mature teratoma to be found at random in the metastases, regardless of the nature of the primary tumor, and for the incidence of mature teratoma in metastatic sites to exceed the incidence of mature teratoma in the testicular primary (which is not exposed to chemotherapy). These findings suggest that the histologic "transformation" to mature tissues that is sometimes a striking feature following chemotherapy is actually the result of selective destruction of chemosensitive, nonteratomatous germ cell components. As a result of this destruction of malignant germ cell tumor, teratomatous foci predominate following chemotherapy.

TERATOMATOUS MALIGNANCIES

We have seen several patients with metastatic testicular or primary mediastinal or retroperitoneal germ cell tumors who developed malignancies of teratomatous derivation within their germ cell tumors following chemotherapy.[16] These neoplasms represented carcinomas or sarcomas derived, we believe, from either atypical teratomatous epithelium or atypical stromal elements of a teratoma. As mentioned previously, many patients had undergone multiple surgical procedures, and it was possible in some of these cases to document a progression from atypical teratomatous elements in tissue resected early in the course of the disease to frankly malignant epithelial or stromal elements in tissue resected at a later date. We wish to emphasize that these malignancies were different from high-grade immature teratomas which are sometimes designated, somewhat confusingly, malignant teratomas. The malignancies of teratomatous origin resembled ordinary carcinomas or sarcomas rather than collections of embryonic-like tissue. They showed infiltrative growth patterns with histologic appearances unlike those of malignant germ cell tumors. The carcinomas that we have seen resembled, at the light microscopic level, either adenocarcinoma, similar to adenocarcinoma of gastrointestinal or respiratory origin, or undifferentiated carcinoma. The sarcomas showed recognizable features of embryonal rhabdomyosarcoma, chondrosarcoma, leiomyosarcoma, myxoid liposarcoma, and others. The situation, we believe, is analogous to the well-described, although unusual, circumstance of a squamous cell carcinoma arising within a cystic teratoma of the ovary.[17]

The development of malignancies derived from teratomatous elements is unusual, but we believe that it represents a phenomenon of increasing incidence. Because of effective chemotherapy, the lives of patients with malignant germ cell tumors have been greatly lengthened. At the same time the teratomatous elements of these patients' tumors, since they are not destroyed by the chemotherapy, have a much longer interval either for the development of malignant transformation or, if initially malignant, for overgrowth of the residual tumor. As a consequence, increased numbers of these neoplasms are to be expected. The diagnosis of a malignancy derived from teratomatous elements should be considered in patients who develop chemorefractory masses following initially successful chemotherapy for a malignant germ cell tumor. While most of the neoplasms in this circumstance will prove to be benign teratomas, a small minority will contain malignancies of teratomatous derivation. This is important to recognize because such tumors do not appear to be responsive to the usual chemotherapy protocols for testicular cancer.[7, 16] The prognosis of patients who have teratomas with malignancies of teratomatous origin is significantly worse than that of patients with teratomas merely containing atypical teratomatous elements. Seventy-eight percent of the former either developed recurrence or died; whereas, only 16 percent of the latter developed recurrence or died[7] (p < 0.005).

There is evidence that in some of the cases of malignancies derived from teratomatous elements the teratomatous malignancy did not develop subsequent to chemotherapy by malignant transformation of epithelial or stromal elements.[16] Instead, it appears that the malignancy of teratomatous derivation represented a minor component of a malignant germ cell tumor that became more prominent with the eradication of the chemosensitive germ cell elements. Review of the original testicular primaries or the initial excisions from those patients with primary mediastinal and retroperitoneal neoplasms showed small foci of malignancy of teratomatous origin in five of nine patients for whom there were slides available.[16]

The most common form of progressive malignancy of teratomatous origin we have encountered is embryonal rhabdomyosarcoma.[16] In four patients with elements of embryonal rhabdomyosarcoma who had one or more additional resections following their initial excision and chemotherapy, the sarcomatous component progressively overgrew the other germ cell components (Fig. 13-8). Three of these patients died of rhabdomyosarcoma: two with massive mediastinal disease and one with mediastinal disease and multiple pulmonary metastases. A fourth patient is apparently cured following radical surgical excision of mediastinal embryonal rhabdomyosarcoma.

Those patients who had other forms of sarcoma did not show as extensive and progressive overgrowth following chemotherapy, probably because of a slower tumor growth rate. Their tumors have acted like recurrent teratoma: they have slowly enlarged and caused problems due to local compression. One patient who developed leiomyosarcoma initially showed atypical stromal elements in a metastasis from a mixed germ cell tumor of the testis (composed of teratoma, embryonal carcinoma, and choriocarcinoma) which was previously treated with chemotherapy (Fig. 13-9A). A subsequent pulmonary metastasis was resected and showed leiomyosarcoma (Fig. 13-9B). The patient is currently alive and well 18 months following orchiectomy. Another patient had an embryonal carcinoma of the testis treated by chemotherapy and followed by a retroperitoneal node dissection. A malignant giant cell tumor, resembling

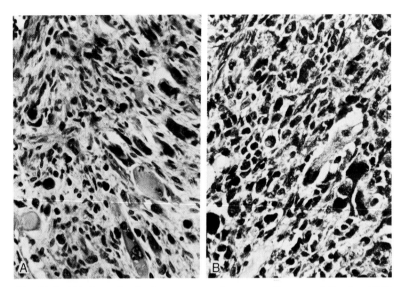

Fig. 13-8. (A) A mediastinal recurrence of a germ cell tumor following PVB chemotherapy shows distinct areas of embryonal rhabdomyosarcoma with numerous strap cells with eosinophilic cytoplasm. H & E. × 160. (B) A subsequent mediastinal recurrence consists of very poorly differentiated sarcoma showing occasional cells with a strap-like configuration. H & E. × 160.

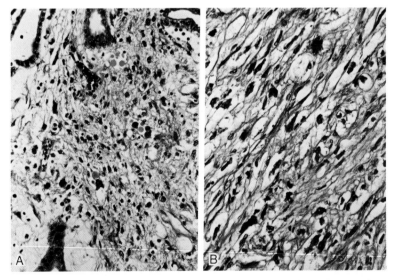

Fig. 13-9. (A) This teratomatous metastasis to the retroperitoneum contains numerous enlarged and hyperchromatic stromal cells scattered between glands lined by bland-appearing epithelial cells. H & E. × 120. (B) A subsequently resected pulmonary metastasis is composed of leiomyosarcoma with a prominent clear-cell histologic appearance. H & E. × 160.

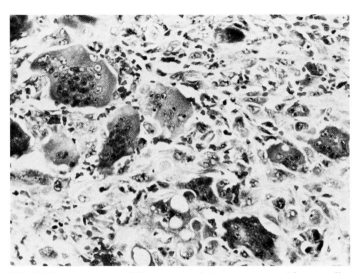

Fig. 13-10. A portion of this metastatic teratoma resembles a malignant giant cell tumor of bone with scattered multinucleated giant cells and single stromal cells having similar atypical nuclear features. An immunoperoxidase stain for HCG was negative. H & E. × 160.

giant cell tumor of bone, was found in conjunction with teratoma in the retroperitoneum (Fig. 13-10). Following lymphadenectomy and additional PVB chemotherapy, the patient has no evidence of disease 14 months after orchiectomy and 8 months after lymphadenectomy. An additional patient showed atypical glandular epithelium in retroperitoneal nodes following PVB chemotherapy (Fig. 13-11A). Because of serologic evidence of relapse he was treated with "salvage" chemotherapy: cisplatin and VP-16. A pulmonary metastasis was subsequently excised and showed immature teratoma intermingled with poorly differentiated adenocarcinoma (Fig. 13-11B) which had, on ultrastructural examination, features of adenosquamous carcinoma (Fig. 13-12). Subsequent mediastinal tumors were excised and consisted of pure adenosquamous carcinoma. The patient has since developed an epidural metastasis and remains alive with disease at 38 months from initial diagnosis.

The diagnosis of a malignancy derived from teratomatous elements is reasonably straightforward when a typical carcinoma or sarcoma is intermingled with benign or atypical teratomatous elements. If there is an absence of intermingled benign elements, the teratomatous malignancy may have replaced the other elements or metastasized to grow in a pure form. However, the possibility of a second primary malignancy should also be considered.

We do not believe that these malignancies of teratomatous origin were caused by the chemotherapy because: (1) in many patients the malignancy was detected in the original specimen before chemotherapy; (2) the time interval from the institution of chemotherapy to the development of overt malignancy of teratomatous origin was usually several months, whereas secondary solid malignancies induced by an agent such as radiation typically occur several years following treatment;[18] and (3) most second malignancies developing in patients treated with chemotherapy have not been solid tumors but usually various forms of leukemia.[19]

PATHOLOGIC EXAMINATION

It is apparent that the pathologic examination of resected metastases following chemotherapy for testicular cancer is a great re-

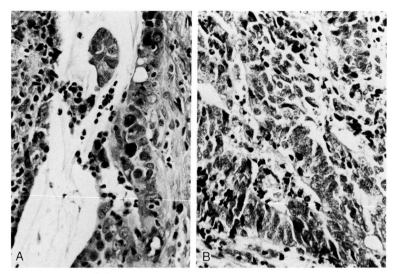

Fig. 13-11. (A) Jumbled, hyperchromatic, and irregularly shaped cells line this gland in a retroperitoneal teratoma which was resected following PVB chemotherapy. H & E. × 160. (B) A subsequent pulmonary metastasis consists of malignant glands lined by epithelium with diffusely clumped chromatin patterns. H & E. × 160.

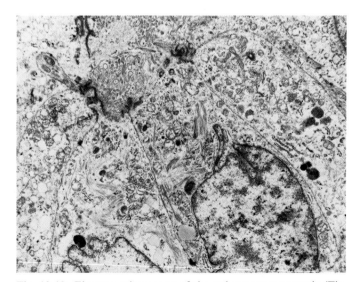

Fig. 13-12. Electron microscopy of the pulmonary metastasis (Fig. 13-11B) shows both glandular and squamous features. The cells are arranged in an acinar grouping with prominent luminal microvilli and junctional complexes. In addition there are prominent bundles of cytoplasmic tonofilaments which occasionally insert on a desmosome (lower center). × 4,200.

sponsibility for the pathologist. Despite seronegativity, viable tumor may be found on pathologic examination. Furthermore, as chemotherapy continues to improve and patients with tumor survive for longer periods of time, it is likely that cancer of teratomatous origin will be found more commonly within the metastases of germ cell tumors. It is incumbent on the pathologist to examine closely the gross specimens resected from patients with metastatic testicular cancer. He or she must carefully sample areas having various gross appearances that occur in these specimens so that residual viable germ cell neoplasm or malignancies of teratomatous origin can be identified, and the patient treated appropriately.

REFERENCES

1. Einhorn LH, Williams SD, Mandelbaum I, Donohue JP: Surgical resection in disseminated testicular cancer following chemotherapeutic cytoreduction. Cancer 48:904, 1981
2. Li MC, Whitmore WF Jr, Golbey R, Grabstald H: Effects of combined drug therapy on metastatic cancer of the testis. JAMA 174:1291, 1960
3. Samuels ML, Howe CD: Vinblastine in the management of testicular cancer. Cancer 25:1009, 1970
4. Blum RH, Carter SK, Agre K: A clinical review of bleomycin—a new anti-neoplastic agent. Cancer 31:903, 1973
5. Samuels ML, Johnson DE, Holoye PY: Continuous intravenous bleomycin (NSC-125066) therapy with vinblastine (NSC-49842) in Stage III testicular neoplasia. Cancer Chemother Rep 59:563, 1975
6. Einhorn LH, Donohue J: *Cis*-diamine-dichloroplatinum, vinblastine, and bleomycin combination chemotherapy in disseminated testicular cancer. Ann Intern Med 87:293, 1977
7. Davey DD, Ulbright TM: The evaluation of teratomas in male patients. A study of 86 cases. Unpublished observations
8. Norris HJ, Zirkin HJ, Benson WL: Immature (malignant) teratoma of the ovary. A clinical and pathologic study of 58 cases. Cancer 37:2359, 1976
9. Donohue JP, Roth LM, Zachary JM et al: Cytoreductive surgery for metastatic testis cancer. Tissue analysis of retroperitoneal masses after chemotherapy. J Urol 127:1111, 1982
10. Willis GW, Hajdu SI: Histologically benign teratoid metastasis of testicular embryonal carcinoma. Report of five cases. Am J Clin Pathol 59:338, 1973
11. Hong WK, Wittes RE, Hajdu SI et al: The evolution of mature teratoma from malignant testicular tumors. Cancer 40:2987, 1977
12. Merrin C, Baumgartner G, Wajsman Z: Benign transformation of testicular carcinoma by chemotherapy. Lancet 1:43, 1975
13. Snyder RN: Completely mature pulmonary metastasis from testicular teratocarcinoma. Case report and review of the literature. Cancer 24:810, 1969
14. Oosterhuis JW, Suurmeyer AJH, Sleyfer DT, et al: Effects of multiple drug chemotherapy (cis-diammine-dichloroplatinum, bleomycin, and vinblastine) on the maturation of retroperitoneal lymph node metastases of non-seminomatous germ cell tumors of the testis. No evidence for de novo induction of differentiation. Cancer 51:408, 1983
15. Fraley EE, Lange PH, Kennedy BJ: Germ-cell testicular cancer in adults (first of two parts). N Engl J Med 301:1370, 1979
16. Ulbright TM, Loehrer PJ, Roth LM et al: The development of non-germ cell malignancies within germ cell tumors. A clinicopathologic study of eleven cases. Cancer 54:1824, 1984
17. Peterson WF: Malignant degeneration of benign cystic teratomas of the ovary. A collective review of the literature. Obstet Gynecol Surv 12:793, 1957
18. Cahan WG, Woodard HW, Higinbothan NL, et al: Sarcoma arising in irradiated bone. Report of eleven cases. Cancer 1:3, 1948
19. Chabner BA: Second neoplasm. A complication of cancer chemotherapy. N Engl J Med 297:213, 1977

14

Effects of Systemic Chemotherapy on Testicular Morphology and Fertility

Maria Paoletti and Francis H. Straus II

The modern use of chemotherapeutic agents in the treatment of cancer has had profound effects upon the natural history of many malignancies, and frequently results in patient survival times much longer than what one would expect without the use of these agents. However, these drugs often have deleterious effects upon the normal physiology of healthy organs in the cancer patient, the testis being one of those organs most frequently adversely affected.

The effects of chemotherapeutic agents on testicular function and morphology will be discussed, particularly with reference to single- and multiple-drug protocols. In addition, a short discussion of the effects of radiation on the testis, which is frequently used as an adjuvant to drug therapy, will be included.

CHEMOTHERAPY AND THE NONHUMAN TESTIS

Numerous experiments have been conducted in laboratory animals to examine the effects of chemotherapeutic agents on testicular germinal epithelium. The goal of these investigations has been to determine whether the toxic effects observed in animal testes could be extrapolated to the human testis. A number of these studies have shown that in many cases it is not possible to predict which drugs will have long-term deleterious effects on human spermatogenesis. This conclusion is based on the fact that, frequently, drugs with minimal cytotoxicity to the animal testis will result in long-term human azoospermia, and vice versa. Also, many of the animal-based studies utilize single injections of single chemotherapeutic agents, which do not realistically reproduce the biology of most multiple dose, multidrug chemotherapy regimens frequently used in humans.

Meistrich et al.[1] examined the toxic effects of 14 different chemotherapeutic drugs on the mouse testis, utilizing single injections of single drugs in varying dosages up to systemic toxic levels. Damage to the various components of the germinal epithelium was noted. Variable toxicity to differentiated spermatogonia was most frequently seen, with relative resistance of spermatocytes and spermatids. The ability of drugs to pass the blood–testis barrier and thus to reach spermatocytes and spermatids has been shown; thus the resistance of these cells cannot be attributed to lack of drug penetration. It is most likely that the greater sensitivity of rapidly dividing differentiated spermatogonia is related to the fact that chemotherapeutic agents selectively damage actively dividing cells.[2] No morphologic evidence of Leydig or Sertoli cell damage was seen.[1]

Attempts to correlate experimental animal data with clinical trials of chemotherapeutic agents showed that, in many cases, the toxicity observed in experimental mouse models could not be extrapolated to humans.[1, 3] The most cytotoxic drug to murine stem cells was adriamycin, which did not produce permanent azoospermia in humans. Conversely, combination chemotherapy with nitrogen mustard, vincristine, vinblastine, and procarbazine often produces irreversible azoospermia in humans, but these individual agents were only slightly cytotoxic to mouse germinal epithelium. Studies in nonhuman primates,[4] however, did show cytotoxic changes in monkey testes after procarbazine administration, similar to those seen in human testes after mechlorethamine, vincristine, procarbazine, and prednisone (MOPP) chemotherapy. These changes consisted of total depletion of germinal epithelium with no evidence of spermatogenesis, and of seminiferous tubules lined exclusively by Sertoli cells (Sertoli-cell only syndrome). Thus, some correlation between animal models, at least nonhuman primates,[4] and clinical observations does exist.

SINGLE CHEMOTHERAPEUTIC AGENTS

One of the first reports on possible gonadal toxicity of chemotherapeutic agents was published in 1956, and documented a group of patients receiving Myleran (busulfan) for chronic granulocytic leukemia. Among these patients were four women, who developed amenorrhea and hypoplastic changes in the endometrium after long-term therapy.[5] Since that time, there have been numerous reports of gonadal toxicity and infertility with single chemotherapeutic drugs, particularly the alkylating agents, such as chlorambucil,[6-8] and cyclophosphamide.[9-12]

Most of the studies on drug-induced infertility have been conducted on men receiving single alkylating agents for malignant lymphoma or renal disease. The alkylating agents primarily affect rapidly multiplying cell populations, and either cross-link or sever strands of DNA. In the testis, the most sensitive cell populations are the spermatogonia and primary spermatocytes, which initially are reduced in numbers, resulting in morphologic hypospermatogenesis. Germ cell elements then become totally depleted, with hyalinization and narrowing of the seminiferous tubules, resulting in azoospermia.[13]

The effects of cyclophosphamide on the testis were first documented[11] in 1972, in a group of 31 male patients receiving cyclophosphamide for varying lengths of time. Decreased sperm counts were noted in men treated with 50 to 100 mg cyclophosphamide daily for as short a period as 3 weeks. All patients who had received treatment for 6 months or longer (with a cumulative dosage of 9 to 18 g) showed azoospermia. Thus, toxicity appeared to be related to the total dosage of the drug. Testicular biopsy was performed in five patients, and no spermatogenesis was seen in patients receiving the drug at the time of biopsy. Most of the seminiferous tubules contained only Sertoli cells, and thus severe testicular atrophy was present in these biopsy specimens. Other studies utilizing cyclophosphamide as a single chemotherapeutic agent have shown similar histologic findings on testicular biopsy specimens.[12]

Chlorambucil is another alkylating agent with deleterious effects on the testicular germinal epithelium. In a study of eight male patients with lymphoma,[6] the degree of tubular damage was dependent upon the total dosage of drug given. The minimum dosage that resulted in azoospermia was 400 mg; in doses of up to 400 mg, a progressive oligospermia developed. In those men exhibiting azoospermia, testicular biopsy specimens revealed slight peritubular fibrosis and hyalinization, absence of germinal cells including spermatogonia, and Sertoli cells attached to the basement membranes. No morphologic evidence of Leydig cell or vascular damage was noted. It was considered that while an individual susceptibility to this drug probably exists, severe testicular damage is a likely consequence of an accumulated dosage in excess of 400 mg of chlorambucil.

COMBINATION
CHEMOTHERAPY

Cytotoxic damage to the germinal epithelium of the testis caused by single chemotherapeutic agents has been described for several drugs, particularly the alkylating agents. With the recent introduction of multiple drug regimens, it is becoming more difficult to assess the cytotoxic effects of individual drugs when used in combination therapies. Several studies have focused on the high rates of infertility produced by these multiple drug regimens, many of which involve combined drug therapies for Hodgkin's disease.

Based on the fact that single alkylating agents produce azoospermia and infertility, it is to be expected that multiple drug therapies that include alkylating agents will also cause severe damage to the germinal epithelium. In one of the first studies on combination chemotherapy and infertility,[14] 16 men with malignant lymphoma in complete remission for 2 months to 7 years after chemotherapy with mechlorethamine, vincristine, procarbazine, and prednisone (MOPP); cyclophosphamide, vinblastine, and prednisone (CVP); or cyclophosphamide alone were studied. Testicular biopsy specimens in 15 patients revealed complete germinal aplasia in 10, scattered spermatogonia with arrest of spermatogenesis in 2, and normal spermatogenesis in 3. Those patients with abnormal biopsy specimens showed either azoospermia or oligospermia on semen analysis.

Chapman et al.,[15] in a retrospective study of 74 male patients with advanced Hodgkin's disease, examined the effects of cyclic combination chemotherapy on fertility. All patients were immediately completely azoospermic after treatment with cyclic mechlorethamine, vinblastine, procarbazine, and prednisone (MVPP); and in a median follow-up period of 27 months, only four of these patients regained spermatogenesis. Testicular biopsies were performed on 16 men 2 to 47 months (median 31 months) after cessation of therapy.

These specimens uniformly showed absence of spermatogenesis, and seminiferous tubules lined only by Sertoli cells (Figs. 14-1 to 14-3). The morphology of Leydig cells was within normal limits (Figs. 14-1 and 14-3). In addition to semen analysis and testicular biopsies, serum gonadotropin and testosterone levels were determined. Median follicle-stimulating hormone (FSH) and luteinizing hormone (LH) levels were consistently abnormally elevated in most patients, and testosterone levels were normal. The interpretation of these hormonal findings is as follows: the persistent elevation of FSH most likely reflects damaged germinal epithelium, (with subsequent loss of inhibin production and loss of negative feedback regulation of FSH secretion) and continuing azoospermia. Levels of LH at the high normal limit probably represent compensated Leydig cell failure, especially in the light of normal testosterone levels. Histologic evidence of Leydig cell damage has not been a described feature of chemotherapy-induced toxicity in the testis. Even so, injury at the organelle level is probable, since elevated LH levels appear to be necessary to maintain testosterone secretion by Leydig cells. No discussion of the electron microscopic features of Leydig cells during chemotherapy is available in the literature; the description of the ultrastructural appearances of these cells would be of interest.

Other studies confirmed the poor prognosis for fertility after chemotherapy for Hodgkin's disease. Whitehead and Shalet[16] examined the effects of MVPP on 74 men with Hodgkin's disease 6 months to 8 years after completion of chemotherapy. Semen samples were obtained from 49 men, which showed azoospermia in 42 patients, and severe oligospermia (with sperm counts less than 1 million/ml) in 7. The mean plasma testosterone level was determined, and was significantly lower than in a group of controls. Median basal serum gonadotropin levels were also measured, and were significantly higher than in a group of age-matched controls. The pituitary gonado-

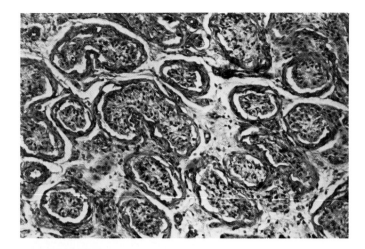

Fig. 14-1. Testis from an autopsy on 26-year-old man with Hodgkin's disease treated with multiple chemotherapeutic agents, including COP and MVPP. There is prominent basement membrane thickening, and severe reduction of spermatogenic elements. H & E. × 100.

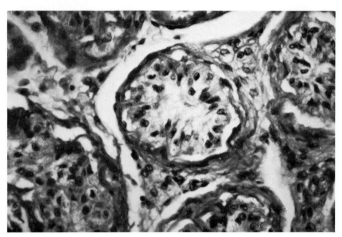

Fig. 14-2. Same patient as in Figure 14-1. Sertoli cells line the seminiferous tubules. Note complete absence of spermatogonia and differentiated elements. H & E. × 250.

tropin reserve was tested via administration of LH-releasing hormone (LHRH), with median serum LH increments significantly higher than those seen in normal controls. This finding also supports the concept that a compensated Leydig cell failure is present in the chemotherapy-damaged testis.

It is interesting to note that other investigators have documented similar exaggerated gonadotropin responses in men with germinal aplasia after LHRH administration. In one study,[17] baseline levels of FSH and LH were significantly elevated in three patients with germinal aplasia, as compared to normals; however, the mean LH level in these patients was in the upper limit of normal range. After administration of LHRH, patients exhibited

a 5.5-fold increase in LH levels, compared to a 3.5-fold increase for the controls. There was a concomitant 1.0-fold increase in FSH levels in patients, and a 0.5-fold increase in controls. Due to the findings of LH and testosterone levels within normal limits with a selective increase in FSH levels, it has been long assumed that the hypothalamic–pituitary–testicular axis was intact in germinal aplasia. The apparently isolated finding of elevated FSH was postulated to be due to loss of production of a specific FSH inhibitor (i.e., inhibin), in the chemotherapy-damaged seminiferous tubule.[17] However, the demonstration of elevated LH and borderline–low or decreased testosterone levels in these studies[17, 19, 20] suggests that there may indeed be derangements

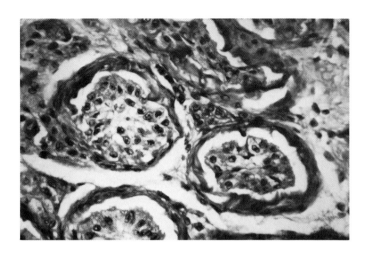

Fig. 14-3. Same case as in Figures 14-1 and 14-2. Note the prominent basement membrane thickening, absence of spermatogonia. Morphologically normal Leydig cells are present in interstitium. H & E. × 250.

of the hypothalamic–pituitary–gonadal axis in men with germinal aplasia, which are manifested as a compensated Leydig cell failure, but with no apparent morphologic manifestation of Leydig cell damage.

Other studies in patients treated with newer combination chemotherapies for testicular cancer and sarcomas have also indicated a dramatic incidence of infertility.[21] In one study, azoospermia was noted in a small group of patients treated with a combination of vincristine, adriamycin, cyclophosphamide, actinomycin-D, and medroxyprogesterone acetate, approximately 12 to 35 months after remission.[22] Another investigation examined the effects of combined vinblastine, bleomycin, and cis-platinum with or without doxorubicin therapy on the fertility of 18 men with germ cell neoplasms.[23] Elevated LH and FSH levels were found, with accompanying azoospermia and normal testosterone levels during the first year after completion of chemotherapy. Further follow-up during a period of 2 years revealed a return of gonadotropin levels to normal in half of the men, as well as a return of spermatogenesis in five of six men 2 years after completing chemotherapy. However, azoospermia was still present in most patients *within* a 24-month period of completion of chemotherapy. These data as well as others[24, 25] suggest that there is a compensated Leydig cell dysfunction with platinum-based

chemotherapies which persists up to 24 months following therapy, based on the elevated LH and normal testosterone values seen in these patients. This study also points to the possible reversibility of infertility in men with chemotherapy-damaged testicular germinal epithelium.[23]

REVERSIBILITY OF INFERTILITY

It has been noted that the administration of chemotherapeutic agents causes extensive damage to the germinal epithelium of the testis, with resultant azoospermia and infertility. Several reports have suggested that there may be some element of reversibility of drug-induced infertility, with eventual recovery of spermatogenesis.[23, 26, 27] Return of fertility seems to be dependent upon several variables, including the type of chemotherapeutic agent employed, the dosage of drug, and the length of time following completion of chemotherapy. Determination of drug regimens that appear to have a poor prognosis for fertility is important, particularly when young cancer patients with a desire for future fertility are being treated.

Single-agent chemotherapeutic regimens are the simplest to evaluate in terms of recovery of fertility, since one does not have to control simultaneously for the different dosage–effect relationships of several drugs in multidrug protocols. As far as the alkylating agents are concerned, reversal of cyclophosphamide-reduced infertility tends to depend upon both the dosage[11, 12] and the length of time of therapy. Buchanan et al.[26] showed that normal spermatogenesis returned in more than half of patients treated for less than 18 months, compared with approximately 25 percent of patients treated for more than 18 months. Even though the number of patients in this study was small (and thus the return of spermatogenesis could not be significantly related to total dosage or duration of therapy) the study suggested that recovery is more likely in patients treated for less than 18 months. Chlorambucil gonadal toxicity is definitely related to dosage; it has been already seen[6] that the minimum total dosage necessary for the production of azoospermia is 400 mg. The time of recovery of spermatogenesis is also related to the accumulated dosage of drug; a patient with a total dosage of chlorambucil of approximately 650 mg recovers normal spermatogenesis in 3 years, while a patient receiving four times that dosage is still oligospermic after 5 years.[8]

Roeser et al.[27] studied 32 patients who received standard combination chemotherapies (CVP, MOPP, or related regimens) for disseminated Hodgkin's and non-Hodgkin's lymphomas. Thirty-one patients had elevated FSH levels during therapy, which were accompanied by azoospermia in the 15 patients who submitted sperm samples. Low testosterone levels were present in five patients, and were associated with elevated LH levels in three. Sixteen patients were available for long-term follow-up after completion of chemotherapy, and recovery of germinal epithelium was markedly different between the CVP-treated group and the MVPP-treated group. In the former group, 7 of 10 patients showed evidence of recovery of spermatogenesis after 34 months of follow-up. Levels of FSH returned to normal in these seven patients; sperm counts were normal in three men, and oligospermia was present in one. Among the MVPP-treated group, only one of six patients showed evidence of recovering germinal epithelium after 52 months of follow-up posttherapy. This patient's sperm count was 1×10^6/ml, and FSH levels were still elevated. The other five patients had persistent azoospermia with elevated FSH levels. It was postulated by this study[27] as well as others[28] that the return of FSH levels to normal seems to be a predictor of recovery of testicular function. These data also suggest that chemotherapy regimens containing procarbazine produce a more lasting toxic damage to testicular germinal epithelium than other drug combinations.

Several other studies confirm the poor prognosis for fertility in Hodgkin's patients receiving MVPP or MOPP chemotherapy.[14, 29] Chapman et al.[15] studied a large group of men who had received this particular drug combination for Hodgkin's disease and who were 1 to 62 months posttreatment. Of 64 men, only 4 regained spermatogenesis. Whitehead et al.[16] found that in long-term (6 to 8 years) follow-up of 11 patients receiving MVPP, 10 were azoospermic. Both of these studies suggest that recovery of fertility is unlikely in patients receiving these particular chemotherapies, but more long-term follow-up studies are needed.

Studies of the return of fertility in patients receiving other combination chemotherapies for other neoplasms are fewer than in those with lymphoma, but appear to show more promising results. Evaluation of the platinum-based chemotherapies for testicular cancer[23, 24] reveals that there is a significant degree of recovery of testicular function 2–3 years after the initiation of chemotherapy. One study[23] showed that after a median of 40 months from the start of cis-platin, vinblastine, and bleomycin with or without adriamycin chemotherapy, 11 of 46 men had normal sperm counts, and 8 had fathered children. Another study[24] showed that 34 months following completion of similar chemotherapy, more than half of the patients evaluated showed normal gonadotropin levels and approximately one-quarter had normal sperm counts, with the remainder of patients showing oligospermia. Thus, it appears that in these patients spermatogenesis may show a slow recovery after a period of months or years following chemotherapy.

IMPAIRED GONADAL FUNCTION BEFORE CHEMOTHERAPY

The role that chemotherapeutic agents play in producing male infertility is clear; however, it is very likely that a preexisting level of gonadal dysfunction is present in many patients with malignancies such as leukemia, lymphoma, and testicular neoplasms. Several prospective studies have examined pretreatment parameters of fertility (such as semen analysis), and have postulated that a significant number of patients with cancer have decreased fertility even before the commencement of chemotherapy. Thus, infertility after chemotherapy cannot be simply attributed to deleterious effects of drugs on the testis, since preexisting spermatozoal defects may be present. The cause of these defects is unclear. In the hematologic malignancies, general poor health and nutritional factors may have some bearing upon spermatogenesis. Preexisting cryptorchidism in the testis containing cancer most certainly affects sperm production,[30] and carcinoma in situ affecting seminiferous tubules may also affect the quality of spermatozoa.[31, 32]

Chapman et al.,[33] in a prospective study of 47 men with Hodgkin's disease, determined that one-third of the patients were subfertile before beginning chemotherapy, as documented by low sperm counts. Abnormal histologic features were present in eight of nine pretreatment testicular biopsy specimens; six showed tubular hyalinization and thickening of the basement membrane, one showed active spermatogenesis with maturation arrest, and one autopsy specimen containing complete hyalinization of tubules, with absence of germinal epithelium and Sertoli cells (Figs. 14-

4 to 14-6). Abnormalities in pretreatment serum hormonal levels were also present, with FSH levels elevated in 6 (15 percent) of 39 men, and LH levels in 16 (40 percent) of 40 men. Testosterone levels were decreased in 5 (19 percent) of 27 men. This study went on to show that after two cycles of MVPP therapy, all of 14 men were persistently azoospermic, with serum FSH levels four to five times normal and posttreatment testicular biopsy specimens that showed complete germinal aplasia, but intact Leydig and Sertoli cells.

Several studies on prechemotherapy fertility in men with testicular cancer have been reported. Jewett et al.,[34] in a prospective study of 42 men with newly diagnosed germ cell tumors of the testis, showed that one-half of the patients had suboptimal sperm counts ($<20 \times 10^6$/ml) at the time of diagnosis, and before treatment other than hemicastration. This was compared to an incidence of 7 percent suboptimal sperm density in a control population. Thus, a high frequency of baseline pretreatment oligospermia was noted.

Similarly, Berthelsen and Skakkebaek[32] showed that spermatogenesis and semen quality were poor before administration of chemotherapy and irradiation in 218 male patients with testicular germ cell neoplasms. Biopsy specimens of the contralateral testis in 24 percent of 200 patients showed severe changes, with 8 percent showing Sertoli-cell-only syndrome, spermatogenic arrest, hyalinized tubules, or carcinoma in situ, and 16 percent showing various degrees of spermatogenic defects. Biopsy specimens from the remaining 76 percent showed all types of spermatogenic cells in all tubules; however, quantitative analysis of 25 biopsies randomly selected from this group showed that 60 percent of these had a reduced number of spermatids. Several theories were postulated to account for the quality of semen, among them cryptorchidism in childhood in 9 percent of patients, carcinoma in situ of the contralateral testis in 5 percent, elevated scrotal temperature (due to testicular tumor), and tumor production

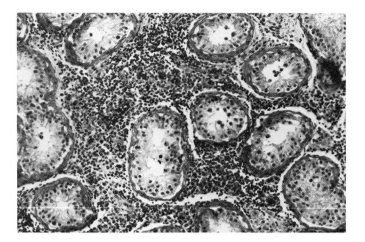

Fig. 14-4. Testis from an autopsy on a 24-year-old man with acute myelogenous leukemia, treated briefly with 6-mercaptopurine, methotrexate, prednisone, and vincristine. Prominent leukemic infiltrates are present in the interstitium. There is severe atrophy of the seminiferous tubular elements. A few residual spermatogonia are present along the basement membrane. H & E. × 100.

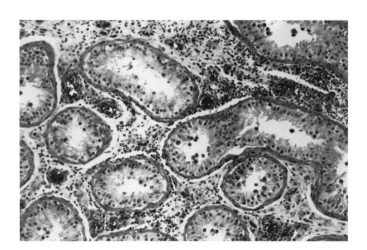

Fig. 14-5. Same case as in Figure 14-4. Leukemic infiltrates, basement membrane thickening, and severe reduction of spermatogenic elements. H & E. × 100.

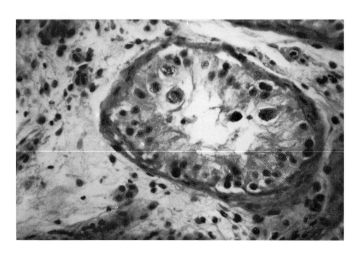

Figu 14-6. Same case as in Figures 14-4 and 14-5. A few surviving spermatogonia along the basement membrane, with a few maturing spermatocytes near the center of the tubular lumen. H & E. × 250.

of human chorionic gonadotropin (HCG), which ostensibly depresses spermatogenesis.[35]

Due to the young age of many cancer patients and the potential for lengthy survival with improved chemotherapeutic regimens, it has been suggested that sperm cryopreservation before chemotherapy should be offered as a means of preserving reproductive capacity in these young patients.[36, 37] The previously mentioned studies as well as others[38, 39] indicate that suboptimal fertility before chemotherapy is frequent in male cancer patients. A study on the feasibility of semen cryopreservation in patients with malignant disease by Sanger et al.[38] revealed that among 22 young men with testicular cancer or lymphoma, only 23 percent met the sperm bank criteria for potential fertility, as opposed to 60 percent in a control population. The deficiencies of semen in these men were manifested by low sperm density and inability of sperm to survive freezing and thawing, thus rendering these patients poor candidates for semen cryopreservation.

EFFECTS OF CHEMOTHERAPY ON THE PREPUBERTAL AND PUBERTAL TESTIS

The prognosis in childhood cancer has been considerably improved by the advent of combination chemotherapy, particularly in acute lymphoblastic leukemia (ALL). As in other young cancer patients, much concern has been expressed about the growth and development of young leukemic patients after receiving chemotherapy. Whether or not reproductive function is preserved in these patients is one of the important questions that has surfaced with the use of multidrug chemotherapy regimens.

It was believed for some time that the prepubertal and the pubertal testis had different susceptibilities to cytotoxic drugs, with the prepubertal testis being relatively resistant to toxic damage. Early studies[40] reinforced this concept, and showed that testicular histologic appearance was often normal in the prepubertal male receiving cytotoxic drugs, and was

accompanied by normal gonadotropin and testosterone levels. Other reports showed normal histologic findings after high dosages of alkylating agents,[41, 42] but the time interval between cessation of chemotherapy and biopsy may have been sufficiently long to allow repair to take place.

The prepubertal testis is indeed damaged by cytotoxic drugs. Lendon et al.[43] examined the testicular morphology of 44 boys who received chemotherapy for ALL while still prepubertal. Interstitial fibrosis was present in half of the sections, while basement membrane thickening and leukemic infiltrates were much less common (Figs. 14-7, 14-8). The mean tubular fertility index (TFI), or percentage of tubules containing identifiable spermatogonia was 50 percent of that in age-matched controls, and roughly one-half of the specimens had a severely depressed TFI of 40 percent or less. No evidence of Leydig or Sertoli cell injury was present in these specimens. These authors reported improvements in TFI with increasing time after completion of chemotherapy, but persistently low TFIs in two patients after 33 and 45 months raised the speculation that irreversible testicular damage may occur in some patients.

Endocrine studies[44, 45] of prepubertal males receiving chemotherapy have failed to show abnormalities in gonadotropin levels and testosterone. The coexistence of normal endocrine profiles and abnormal testicular morphology has led some authors to postulate that measurements of endocrine parameters are not reflective of the often severe gonadal damage caused by chemotherapeutic agents.

Studies of the effects of chemotherapy on the pubertal testis have revealed both morphologic and hormonal abnormalities. In a group of pubertal boys treated with MOPP for Hodgkin's disease,[46] gynecomastia developed in the majority of patients, and was accompanied by elevated LH and FSH levels and low testosterone levels. Testicular biopsy specimens in the patients with gynecomastia revealed complete germinal aplasia. The endocrine and gonadal status of many of these

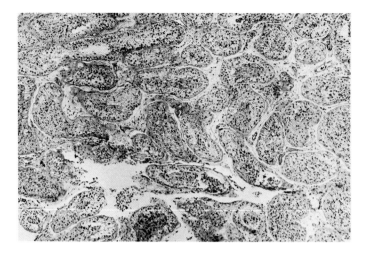

Fig. 14-7. Testicular biopsy specimen from 16-year-old boy with acute lymphocytic leukemia receiving chemotherapy. Mild interstitial fibrosis is present. Many tubules contain active spermatogenesis. H & E. × 40.

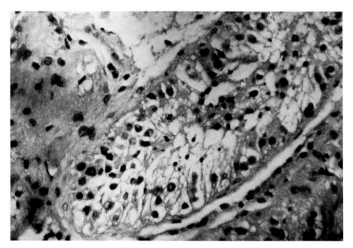

Fig. 14-8. Same patient as in Figure 14-7. Residual spermatogenesis with maturation from spermatogonia to spermatids, is apparent. H & E. × 250.

patients is similar to that seen in adult men receiving combination chemotherapy, that is, compensated Leydig cell failure characterized by elevated LH and low testosterone levels, accompanied by absence of spermatogenesis. The cause of gynecomastia in these patients is unclear, and needs to be further characterized.

THE EFFECTS OF RADIATION THERAPY ON THE HUMAN TESTIS

Much information is present in the literature on the effects of chemotherapeutic agents on male fertility. With current multimodal cancer treatment protocols, the effects of radiation on the testis must be considered, particularly in young patients who will enjoy prolonged survival and desire fertility.

Numerous experiments have been conducted in animals on the effects of radiation, and the dosages required to cause sterility in different species have been determined.[47, 48] In humans, data on spermatogenesis after radiation treatment have been derived from two principal sources.[49] These include men who have received gonadal radiation as a consequence of radiotherapy for malignant tumors, and men who have volunteered to receive graded doses of gonadal radiation as part of controlled experiments. Case reports regarding the effects of accidental radiation exposure on the gonads are also described in the literature.[50]

It has been shown that a single dose of radiation as little as 15 rad can produce oligospermia, and a single dose of 100 rad consistently produces azoospermia. A single total dose of 300 rad produces no significant effect before 46 days following radiation, whereas a single total dose of 600 rad causes an immediate decrease in sperm count.[34]

Recovery from testicular irradiation is also dosage-related. A dose of 100 to 300 rad usually results in slow but complete recovery of spermatogenesis, while doses of 400 to 600 rad are followed by a prolonged unpredictable restoration of sperm production.[34] Fractionated doses of radiation also cause unpredictable recoveries, and in some instances are more lethal to stem cells than single doses of radiation.[51]

The various components of testicular germinal epithelium differ in their susceptibilities to radiation therapy.[49] In experimental situations, premeiotic spermatogonia were found to be the most radiosensitive cell population, and showed decreased numbers after dosages as low as 8 rad. Spermatocytes were damaged after 200 to 300 rad; maturation division could not be completed, and spermatid numbers were reduced as a result. Spermatids were damaged after 400 to 600 rads (manifested by decreased numbers of spermatozoa), and mature sperm were relatively radioresistant.[52] It was found that spermatogonia repopulate the seminiferous tubules in an unpredictable fashion, and produce additional spermatogonia or spermatocytes at random. Thus, biopsy specimens obtained during early recovery of spermatogenesis may show some seminiferous tubules containing spermatogonia and/or spermatocytes, while adjacent tubules may be devoid of germ cell elements other than a single spermatogonium. This is in contradistinction to the mouse testis, where spermatogonia uniformly repopulate themselves before beginning differentiation into spermatocytes. Leydig and Sertoli cells were also relatively im-

mune to radiation; however, large dosages of radiation (600 rad) did result in increased numbers of Leydig cells.

REFERENCES

1. Meistrich ML, Finch M, de Cunha MF et al: Damaging effects of fourteen chemotherapeutic agents in mouse testis cells. Cancer Res 42:122, 1982
2. Drewinko B, Patchen M, Yang L-Y, Barlogie B: Differential killing efficacy of twenty antitumor drugs on proliferating and non-proliferating human tumor cells. Cancer Res 41:2328, 1981
3. Lu CC, Meistrich ML: Cytotoxic effects of chemotherapeutic drugs on mouse testis cells. Cancer Res 39:3575, 1979
4. Sieber SM, Correa P, Dalgard W, Adamson RH: Carcinogenic and other adverse effects of procarbazine in non-human primates. Cancer Res 38:2125, 1978
5. Louis J, Limarzi LR, Best WR: Treatment of chronic granulocytic leukemia with Myleran. Arch Intern Med 97:299, 1956
6. Richter P, Calamera JC, Morgenfeld MC et al: Effect of chlorambucil on spermatogenesis in the human with malignant lymphoma. Cancer 25:1026, 1970
7. Miller DG: Alkylating agents and spermatogenesis. JAMA 217:1662, 1971
8. Cheviakoff S, Calamera JC, Morgenfeld M, Mancini RE: Recovery of spermatogenesis in patients with lymphoma after treatment with chlorambucil. J Reprod Fertil 33:155, 1973
9. Miller JJ, Williams GF, Leissring JC: Multiple late complications of therapy with cyclophosphamide, including ovarian destruction. Am J Med 50:530, 1971
10. Warne GL, Fairley KT, Hobbs JB, Martin FIR: Cyclophosphamide-induced ovarian failure. N Engl J Med 289:1159, 1973
11. Fairley KF, Barrie JU, Johnson W: Sterility and testicular atrophy related to cyclophosphamide therapy. Lancet 1:568, 1972
12. Kumar R, McEvoy J, Biggart JD, McGeown MG: Cyclophosphamide and reproductive function. Lancet 1:1212, 1972
13. Straus FH II: The testis. p. 279 In Riddell

RH (ed): Pathology of Drug-Induced and Toxic Diseases. Churchill Livingstone, New York, 1982

14. Sherins RJ, DeVita VT Jr: Effects of drug treatment for lymphoma on male reproductive capacity: studies of men in remission after therapy. Ann Intern Med 79:216, 1973

15. Chapman RM, Rees LH, Sutcliffe SB, et al: Cyclical combination chemotherapy and gonadal function. Lancet 1:285, 1979

16. Whitehead E, Shalet SM, Blackledge G et al: Effects of Hodgkin's disease and combination chemotherapy on gonadal function in the adult male. Cancer 49:418, 1982

17. Mecklenburg RS, Sherins RJ: Gonadotropin response to luteinizing hormone-releasing hormone in men with germinal aplasia. J Clin Endocrinol Metabol 38:1005, 1974

18. Van Thiel DU, Sherins RJ, Meyers GH, DeVita VT: Evidence for a specific seminiferous tubular factor affecting follicle stimulating hormone secretion in man. J Clin Invest 51:1009, 1972

19. Dunzendorfer U, Weber W: Testosterone, LH and FSH in patients with treated testicular carcinomas. Horm Metab Res 10:156, 1978

20. Fossa SD, Klepp O, Aakvaag A: Serum hormone levels in patients with malignant testicular germ cell tumors without clinical and/or radiological signs of tumor. Br J Urol 52:151, 1980

21. Shamberger RC, Sherins RJ, Rosenberg SA: The effects of post-operative adjuvant chemotherapy and radiotherapy on testicular function in men undergoing treatment for soft tissue sarcoma. Cancer 47:2368, 1981

22. Fossa SD, Klepp O, Aakvaag A, Molne K: Testicular function after combined chemotherapy for metastatic testicular cancer. Int J Androl 3:59, 1980

23. Johnson DH, Hainsworth JD, Linde RB, Greco FA: Testicular function following combination chemotherapy with cis-platin, vinblastine, and bleomycin. Med Pediatr Oncol 12:233, 1984

24. Drasga RE, Einhorn LH, Williams SD et al: Fertility after chemotherapy for testicular cancer. J Clin Oncol 1:179, 1983

25. Trump DL: Serial assessment of follicle stimulating hormone, luteinizing hormone, testosterone, and estradiol during chemotherapy for advanced testis cancer. Proc Am Soc Clin Oncol 1:122, 1982

26. Buchanan JD, Fairley KF, Barrie JU: Return of spermatogenesis after stopping cyclophosphamide therapy. Lancet 2:156, 1975

27. Roeser HP, Stocks AE, Smith AJ: Testicular damage due to cytotoxic drugs and recovery after cessation of therapy. Aust NZ J Med 8:250, 1978

28. Lange PH, Narayan P, Vogelzang NJ, et al: Return of fertility after treatment for non-seminomatous testicular cancer. J Urol 129:1131, 1983

29. Waxman JHX, Terry YA, Wrigley PFM et al: Gonadal function in Hodgkin's disease: long term follow-up of chemotherapy. Br Med J 285:1612, 1982

30. Farrington GH: Histologic observations in cryptorchidism: congenital germinal cell deficiency of undescended testes. J Pediatr Surg 4:606, 1969

31. Berthelsen JG, Skakkebaek NE, Mogensen P, Sorensen BC: Incidence of carcinoma in situ of germ cells in contralateral testis of men with testicular tumors. Br Med J 2:363, 1979

32. Berthelsen JG, Skakkebaek NE: Gonadal function in men with testis cancer. Fertil Steril 39:68, 1983

33. Chapman RM, Sutcliffe SB, Malpas JS: Male gonadal dysfunction in Hodgkin's disease. JAMA 245:1323, 1981

34. Jewett MAS, Thachil JV, Rider WD: The effects of cancer and cancer therapy on male fertility. J Urol 126:141, 1981

35. Weissbach L, Vahlensieck W, Figge M, Granthoff H: Diagnostik bei hodentumoren. Urologe [Ausg B] 20:106, 1980

36. Beck WW Jr: Artificial insemination and semen preservation. Clin Obstet Gynecol 17:115, 1974

37. Ackerman DR, Behrman SJ: Artificial insemination and preservation of human semen. p 765. In Behrman SJ, Kistner RW (eds): Progress in Infertility, ed. 2. Boston, Little, Brown and Co., 1975

38. Sanger WG, Armitage JO, Schmidt MA: Feasibility of semen cryopreservation in patients with malignant disease. JAMA 244:789, 1980

39. Bracken RB, Smith KD: Is semen cryopreservation helpful in testicular cancer? Urology 15:581, 1980

40. Pennisi AJ, Grushkin CM, Lieberman E: Gonadal function in children with nephrosis treated with cyclophosphamide. Am J Dis Child 129:315, 1975

41. Arneil GC: Cyclophosphamide and the prepubertal testis. Lancet 2:1259, 1972

42. Berry CL, Cameron JS, Ogg CS et al: Cyclophosphamide and the prepubertal testis. Lancet 2:1033, 1972

43. Lendon M, Palmer MK, Hann LM et al: Testicular histology after combination chemotherapy in childhood for acute lymphoblastic leukemia. Lancet 2:439, 1978

44. Blatt J, Poplack DG, Sherins RJ: Testicular function in boys after chemotherapy for acute lymphoblastic leukemia. N Engl J Med 304:1121, 1981

45. Shalet SM, Hann IM, Lendon M et al: Testicular function after combination chemotherapy in childhood for acute lymphoblastic leukemia. Arch Dis Child 56:275, 1981

46. Sherins RJ, Olweny CLM, Ziegler JL: Gynecomastia and gonadal dysfunction in adolescent boys treated with combination chemotherapy for Hodgkin's disease. N Engl J Med 299:12, 1978

47. Carter TC, Lyon MF, Phillips RJS: Induction of sterility in male mice by chronic gamma irradiation. Br J Radiol 27:418, 1954

48. Withers HR, Hunger N, Barkley HT, Reid BO: Radiation survival and regeneration characteristics of spermatogenic stem cells of mouse testis. Radiat Res 57:88, 1974

49. Ash P: The influence of radiation on fertility in man. Br J Radiol 53:271, 1980

50. Oakes WR, Lushbaugh CC: Cause of testicular injury following accidental exposure to nuclear radiations; report of a case. Radiology 59:737, 1952

51. Speiser B, Rubin P, Casarett G: Aspermia following lower truncal irradiation in Hodgkin's disease. Cancer 32:692, 1973

52. Rowley MJ, Leach DR, Watner GA, Heller CG: Effect of graded doses of ionizing radiation on the human testis. Radiat Res 59:665, 1974

INDEX